Images in Clinical Medicine

Selections from

The New England Journal of Medicine

ISBN 0-910133-41-7

Library of Congress Catalog Card No. 97-73446

Printed in Canada
10 9 8 7 6 5 4 3 2 1

Preface

Since we introduced the Images in Clinical Medicine feature in the *New England Journal of Medicine* in early 1992, we have published more than 250 images. In scope they represent a multitude of medical disciplines as well as a wide variety of types of clinical images. Photographs of skin lesions, MRIs, CT scans, electrocardiograms, histologic specimens, graphs of fever curves, photographs taken through endoscopes, images of curious-looking cells, parasites, and the like — they have run the gamut of the types of visual evidence physicians encounter in the practice of medicine. The popularity of this feature has been gratifying. Many of the images have been hung on walls, converted into slides, and used to illustrate important clinical principles. Many subscribers have told us that they turn to the "Images" page first. The allure of a visual image standing by itself on a journal page is irresistible.

Some readers have wondered how we select an image for an issue of the *Journal.* Often we try to match an image in our unpublished collection with some article in the same issue. We used an image of sickle cells in an issue featuring a study of the efficacy of butyrate in the treatment of hemoglobinopathies. We chose a classic example of gallstone ileus for the issue in which a study of the complications of endoscopic biliary sphincterotomy appeared, and an image of the use of a stent to treat inoperable cancer of the esophagus in the same issue as a study of combined chemotherapy and surgery for carcinoma of the esophagus. Often the relevance of the image was indirect or seasonal. We published an electron micrograph of ragweed pollen one month before the beginning of the hay fever season, photographs of the tick that causes Lyme disease in the late summer, a photograph of head lice just after Labor Day (in time for the return to school), an electron micrograph of the influenza virus in the early fall, and a terrifying coronal CT scan of the head showing carotid-artery dissection on Halloween.

Sometimes, though, we got more credit for planning than we deserved. When we published an image of a primary syphilitic lesion, it happened to show up on page 1492, the year that Columbus' sailors were reputed to have first been exposed to syphilis, before bringing it back to Europe. When we published a photograph of one of the last patients to have smallpox, by chance we did so two days after the 200th anniversary of Jenner's famous vaccination experiment. We would like to claim credit for these coincidences, but we cannot. When we had no particular reason for selecting an image, we simply chose the one that had been accepted for publication first. From time to time, we chose an image purely for aesthetic reasons: a photograph of the flowers of the foxglove plant, one of multicolored uric acid crystals in urine, and another of cholesterol crystals in a bursa. Once in a while, to amuse our readers and ourselves, we chose a funny-looking cell that resembled a footprint or a question mark.

From the beginning, subscribers have asked when we were going to collect the images in a book. I hesitated to do so until we had at least several examples from each of the major medical disciplines, such as cardiology, neurology, and gynecology. The collection we present here is not intended to be either comprehensive or balanced, however. Because the material was submitted for publication in no special order and images were accepted without regard for discipline, some specialties are represented by more images than others. In addition, some disciplines (cardiology, for example) are likely to yield a wider variety of images than others because of the advanced nature of their imaging technology — for visualizing the heart and blood vessels, for example. Though the collection here is far from complete, neither is it a hodgepodge. Many common conditions and types of images are represented, as well as many unusual ones that convince us of the validity of the saying, A picture is worth 1000 words.

The editorial I wrote in 1992 to accompany the first installment of Images in Clinical Medicine is reprinted here. We believe that we have accomplished much of what we set out to do. We continue to believe that a single example of a classic x-ray film, a gross tissue or organ specimen, or a coronary arteriogram is a powerful teaching tool. It simply is not possible for a student, a house officer, or even an experienced physician to be exposed to all the different kinds of images that are encompassed by the many areas of clinical medicine, and we hope our images fill in some of the gaps. Furthermore, the feelings evoked by the sight of leukemic cells in the blood or bone marrow, the results of a successful surgical treatment, or a budding human immunodeficiency virus as seen on electron microscopy represent the wide range of emotional responses entailed in being a physician. Scientific wonder, the anguish of identifying a fatal disease, and the triumph of making a diagnosis or seeing the results of successful treatment — these define not only what we do but in some sense who we are.

Fortunately, even as these images from past issues are collected in book form, we still have dozens of superb unpublished images. We plan to continue the series as long as we have material that is interesting, educational, and high in quality.

Finally, we wish to express our deep gratitude to the hundreds of reviewers who rendered their judgment over the past few years on the quality of the prints and the adequacy of the legends. Almost all are academic specialists from the Boston area. With rare exceptions, they performed this task efficiently and treated this short teaching exercise as seriously as they would a full-length scientific manuscript.

Jerome P. Kassirer, M.D., Editor-in-Chief

Kim Eagle, M.D., Series Editor

Acknowledgment

We are grateful to many people in the Editorial Offices and Publishing Division of the Massachusetts Medical Society for their help in preparing and producing this book. Kathy Stern deserves a special commendation for her superb design. Marie Chieppo patiently helped to organize the component images. Stephen Cinto and Ellen Duff shepherded the book through its production. In addition, we wish to thank Frank Bourret, Debbie Brooks, Joan Graham, Mark LeBlanc, Mary E. Tanner, Mike Tomases, and Richard Waring for their help in the production process.

Images in Clinical Medicine

Visual images are a rich source of the information we use in clinical medicine, yet we expend little effort to enhance our perception and recognition of these images. A new feature introduced in this issue of the *Journal,* Images in Clinical Medicine, will present a broad representation of useful and clinically important visual images. We believe that exposure to these photographs will help sharpen the reader's ability to identify common forms. As doctors we encounter an enormous variety of images from day to day, including skin lesions, funduscopic views, blood smears, bone marrow smears, urine sediments, microbiologic specimens, joint aspirates, x-ray studies (chest, abdomen, pelvis, limbs, skull), recordings of electrical potentials (electrocardiograms, electroencephalograms, and electromyograms), gross pathology specimens, histologic sections (routine, immunofluorescent, electron microscopy, special stains), endoscopic views, scans (CT, magnetic resonance imaging, radionuclide), sonograms, arteriograms, and venograms.

We will solicit from our readers original, unpublished, high-quality color or black-and-white photographs of typical images, accompanied by a brief descriptive legend. We will review them and, when necessary, send them out for peer review just as we do original manuscripts. Each published image will include the name of the person who submitted it. The editor of the series, Dr. Kim Eagle, is an outstanding clinician with a broad view of clinical medicine. We intend to emphasize images a doctor might encounter in an average day at the office, in the emergency ward, or in the hospital.

Although our intention is to present prototypes, we recognize that an image considered typical by one expert may seem atypical to another. Such discrepancies derive partly from differences in judgment, training, and experience, but differing interpretations can also be explained by the natural polymorphism of many biologic phenomena. Some diagnostically important objects vary little in their physical appearance, whereas others vary considerably. Blast cells in a blood smear or tubercle bacilli in a sputum specimen, for example, are rather monomorphic, but CT scans of a small-cell lung cancer vary substantially depending on the location and size of the tumor, the structures involved, and other variables. Yet even among polymorphic objects, some examples are likely to be more typical of the category than others. One might expect, however, that the more polymorphic the category, the more disagreement about what is typical and what is not. Editorial peer review will not guarantee that all the images we select will be prototypes, but it will help.

The perception of images is initiated by physicochemical events, including the activation of retinal cells, transmission of impulses to the hemispheres, and registration of impulses in the cerebral cortex. This message transfer is but the beginning of a complex function, one that involves a rich internal representation of reality and requires considerable cognitive processing. To interpret an image, we use information from experience and memory to create a model of reality. The layers of imagery go even deeper; many of the images we use in medicine are already models. Microscopical slides are not living cells; CT scans of adrenal tumors are only representations of the actual tumor; ultrasound representations of a septal defect are sound waves converted into a video or film image, not the defect itself. Often, therefore, we are creating mental models of physical models, a process somewhat removed from classical hands-on auscultation, percussion, and palpation. Nevertheless, such models, whether once or even twice removed from reality, are invaluable aids to perception and interpretation, functions critical to the performance of doctors.

Visual clues yield hypotheses for further data gathering or further testing. A patient's stare evokes palpation of the neck, a purpuric rash invites a prompt platelet count, and plump hilar vessels on a chest film send us scurrying back to the bedside to recheck a patient's neck veins and listen to the cardiac sounds. Images evoke even more than hypotheses. They evoke predictions, decision making, and planning. Erythema chronicum migrans not only suggests the possibility of Lyme disease but also provokes immediate testing to assess exposure. Free air under the diaphragm on an abdominal plain film often evokes the decision to explore the abdomen, and certain characteristics of a mole prompt decisions to remove it or leave it alone. The interpretation of images generates expectations and predictions: the location and appearance of a lesion on a barium enema x-ray film may immediately suggest not only the patient's long-term prognosis but also a detailed therapeutic plan for the lesion's biopsy or removal. What at first glance appears to be simple perception of images, then, is a complex stimulus to reasoning that leads to appropriate patient care.

Given these complex relations between perception and cognition, exposure to the classic images that we encounter in the course of a day's rounds should help not only to anchor the appearance of these objects in memory, but also to remind us of their clinical importance. We invite readers to submit material for this series.

Jerome P. Kassirer, M.D.

March 19, 1992

Infectious Diseases

Cardiology

Hematology and Oncology

Gastroenterology

Nephrology

Pulmonary Diseases

Parasites and Insects

Miscellaneous

Infectious Diseases

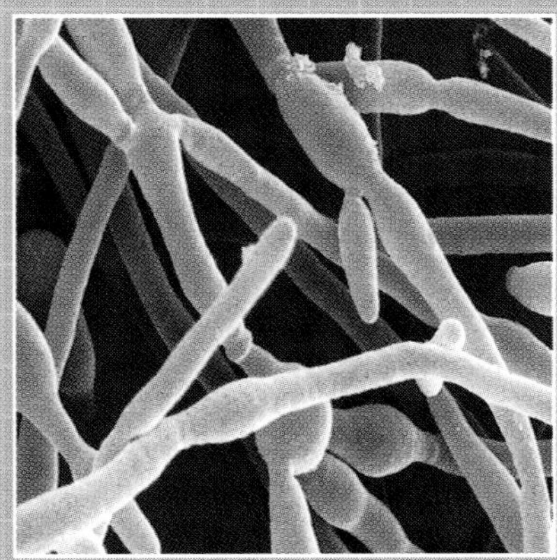

The Vector of the Lyme Disease Spirochete

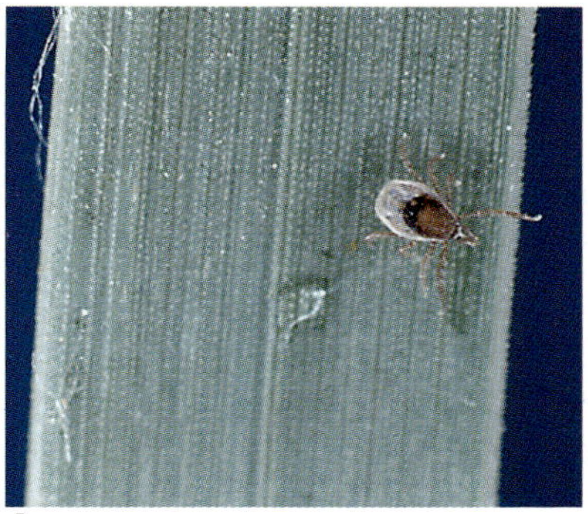
A

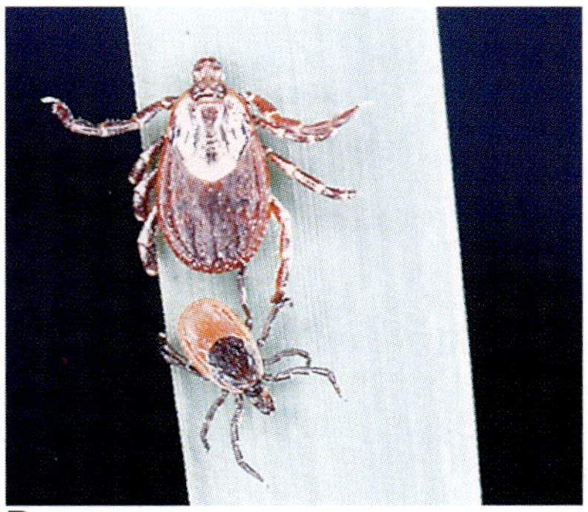
B

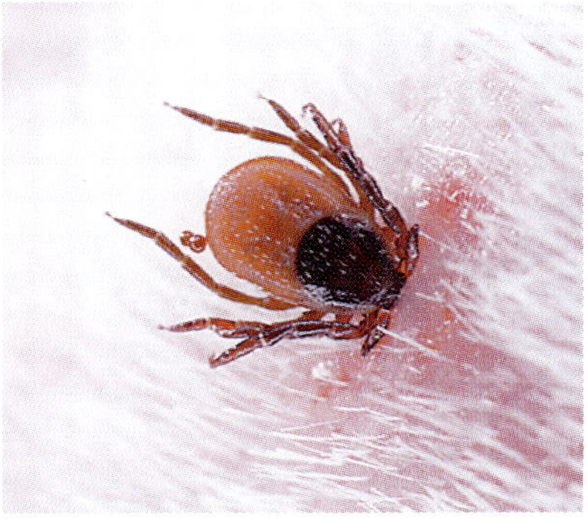
C

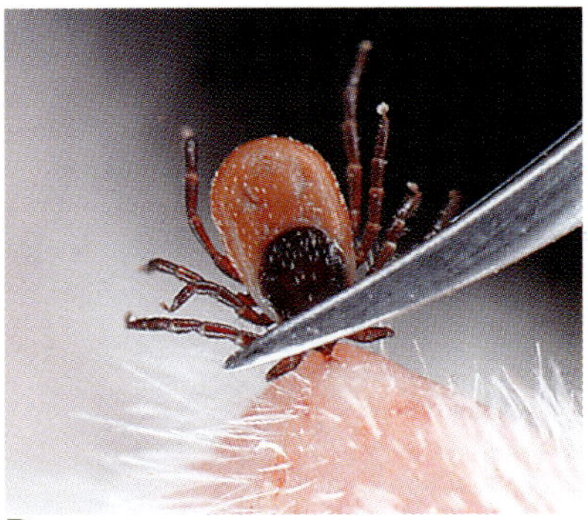
D

The deer ticks (*Ixodes dammini*) that transmit the Lyme disease spirochete (*Borrelia burgdorferi*) in the northeastern United States are members of a morphologically similar group of "black-legged ticks" that includes the wood tick (*I. ricinus*) of Europe and the taiga tick (*I. persulcatus*) of Asia. The same ticks also transmit human babesiosis (*Babesia microti*) in the United States and tick-borne encephalitis in Europe and Asia. The adult ticks are parasites of deer, but the spirochete is acquired when the larval stage feeds on a mouse.

The small nymph (shown on a blade of grass in Panel A) is found on low vegetation between early May and mid-July. It is only about the size of a poppy seed. When brushed onto a passing mouse or a person's feet, nymphs attach and feed for a few days (but only once). Spirochetes may infect about a third of nymphs, which are the stage of the deer tick that most often transmits the agent of Lyme disease to humans.

The posterior portion of the apple-seed-sized adult female deer tick (Panel B) is marked by an orange-red crescent. More than half the ticks in this winter-feeding stage may be infected. These adult deer ticks are found on grass or brush at the height of a person's knees. Shown for comparison is the adult stage of the more familiar dog tick (*Dermacentor variabilis*), which is larger than *I. dammini*. The dog tick does not transmit the agent of Lyme disease.

Adult deer ticks attach to their hosts for a week or more. They feed by inserting their mouthparts deep into the skin of their hosts, as shown here on the skin of an albino hamster (Panels C and D). As soon as they are discovered, and without prior treatment, ticks should be removed with forceps placed close to the point of attachment.

Franz-Rainer Matuschka

Free University of Berlin
Berlin, Germany

Andrew Spielman

Harvard School of Public Health
Boston, MA 02115

August 20, 1992

Lyme Disease

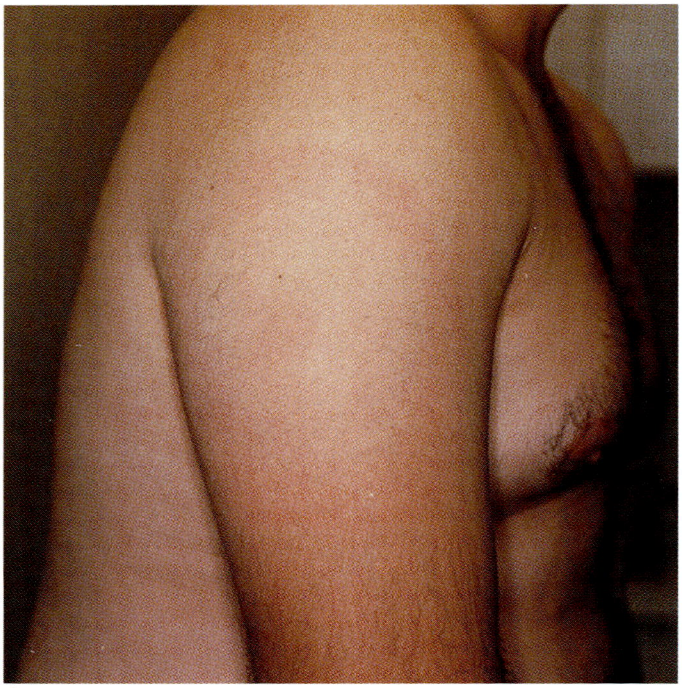

A

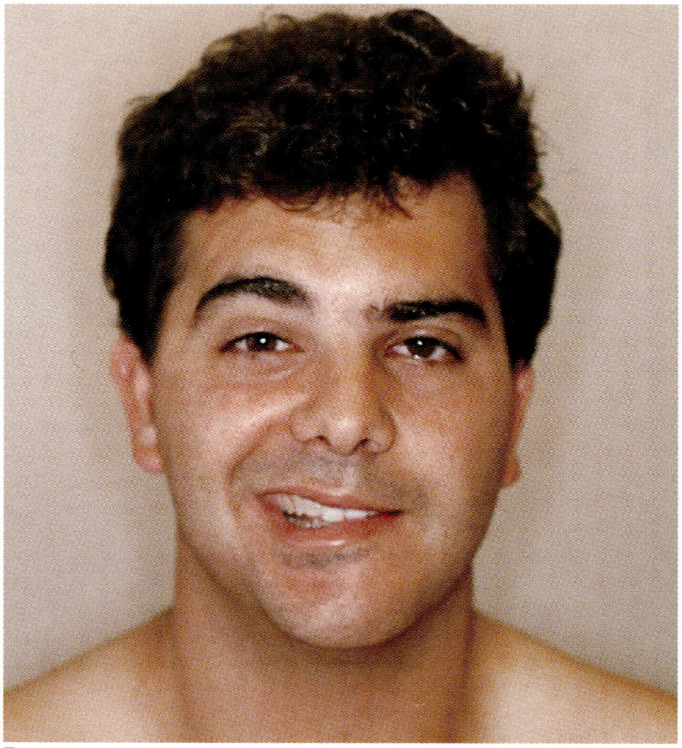

B

A young man presented with two common manifestations of early Lyme disease: the skin lesion on his arm, termed erythema chronicum migrans (Panel A), and Bell's palsy, causing left facial droop (Panel B).

Mark S. Klempner, M.D.

New England Medical Center
Boston, MA 02111

Philip J. Molloy, M.D.

Tufts University School of Medicine
Boston, MA 02111

December 17, 1992

Correspondence

Facial Palsy in Lyme Disease

May 27, 1993

To the Editor: In Images in Clinical Medicine, Klempner and Molloy (Dec. 17 issue)[1] showed a young man with Lyme disease who had erythema chronicum migrans and "Bell's palsy." The term "Bell's palsy," from the Scottish anatomist and surgeon,[2] is reserved for an idiopathic lower-motor-nerve lesion ("peripheral") of the seventh cranial nerve.[3] Lower-motor-nerve facial palsies are a common manifestation of Lyme disease, with a presumed pathophysiology intimately related to the infection itself; therefore, the use of "Bell's palsy" in this setting is incorrect. Rather, this manifestation should merely be referred to as a lower-motor facial paresis associated with Lyme disease, thus reserving "Bell's palsy" for facial paresis of truly unknown cause.

Eric R. Eggenberger, D.O.
Johns Hopkins Hospitals
Baltimore, MD 21287

1. Klempner MS, Molloy PJ. Lyme disease. N Engl J Med 1992;327:1793.
2. Bell C. On the nerves of the face, being a second paper on that subject. Phil Trans 1829; 111:317-30.
3. Diseases of the cranial nerves. In: Adams RD, Victor M. Principles of neurology. 4th ed. New York: McGraw-Hill, 1989:1081-3.

Primary Syphilis

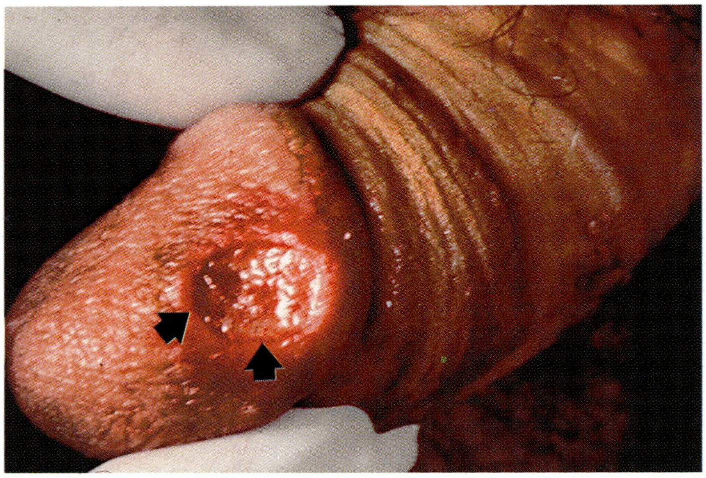

A

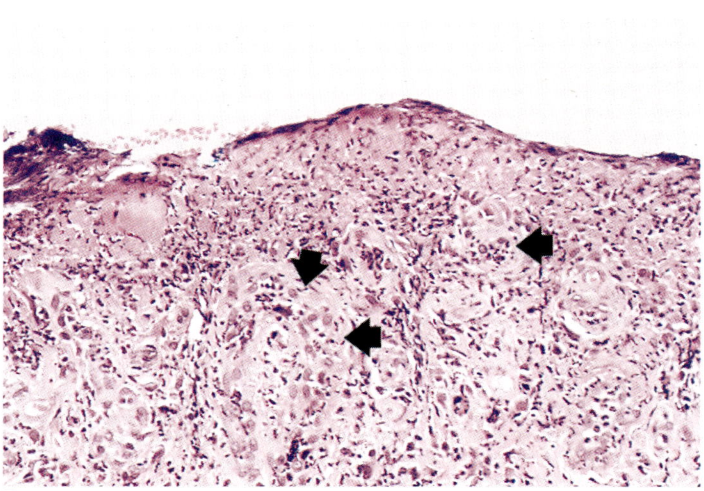

B

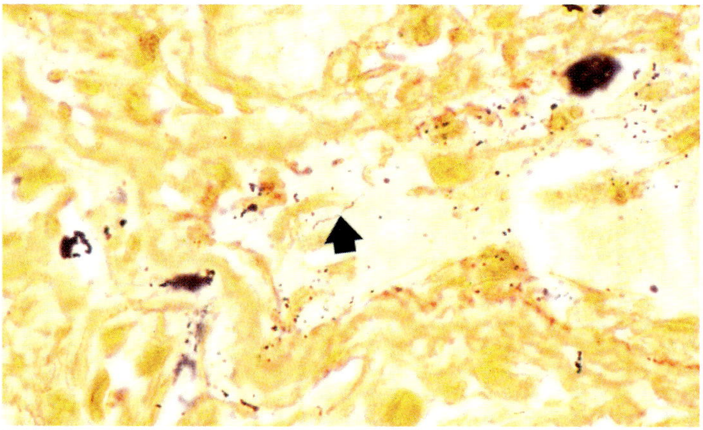

C

Panel A shows a primary chancre of syphilis, which began as a papule, eroded and developed into a painless ulcer (arrows) with raised, firm, indurated borders and a clean smooth base. Histologically, it is characterized by superficial ulceration, plasma-cell infiltrates, endarteritis, and endothelial proliferation (Panel B, arrows). In Panel C silver staining reveals a spirochete 6 to 15 μm in length with regularly spaced spiral coils (arrow).

Tai-Yuen Wong, M.D.
Martin C. Mihm, Jr., M.D.

Massachusetts General Hospital
Boston, MA 02114

December 1, 1994

Correspondence

Syphilis and Coincidence

April 27, 1995

To the Editor: It is instructive to see the vivid illustrations in the Images in Clinical Medicine series, especially Wong and Mihm's images of primary syphilis (Dec. 1 issue).[1]

The photograph showing the hunterian chancre is superb. Also, Wong and Mihm have demonstrated classic histologic techniques with the hematoxylin-and-eosin staining and the spirochetes visualized with silver staining.

The evaluation of this disease would be enhanced, and an immediate diagnosis of a treatable disorder provided, if direct dark-field microscopy was performed on a serum specimen obtained directly from the edge of the chancre by touching a cover-slip to the lesion and pressing the edge. The presence of treponema organisms, which look like twirling, spinning corkscrews, establishes the diagnosis of primary syphilis. This procedure is readily performed with a microscope and a dark-field adapter.

Dark-field microscopy must not be pushed aside when it can offer the most immediate and definite diagnosis, as in this remarkable case, thereby permitting prompt treatment for a potentially destructive systemic disease.

Robert Lee Carter, M.D.
1515 Chain Bridge Rd., McLean, VA 22101

1. Wong T-Y, Mihm MC Jr. Primary syphilis. N Engl J Med 1994;331:1492.

To the Editor: With two articles on syphilis[1,2] and an editorial on the same topic,[3] the December 1 issue might be said to be truly venereal. Appropriately, the Images in Clinical Medicine section also concerns syphilis. The master stroke, however, was to place these illustrations on page 1492. Was this inadvertent, or was it a sly reference to the belief — possibly erroneous — that it was the sailors on Columbus's expedition who brought syphilis back from the New World, whereupon the disease ravaged Europe? If the page allocation was inadvertent, it was certainly felicitous.

Alexander S.D. Spiers, M.D., Ph.D.
University of South Florida, Tampa, FL 33682

1. Gordon SM, Eaton ME, George R, et al. The response of symptomatic neurosyphilis to high-dose intravenous penicillin G in patients with human immunodeficiency virus infection. N Engl J Med 1994;331:1469-73.
2. Horowitz HW, Valsamis MP, Wicher V, et al. Cerebral syphilitic gumma confirmed by the polymerase chain reaction in a man with human immunodeficiency virus infection. N Engl J Med 1994;331:1488-91.
3. Musher DM, Baughn RE. Neurosyphilis in HIV-infected persons. N Engl J Med 1994; 331:1516-7.

To the Editor: There is strong evidence that syphilis was introduced into the Old World after Columbus's expedition to the New World in 1492. I am therefore delighted to note the sense of history reflected in the coincidental publication of the images of syphilis on page 1492.

Peter K. Lewin, M.D.
Hospital for Sick Children, Toronto, ON M5G 1X8, Canada

To the Editor: Is it a curious coincidence that the images of primary syphilis are on page 1492?

Darryl A. Robbins, D.O
3341 E. Livingston Ave., Columbus, OH 43227

Dr. Kassirer replies: Pure coincidence.

Jerome P. Kassirer, M.D.

Secondary Syphilis

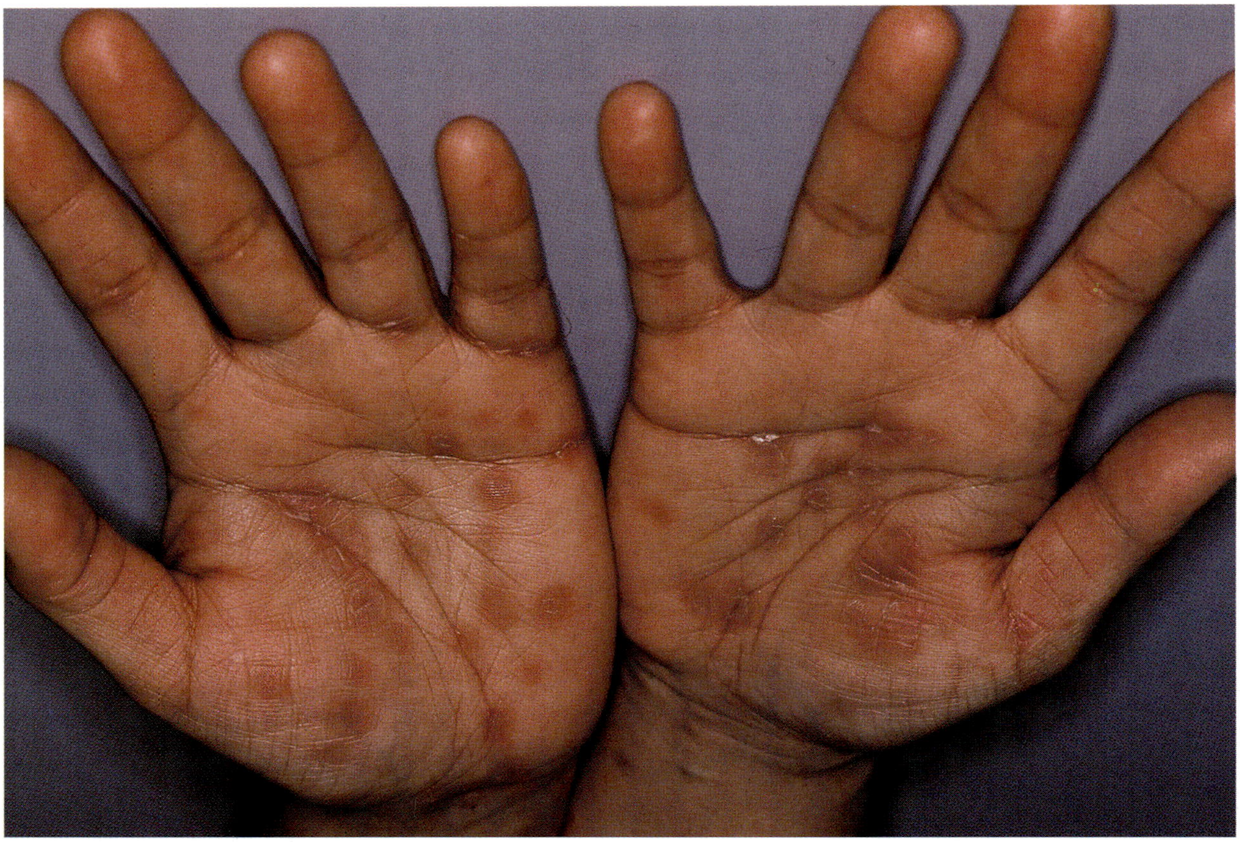

The hands of a 41-year-old woman with secondary syphilis show a symmetric, dusky red, and polymorphic papulosquamous rash, also present on her soles.

Steven R. Potts, D.O.

Northwestern University Medical School
Chicago, IL 60611

July 15, 1993

Purpura Fulminans in Neisseria meningitidis *Sepsis*

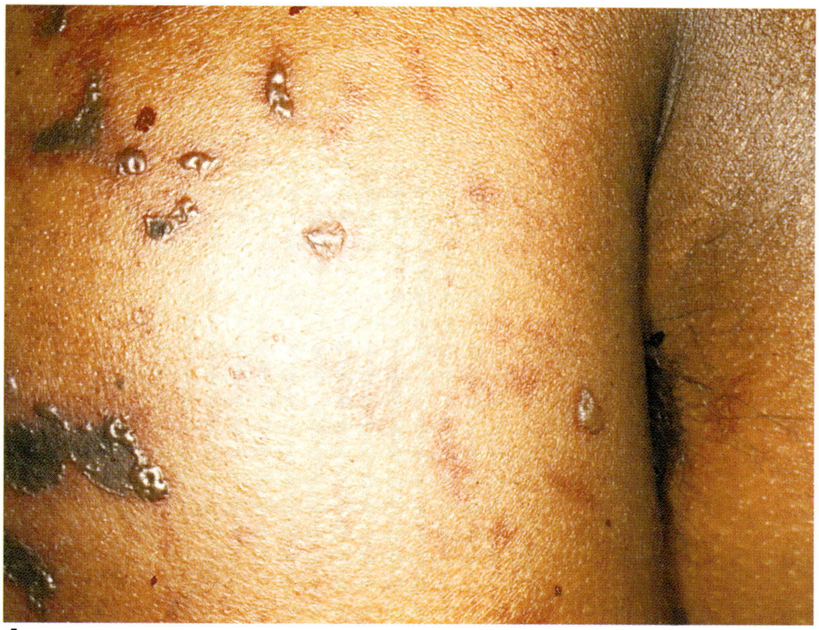

A

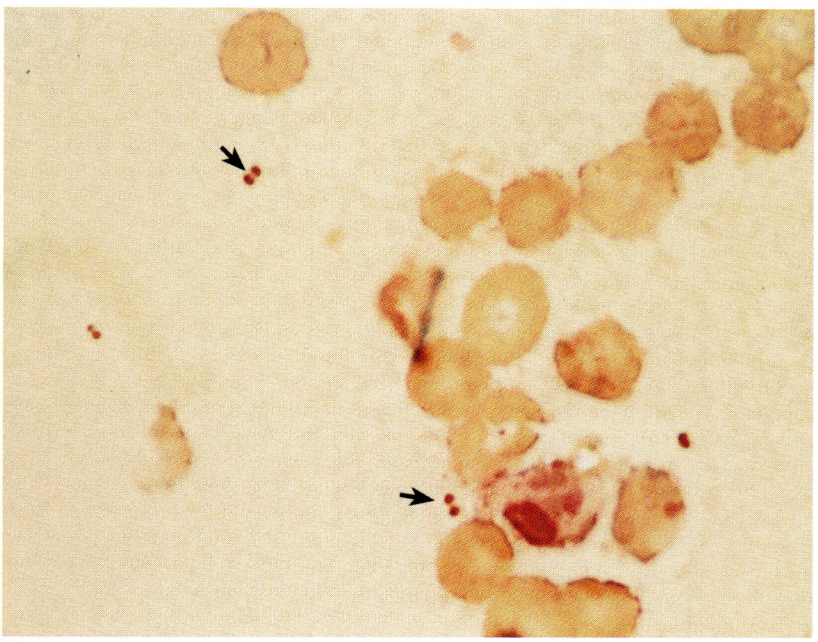

B

A 26-year-old man with a one-day history of mild headache and fever was admitted to the hospital after having a seizure at home. He had had no contact with other sick people. On admission the patient's consciousness was impaired (score on the Glasgow coma scale, 10), but he had no neck stiffness. He was febrile (temperature, 41°C), with hypotension, leukopenia, and thrombocytopenia. Shortly after admission he had another seizure. The cerebrospinal fluid contained 165 red cells and 18 white cells per cubic millimeter, with 60 percent neutrophils, 5 percent band forms, 29 percent lymphocytes, and 6 percent monocytes. A Gram's stain showed no organisms, and antigen tests of the cerebrospinal fluid for *Haemophilus influenzae, Streptococcus pneumoniae, Neisseria meningitidis,* and *S. agalactiae* (group B streptococci) were negative. The patient was intubated and treated with intravenous fluids and ceftriaxone.

Within hours of admission, petechiae developed on the chest, arms, and legs and were quickly replaced by bullous, purpuric lesions (Panel A). On the second day of hospitalization blood cultures obtained on admission were positive for *N. meningitidis* (shown as gram-negative diplococci [arrows] in Panel B; ×1500). Cultures of cerebrospinal fluid were negative. Despite the addition of aztreonam, penicillin G, and corticosteroids to the treatment regimen as well as other supportive measures, disseminated intravascular coagulation and multiorgan failure developed and the patient died on the 19th day of hospitalization.

Luis M. de la Maza, M.D., Ph.D.
Marie Pezzlo, M.A.

University of California, Irvine
Orange, CA 92668-4805

June 27, 1996

Relapsing Fever

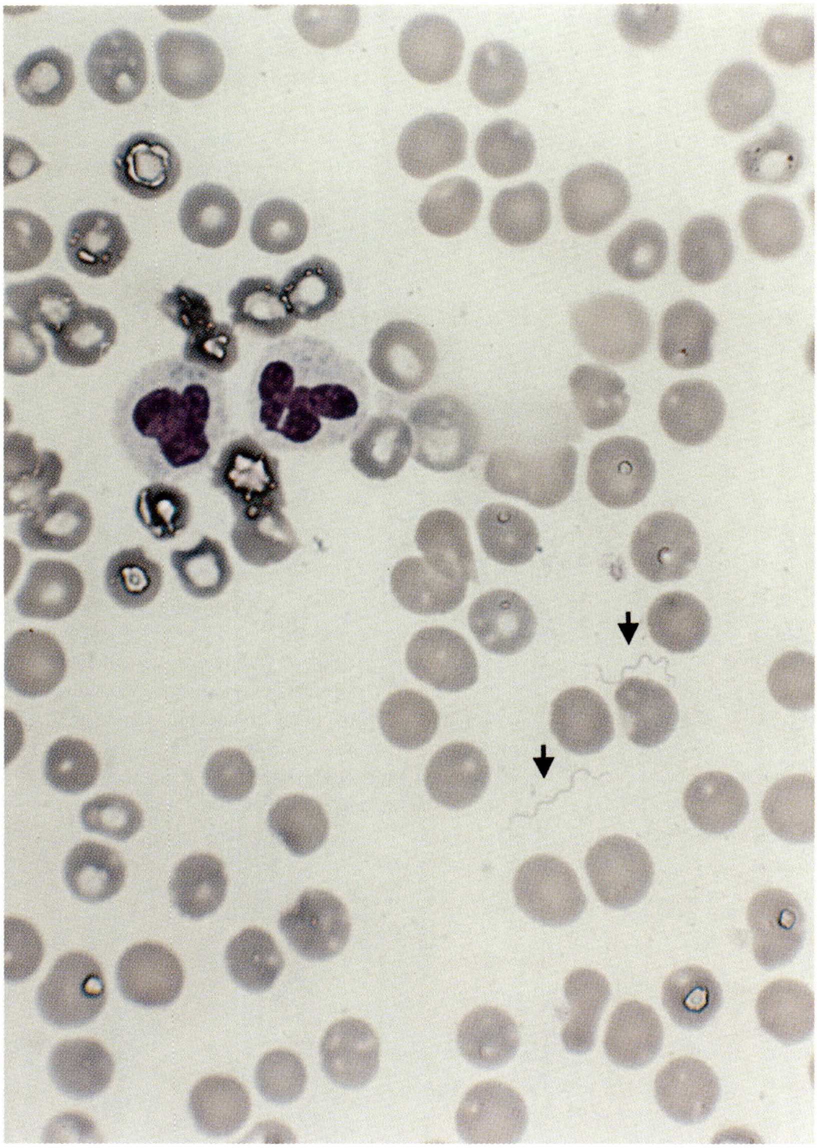

A 41-year-old woman presented with a four-week history of recurring fever (temperature, 40.5°C), headache, and diffuse myalgias. She was one of three family members in whom relapsing fever developed after they vacationed in a rustic, rodent-infested cabin in northeast Washington State. A Wright's-stained peripheral-blood smear contains two borrelia spirochetes (arrows). The patient was treated with 100 mg of doxycycline orally twice a day and had no further symptoms.

James A. Newton, M.D.

Naval Medical Center
Portsmouth, VA 23708

Patricia V. Pepper, M.D.

Naval Medical Center
San Diego, CA 92134

October 17, 1996

Skin and Nail Lesions in Endocarditis

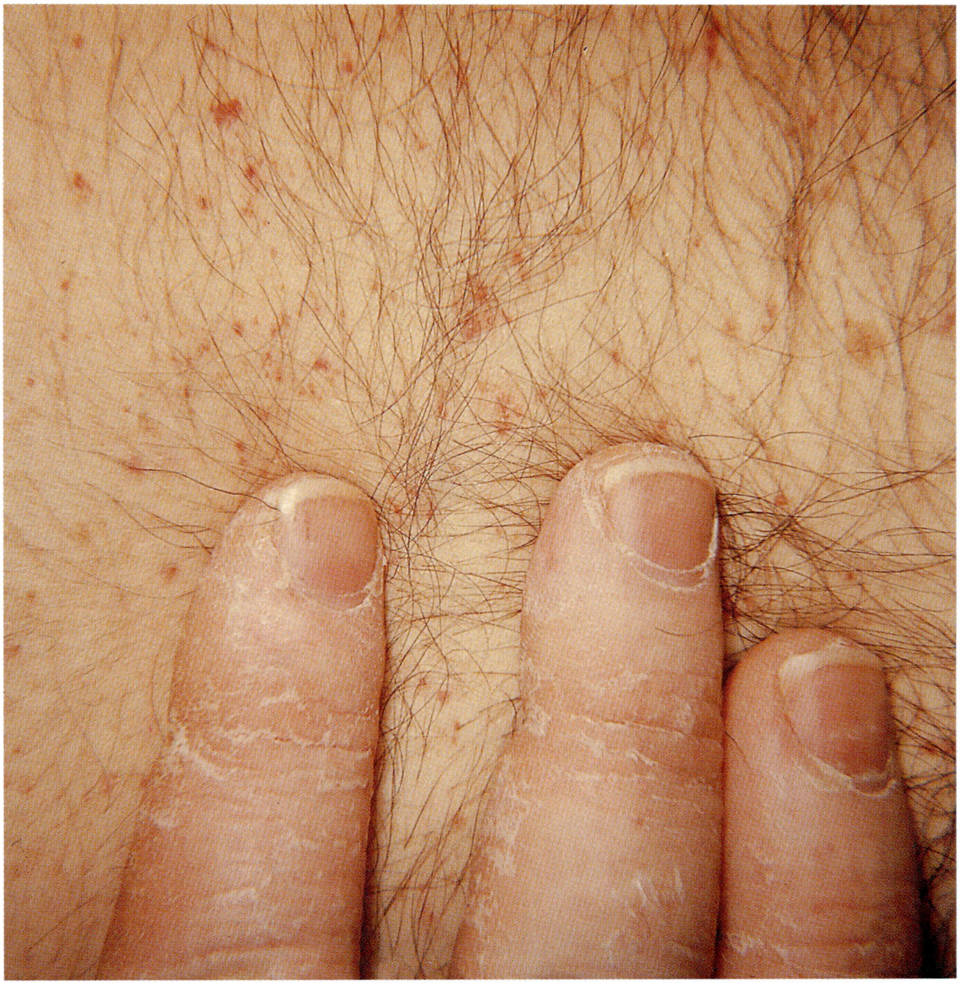

Typical subungual ("splinter") hemorrhage and numerous petechiae on the skin of the abdomen are seen in a patient with staphylococcal endocarditis.

Michael Barza, M.D.

New England Medical Center
Boston, MA 02111

November 25, 1993

Vertebral Osteomyelitis

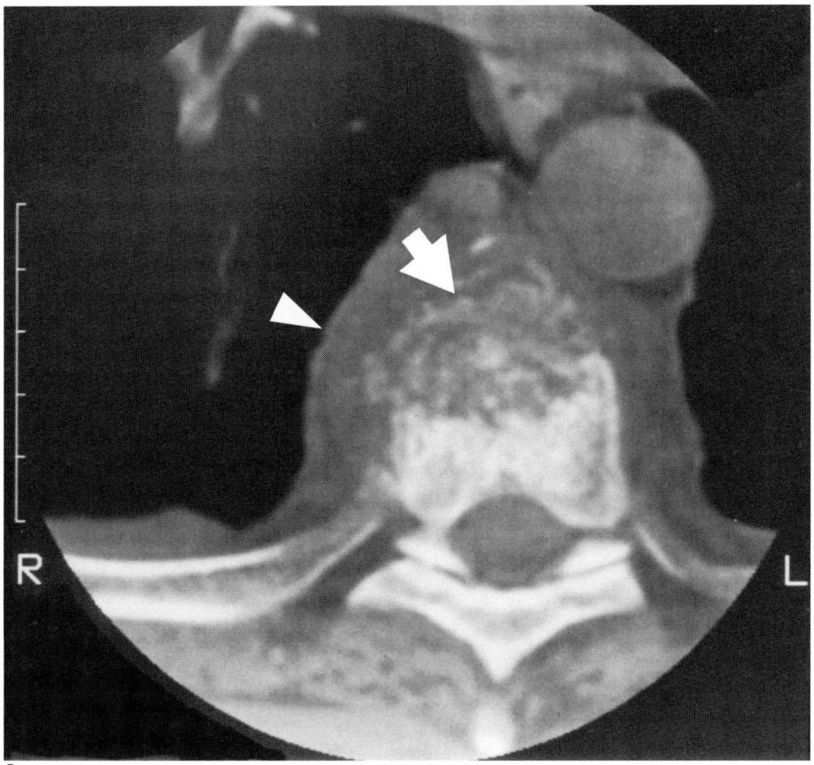

A

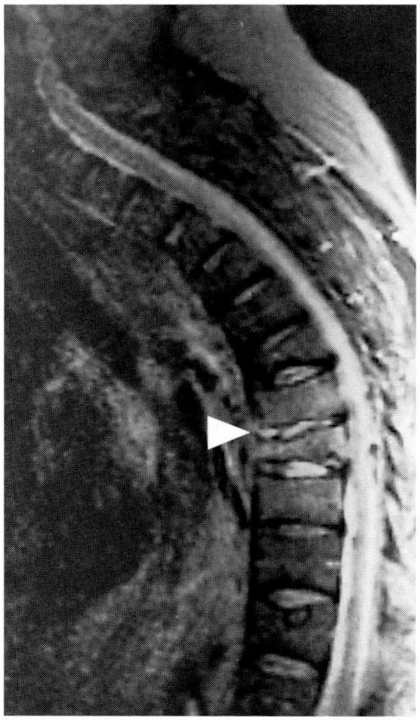

B

A 63-year-old man, admitted to the hospital for an exacerbation of chronic lung disease, had blood cultures that were positive for *Staphylococcus aureus.* Imaging studies of the spine showed that he had vertebral osteomyelitis, diskitis between T8 and T9, and a paravertebral inflammatory mass. Panel A is an unenhanced computed tomogram of the spine at T8. The inferior end-plate of the vertebral body is eroded (arrow), with a large surrounding area of paraspinal soft-tissue density (arrowhead). Panel B is a sagittal T_2-weighted magnetic resonance image of the thoracic spine. An increased signal is seen at the intervertebral disk between T8 and T9, a finding consistent with diskitis (arrowhead). The body of T8 also shows anterior wedging and the loss of normal height.

Mihran A. Artinian, M.D.
Albert T. Leung, M.D.
Peter V. Tishler, M.D.

Brockton–West Roxbury Veterans Affairs Medical Center
Brockton, MA 02401

August 5, 1993

Acute Bacterial Endocarditis

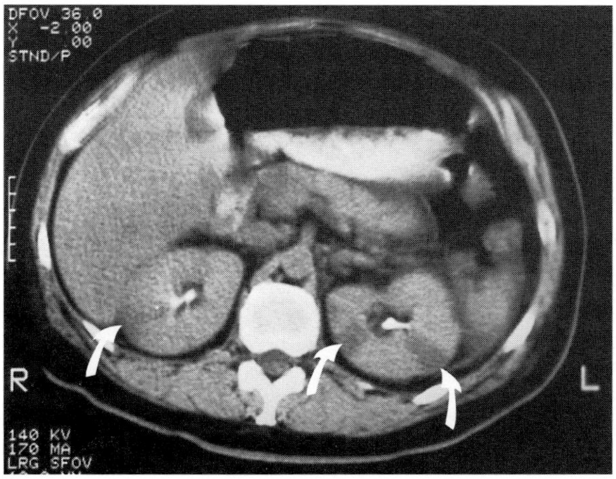

A

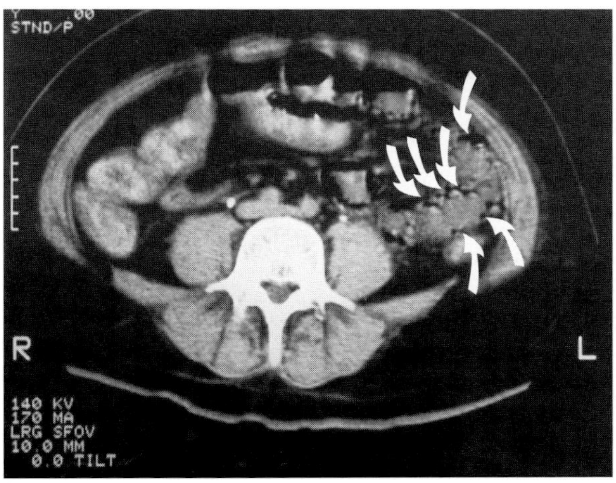

B

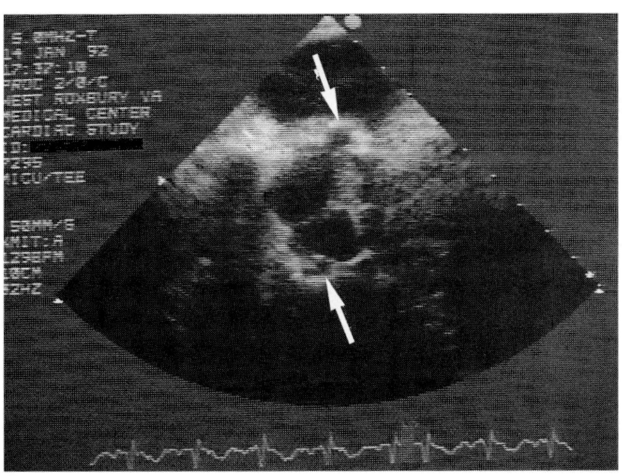

C

Lesions of acute bacterial endocarditis are shown in a 40-year-old male intravenous drug user with sudden fever, severe crampy, left-sided abdominal pain, nausea, and vomiting. A contrast-enhanced abdominal CT scan demonstrates bilateral wedge-shaped low-density areas (curved white arrows, Panel A) in both kidneys that are consistent with embolic infarcts. A lower section (Panel B) shows mildly dilated small-bowel loops on the left, with air in the wall of the small bowel (white arrows), that are consistent with pneumatosis intestinalis and bowel infarction. Transesophageal echocardiographic imaging of the aortic valve and aortic root (Panel C) identified a 1-cm aortic-valve vegetation (not shown), as well as two echolucent spaces at the anterior and posterior walls of the aortic root (white arrows), consistent with localized abscess cavities. The line drawing (Panel D) corresponds to the real-time two-dimensional image shown in Panel C. Multiple blood cultures grew *Staphylococcus aureus.* The presence of aortic-valve ring abscesses led to prompt surgical intervention.

Michael E. Jay, M.D.

Brockton–West Roxbury Veterans Affairs Medical Center
West Roxbury, MA 02132

Marc T. Silver, M.D.

Massachusetts General Hospital
Boston, MA 02114

December 10, 1992

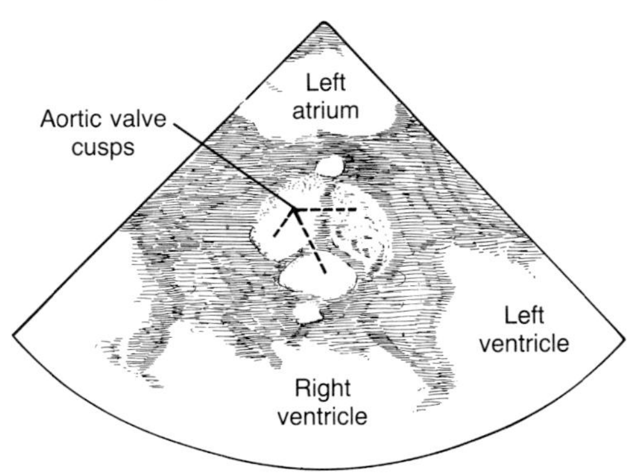

D

Acid-Fast Organisms

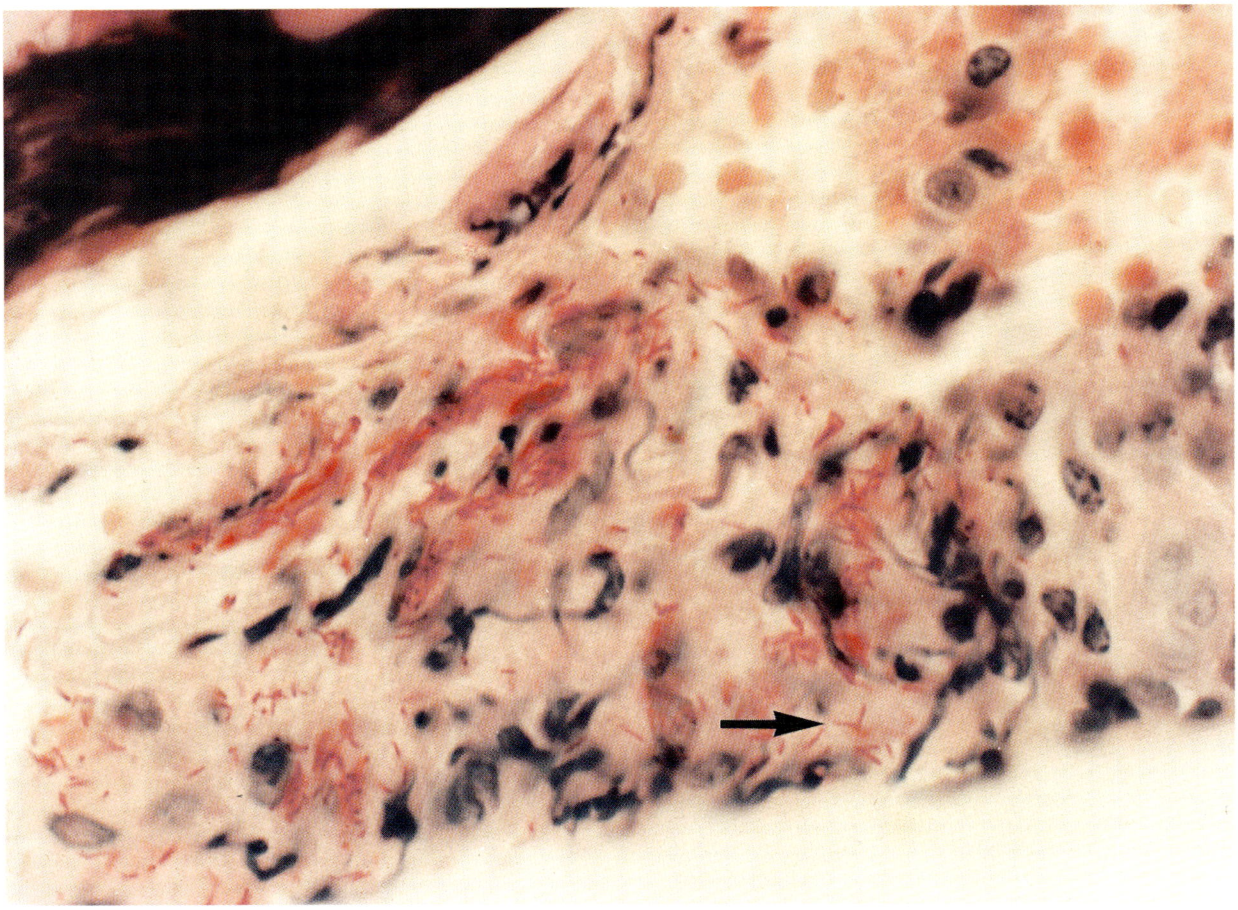

A bone marrow–biopsy specimen, stained by the Ziehl–Neelsen technique (×1000), was obtained from a 47-year-old man with the acquired immunodeficiency syndrome who presented with a high fever and pancytopenia. The small bright-red, rod-shaped cells (arrow) are acid-fast organisms. The larger bright-red areas are clumps of the same organisms. Despite therapy with a combination of ethambutol, clofazimine, rifampin, and ciprofloxacin, the patient died 11 days after the biopsy was performed. Bone marrow cultures subsequently grew *Mycobacterium xenopi.*

Scott Saxman, M.D.

Indiana University School of Medicine
Indianapolis, IN 46202

Ruth Ann Portman, M.T.

University of Oklahoma
Oklahoma City, OK 73104

April 14, 1994

Cytomegalovirus Retinitis in AIDS

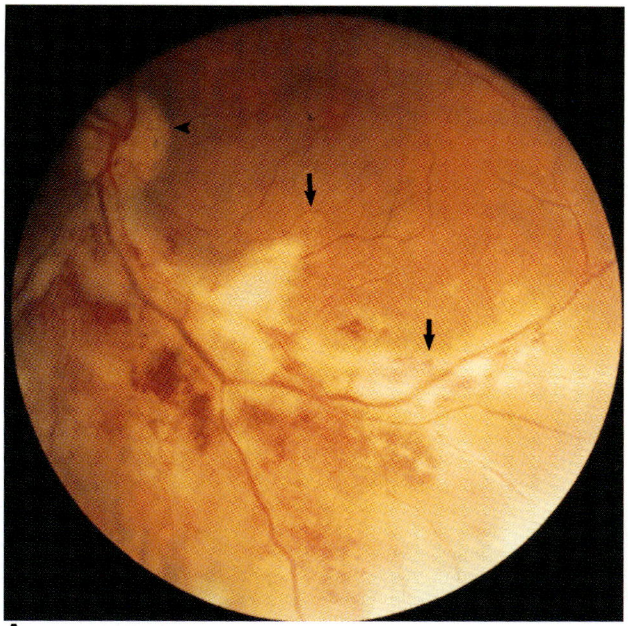

A

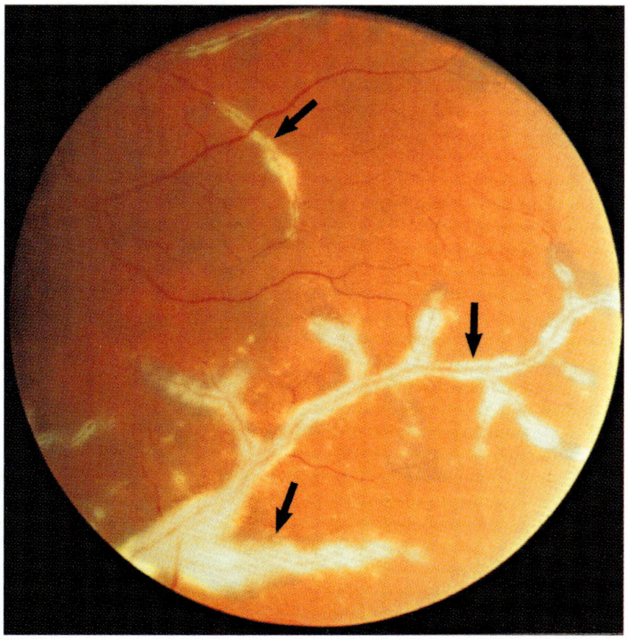

B

A 35-year-old man with the acquired immunodeficiency syndrome presented with floaters and blurred vision in both eyes. In the left eye (Panel A), the white wedge-shaped areas with accompanying hemorrhage along the inferior vascular arcade (arrows) represent necrosis of the retina. The arrowhead points to the optic disk. In the right eye (Panel B), the peripheral retina shows white sheathing along the blood vessels, so-called frosted-branch sheathing (arrows), a finding characteristic of vasculitis but not pathognomonic for cytomegalovirus retinitis.

The patient was treated with intravenous ganciclovir. The retinal lesions regressed, and vision improved. Six months later, the patient died of multiple opportunistic infections.

Jan E.E. Keunen, M.D., Ph.D.
Aniki Rothova, M.D., Ph.D.

Academisch Ziekenhuis Utrecht
3584 CX Utrecht, the Netherlands

September 7, 1995

Zidovudine Myopathy

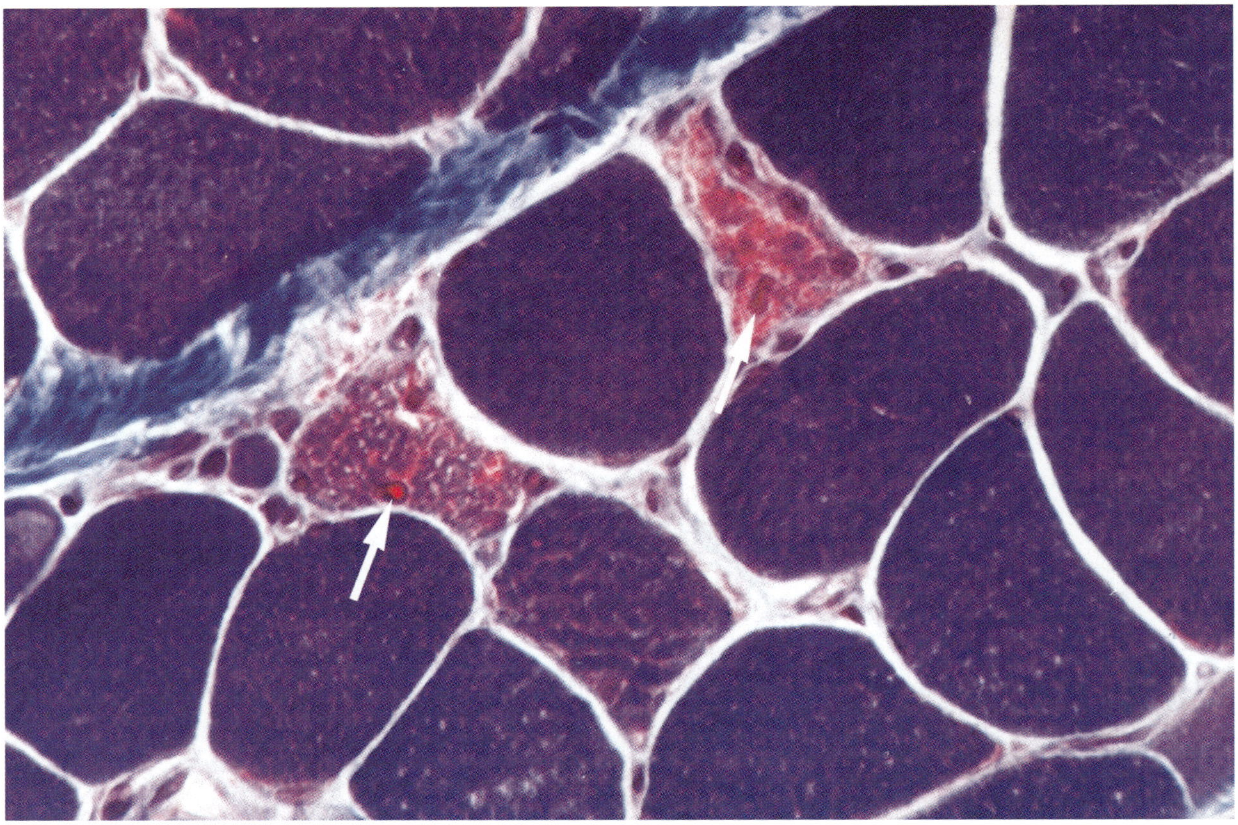

A muscle-biopsy specimen from a 33-year-old man who had been treated with zidovudine for 24 months shows an accumulation of fine reddish granules in the sarcoplasm, corresponding to mitochondria in atrophic fibers (trichrome, ×600). In addition to mitochondrial accumulation, the fibers show marked myofilamentous abnormalities that include myofibrillar loss and cytoplasmic-body formation (arrows).

Patrick Chariot, M.D.

Hôpital Henri-Mondor
94000 Créteil, France

June 10, 1993

Kawasaki's Disease

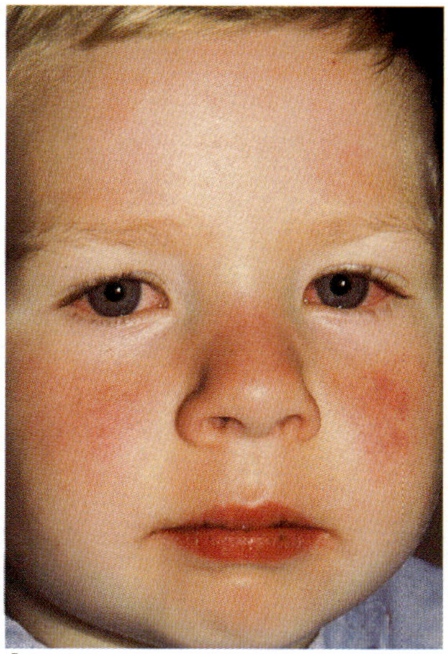

A

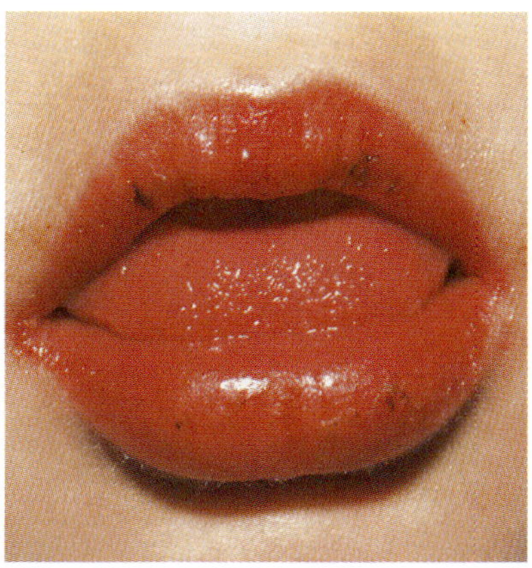

B

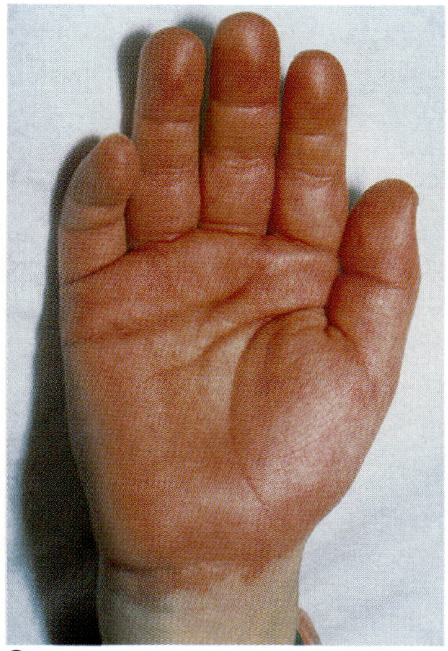

C

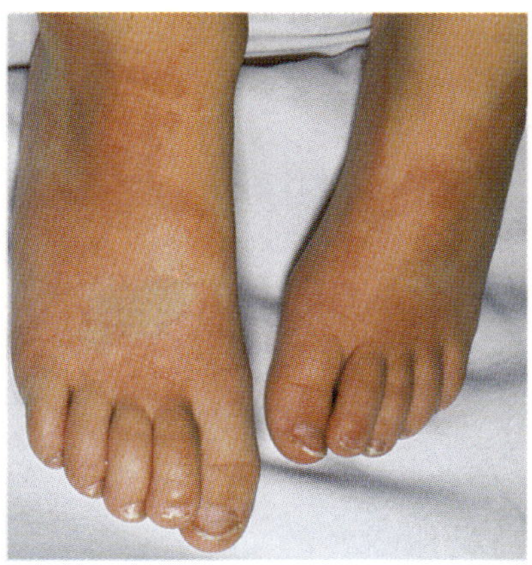

D

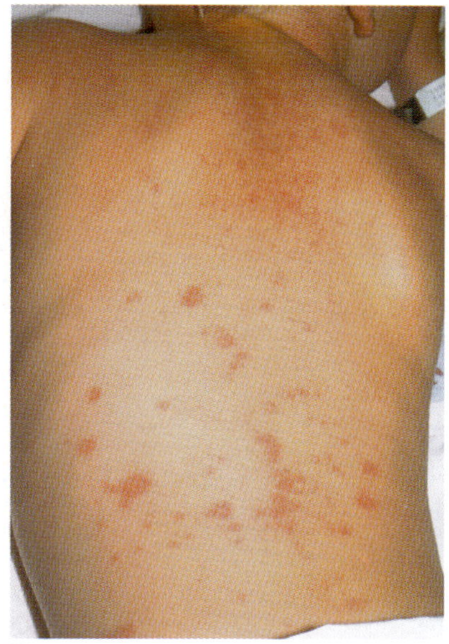

E

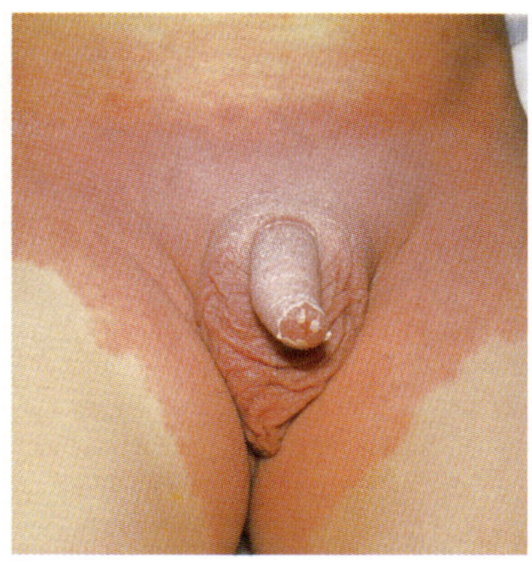

F

Photographs of a four-year-old boy show the typical features of Kawasaki's disease. These features include bilateral nonexudative conjunctivitis (Panel A); dry, fissured, erythematous lips and a "strawberry" tongue (Panels A and B); erythematous and edematous hands and feet (Panels C and D); an erythematous truncal rash (Panel E); and a desquamating perineal rash (Panel F). The patient also had anterior cervical lymphadenopathy and sterile pyuria but none of the other complications of the disease. The child recovered uneventfully after receiving treatment with intravenous immune globulin and aspirin.

Jonathan D.K. Trager, M.D.

Children's Hospital of Pittsburgh
Pittsburgh, PA 15213

November 23, 1995

Rabies

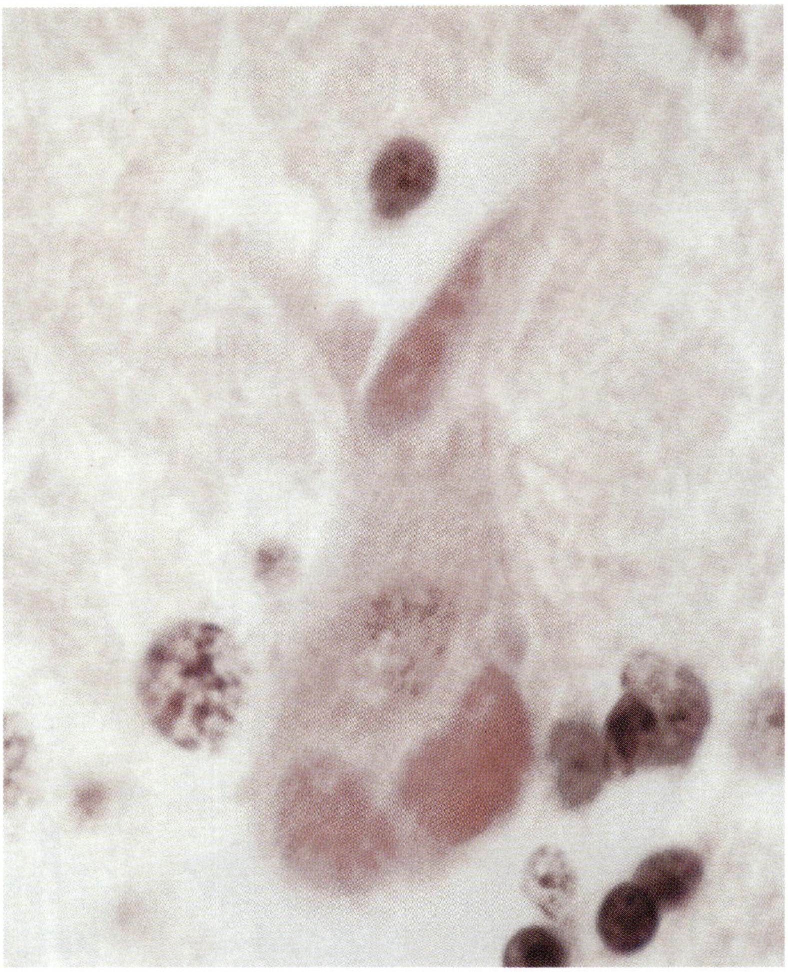

Three large Negri bodies, which are eosinophilic viral inclusion bodies, can be seen in the cytoplasm of a cerebellar Purkinje cell obtained at autopsy from an eight-year-old boy in Mexico City (hematoxylin and eosin, ×2300). These viral inclusions are the pathological hallmark of rabies. The boy, bitten on the forearm by a dog that died of rabies 15 days later, had numbness and tingling at the site of the bite several days later. He presented at a clinic one month after the bite, and rabies vaccination with Fuenzalida vaccine (suckling-mouse-brain vaccine) was initiated. Two days later he was admitted to the hospital with agitation, aggressive behavior, and hydrophobia. He was treated with sedation, antiepileptic therapy, immune globulin, and ribavirin. His condition progressively deteriorated, and he died 10 days after admission. In the United States, recommendations for post-exposure rabies prophylaxis include prompt local cleaning of the wound with soap and water, administration of human rabies immune globulin by infiltration about the wound and intramuscularly (gluteal region), and initiation of a course of rabies vaccination with human diploid-cell vaccine or rhesus-monkey diploid-cell vaccine (rabies vaccine, adsorbed).

Alan C. Jackson, M.D.

Queen's University
Kingston, ON K7L 3J7, Canada

Eduardo Lopez-Corella, M.D., Ph.D.

Instituto Nacional de Pediatria
04530 Mexico DF, Mexico

August 22, 1996

Fifth Disease

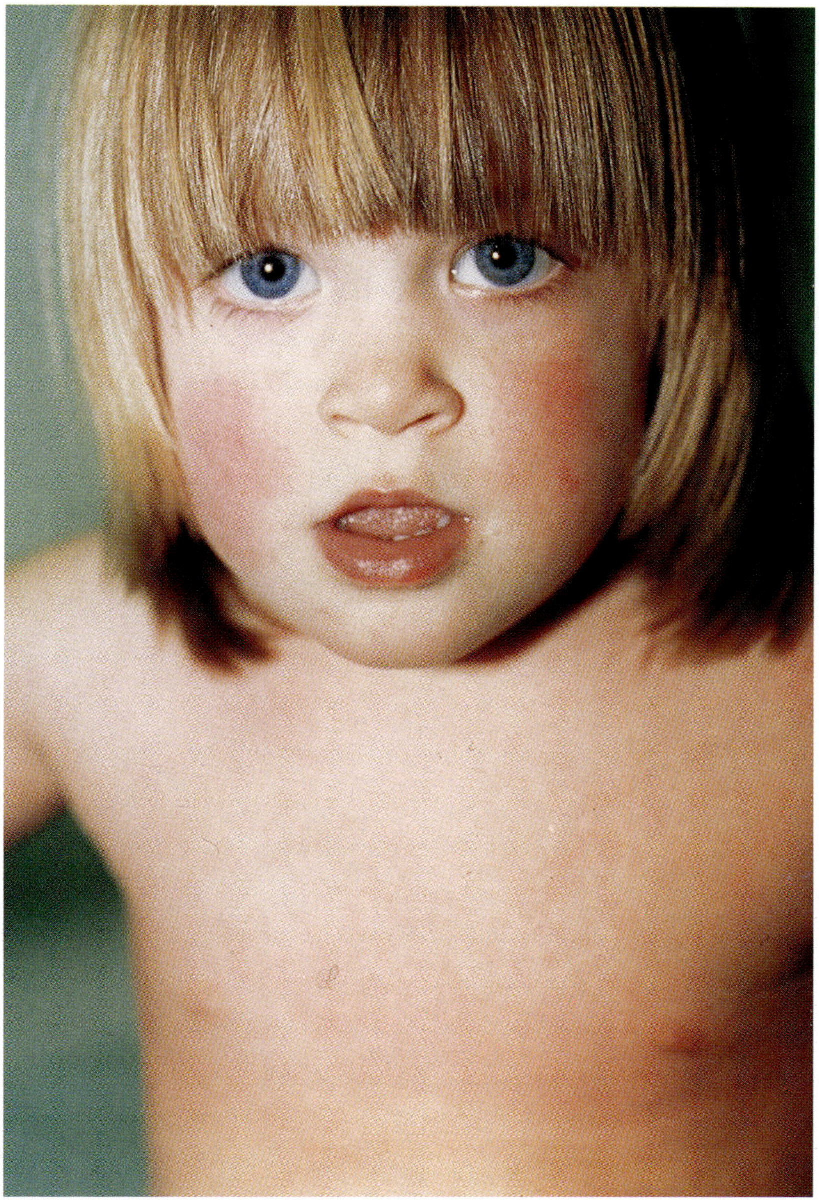

Typical "slapped cheek" rash is apparent in a two-year-old child with fifth disease (erythema infectiosum), caused by parvovirus B19 infection. The common lacelike erythema of the trunk is also present but not clearly in focus. This disease, which is usually self-limited, is one of the six classic childhood exanthems, which include measles (rubeola), scarlet fever, German measles (rubella), Filatov–Dukes disease (not a separate exanthem but a variant of scarlet fever or toxin-producing staphylococcus infection), and exanthema subitum, or roseola (human herpesvirus 6 infection).

Henry M. Feder, Jr., M.D.

University of Connecticut
Health Center
Farmington, CT 06030

October 20, 1994

Vulvar Herpes Simplex Infection

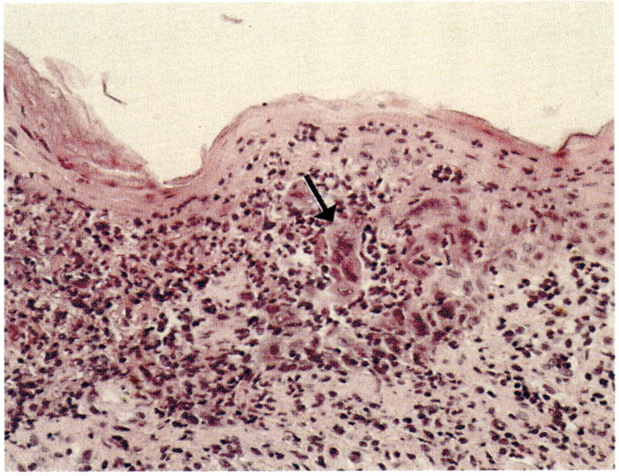

A

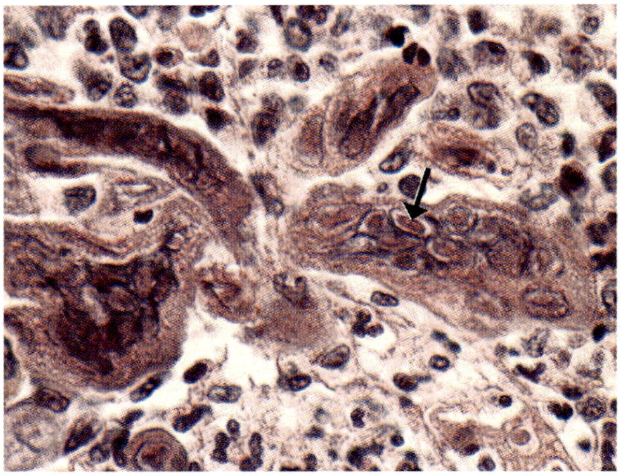

B

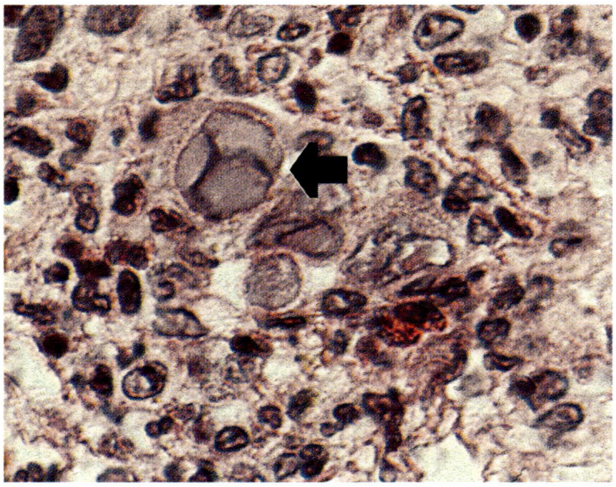

C

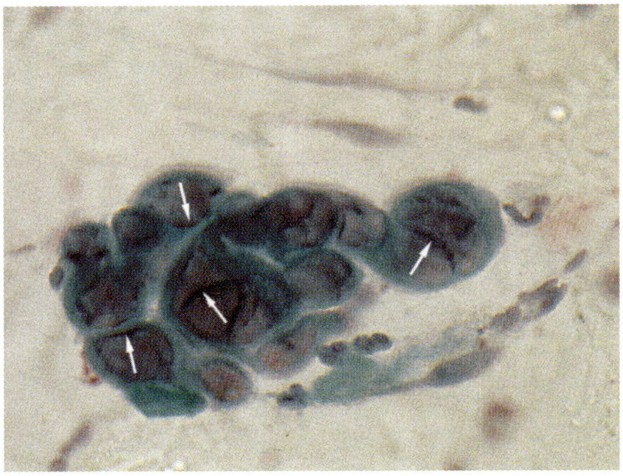

D

Characteristic histologic changes are seen in herpes simplex virus infection of the vulva. Panel A shows necrosis of the epidermis and dermis, with acute inflammation and nuclear debris on the left, viable mucosal keratinocytes on the right, and multinucleated giant cells in the center (arrow) (hematoxylin–eosin, ×90). Panel B shows multinucleated cells with Cowdry type A intranuclear viral inclusions (arrow) (hematoxylin–eosin, ×220). Panel C shows nuclear molding (the contours of adjacent nuclei conform to one another) with a ground-glass chromatin pattern (arrow) in an enlarged, multinucleated cell (hematoxylin–eosin, ×480). In Panel D, a vaginal smear shows margination by nuclear chromatin (arrows) (Papanicolaou's stain, ×550).

Jeoffry Brennick, M.D.
Lyn Duncan, M.D.

Massachusetts General Hospital
Boston, MA 02114

December 9, 1993

Herpes Simplex Virus Corneal Dendrite

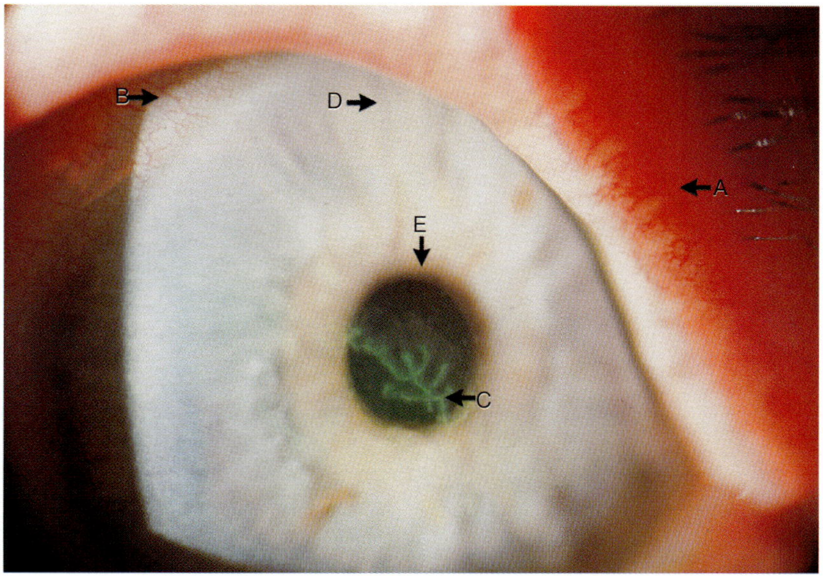

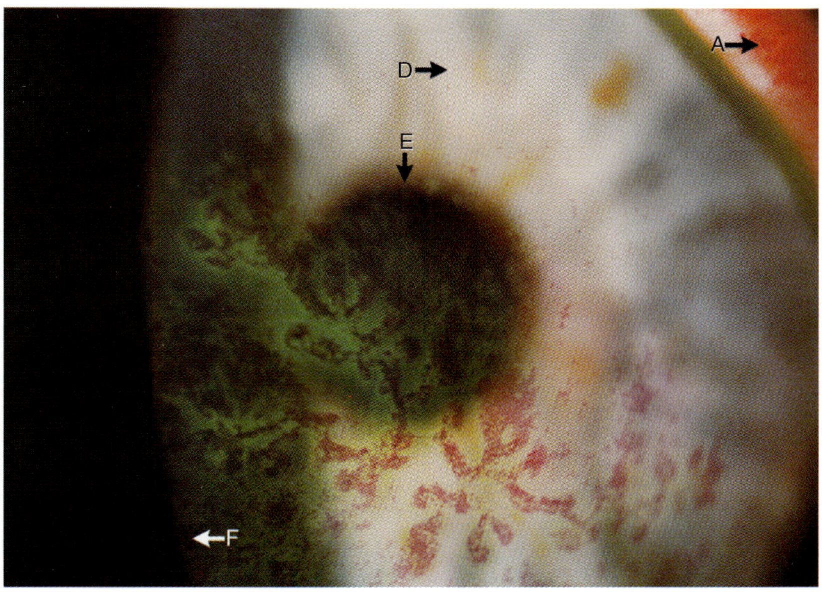

A herpes simplex virus corneal dendrite is revealed by slit-lamp examination with fluorescein (upper panel) and fluorescein plus rose bengal (lower panel, high power) in a 70-year-old man who reported two days of pain and redness in his right eye. His visual acuity was minimally diminished. The lids (A) are normal; the conjunctiva (B) is injected; the diagnostic dendrite (C) results from a branching pattern of desquamation of infected corneal epithelial cells. Desquamated cornea stains with fluorescein, whereas the remaining infected epithelial cells at the margin of the dendrite stain brilliantly with rose bengal. This epithelial infection differs from a corneal ulcer, which involves infection and erosion of the corneal stroma. The iris (D) and pupil (E) are normal. The leading edge of the slit-lamp beam (F) reveals the sloping contour of the corneal surface and suggests that the depth of the anterior chamber is normal. The patient was successfully treated with a 14-day course of topical trifluridine, an antiviral agent, and had no permanent visual impairment.

Thomas A. Ciulla, M.D.
Kit Johnson

Massachusetts Eye and
Ear Infirmary
Boston, MA 02114

December 28, 1995

Herpes Zoster

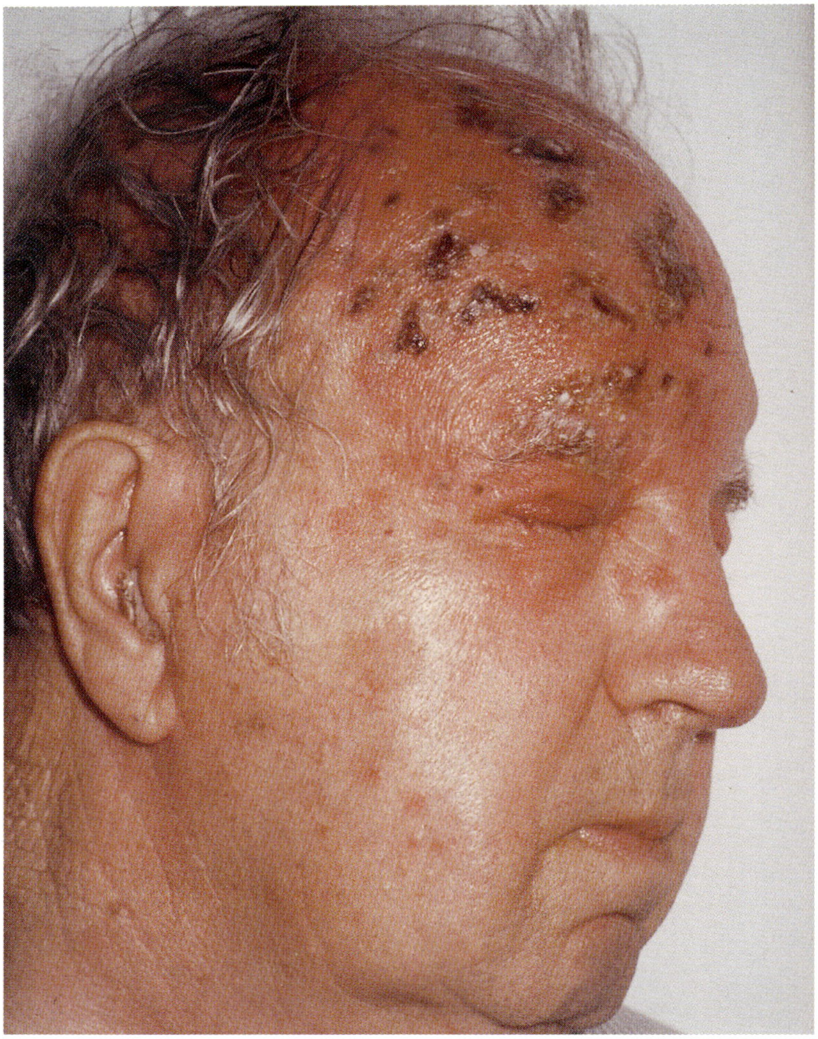

A 78-year-old man had numerous crusts and erosions on the right side of his face and scalp. Staining with a monoclonal-antibody stain (Syva Microtrak, Palo Alto, Calif.) conjugated with fluorescein isothiocyanate specific for varicella–zoster virus glycoproteins was performed on fluid from lesions on the patient's back and was positive. An ophthalmologic examination also revealed keratitis. The only risk factor identified for dissemination was the daily use of 1 percent hydrocortisone cream when the facial lesions first appeared. The patient was treated with intravenous acyclovir along with trifluridine and sulfacetamide–prednisolone eye drops. After the lesions disappeared, postherpetic neuralgia developed.

Greg Rosencrance, M.D.

West Virginia University Health
Sciences Center
Charleston, WV 25304

March 31, 1994

Correspondence

Trifluridine for Herpes Zoster

August 18, 1994

To the Editor: In the Images in Clinical Medicine section (March 31 issue),[1] Rosencrance presents an excellent clinical photograph of herpes zoster involving the right trigeminal nerve. He mentions that the patient was treated with intravenous acyclovir, as well as trifluridine and sulfacetamide–prednisolone eyedrops. I am aware of no study supporting the use of trifluridine for the treatment of herpes zoster keratitis.[2] Topical trifluridine is extremely expensive, causes side effects such as superficial punctate keratopathy and epithelial defects, and is indicated only for the treatment of external eye infections caused by herpes simplex virus. Although herpes zoster uveitis and keratitis may respond to topical steroids, the need for sulfacetamide (presumably to prevent superinfection by sulfa-sensitive bacteria) is also questionable in this case.

David J. Harris, Jr., M.D.
University of Tennessee Medical Center
Knoxville, TN 37920

1. Rosencrance G. Herpes zoster. N Engl J Med 1994;330:906.
2. Karbassi M, Raizman MB, Schuman JS. Herpes zoster ophthalmicus. Surv Ophthalmol 1992;36:395-410.

Dr. Rosencrance and a colleague, Dr. Frances, reply:

To the Editor: Dr. Harris is correct in stating that there is no study supporting the use of trifluridine eyedrops for the treatment of herpes zoster keratitis. However, to classify trifluridine as extremely expensive is misleading. The cost at our institution for a 7.5-ml bottle is $26.50. During the acute phase of herpes zoster ophthalmicus, topical steroids are clearly indicated and effective in suppressing the inflammatory response.[1] They are also effective in reducing corneal infiltrates and keratic precipitates.[2] Since the risk of superinfection is present, we think simultaneous topical antibiotics are indicated.

Greg Rosencrance, M.D.
Charles Frances, M.D.
West Virginia University
Charleston, WV 25304-1299

1. Mader TH, Stulting RD. Viral keratitis. Infect Dis Clin North Am 1992;6:831-49.
2. Bergaust B, Westby RK. Zoster ophthalmicus: local treatment with cortisone. Acta Ophthalmol 1967;45:787-93.

Smallpox — 26 Years Ago

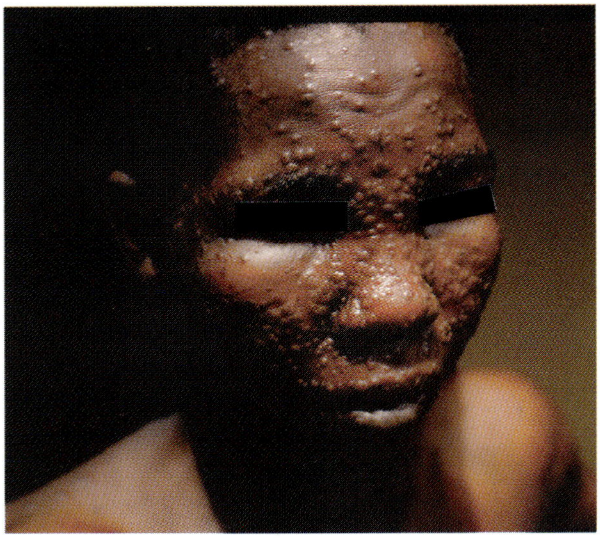

A

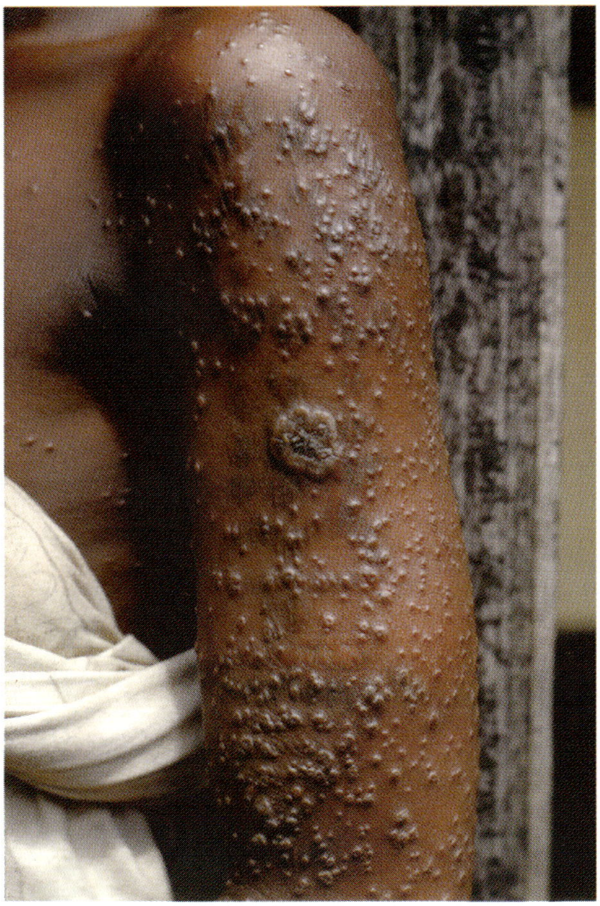

B

The last case of smallpox within a 20-nation area of west and central Africa was found in Nigeria on May 21, 1970. This event marked the success of a five-year program to eradicate smallpox from a large area in which it was endemic. The 27-year-old patient was the last victim in an epidemic of about 86 documented cases. She had been vaccinated about 10 days before these photographs were taken, as part of activities to control the outbreak after the discovery of smallpox in one other resident of her village a week previously.

These figures illustrate some classic features of smallpox: the patient appears weak or fatigued, the lesions have a peripheral distribution, there is facial edema, and the lesions are deep-seated, firm in appearance, and uniform in terms of stage of development (Panel A). The relatively small and variable size of the lesions on the left arm and the large pustule consistent with a successful primary vaccination (Panel B), as well as a relatively rapid course of illness (the photographs were taken on day 3 of the rash), suggest that this last case was modified (and almost prevented) by vaccination. This program's successful techniques were later used in the parts of the world where the disease was still endemic, ultimately leading to the complete cessation of natural transmission of smallpox in October 1977.

Charles Herron, M.D.

10014 Edgewater Dr.
Cleveland, OH 44102

May 16, 1996

Correspondence

Smallpox

September 19, 1996

To the Editor: Herron provides striking photographs of a patient with smallpox in the May 16 issue.[1] Of course, 1996 is the 200th anniversary of Edward Jenner's first use of vaccination against smallpox, in Berkeley, England. Jenner's courageous act was not inoculating pus from a cowpox lesion into a small boy, but later inoculating pus from a smallpox lesion into that boy to prove his immunity. This would certainly be a controversial experiment today.

James Magner, M.D.
East Carolina University
Greenville, NC 27858-4354

1. Herron C. Smallpox — 26 years ago. N Engl J Med 1996;334:1304.

To the Editor: The photographs of the patient with smallpox brought back images of tropical medicine and "people-to-people" public health programs from my early Vietnam War experiences. They also raised doubt about the precise diagnosis: smallpox modified by vaccination.

In 1962, before the main U.S. military escalation in Vietnam and before the fall of the Diem regime, a civilian physician from the U.S. Operations Mission and I were dispatched in a convoy through the jungles to verify reports of a smallpox outbreak among Montagnard villagers.

What we found at the end of our journey was a small village with half a dozen fresh graves (allegedly of smallpox victims, but during war, who knows?). Of the villagers who came out to greet us, fully 40 percent looked exactly like the patient in Dr. Herron's photographs. However, there was a major difference. Questioning revealed that a French medical team had been through the area nine days earlier and had inoculated one third of the villagers, using the old French method of scarification. Drops of smallpox vaccine were placed on the upper arm and scarified with the tip of a lancet, so that the skin was cut and blood appeared in the X-shaped scar through each droplet.

In those days, French textbooks described the technique for "vaccination antivariolique" as follows: "Scarification must be epidermal; it is necessary to avoid reaching the dermis and causing bleeding. . . . A simple linear incision 3 to 5 mm long is sufficient."[1]

Despite the warning, the result in Vietnam was iatrogenic generalized vaccinia in most patients. The resultant shedding of the virus generated numerous secondary cases throughout the village, thus increasing the overall herd immunity.

According to Henderson:

> Generalized vaccinia represents a secondary eruption resulting from bloodborne dissemination of vaccinia virus. Almost all cases occur after primary vaccination. The lesions become evident between six and nine days after vaccination. The number of lesions may range from a few to a generalized involvement of the skin. It is a self-limited illness, and complete recovery occurs without a specific therapy.[2]

Benenson also notes that the vesicles of generalized vaccinia appear 5 to 10 days after vaccination and that the condition is benign and self-limited.[3]

It seems to me that the information on timing, as well as the clinical description accompanying the photographs, may well be consistent with the above description.

John P. Maher, M.D., M.P.H.
Chester County Health Department
West Chester, PA 19382-4542

1. Fattorusso V, Ritter AO. Vademecum clinique du médecin practicien du symptôme à l'ordonnance. 3rd ed. Paris: Masson et Cie, 1958.

Correspondence Continued

2. Henderson DA. Variola and vaccinia. In: Wyngaarden JB, Smith LH Jr, eds. Cecil textbook of medicine. 18th ed. Vol. 2. Philadelphia: W.B. Saunders, 1988:1791-3.
3. Benenson AS. Smallpox. In: Wehrle PF, Top FH, eds. Communicable and infectious diseases. 9th ed. St. Louis: Mosby, 1981:577-88.

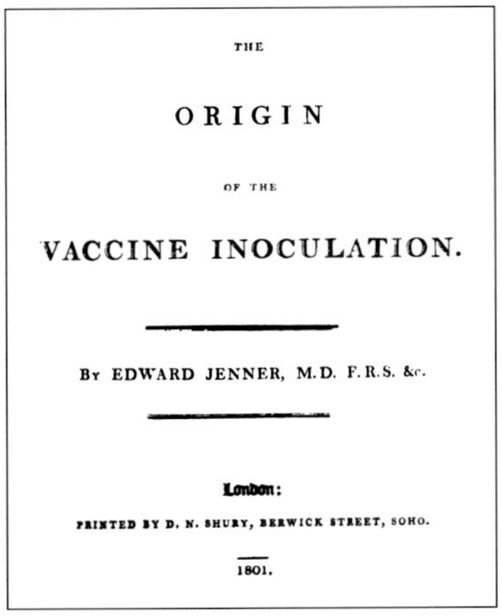

THE

ORIGIN

OF THE

VACCINE INOCULATION.

By EDWARD JENNER, M.D. F.R.S. &c.

London:

PRINTED BY D. N. SHURY, BERWICK STREET, SOHO.

1801.

Figure 1. Edward Jenner's Report on Cowpox Inoculation, Published Five Years after His First Experiment on May 14, 1796.

To the Editor: The photographs of a patient with smallpox in Nigeria in 1970 remind us of the modifying effect of smallpox vaccination on the natural course of smallpox and, more important, of the eradication of this dreadful disease due to the successful program started in 1958 by the World Health Organization.

Is it a coincidence that you published this image on nearly the same day, though 200 years later, that Edward Jenner performed the famous inoculation of cowpox virus into the young James Phipps, on May 14, 1796?

The successful eradication program is based on Jenner's experiments and on his lifelong promotion of vaccine inoculation. In 1801 he summarized his experiences with cowpox inoculation (Fig. 1) and stated, "The numbers who have partaken of its benefits throughout Europe and other parts of the Globe are incalculable: and it now becomes too manifest to admit of controversy, that the annihilation of the Small Pox, the most dreadful scourge of the human species, must be the final result of this practice."[1] He got it right, 200 years later. The most recent Swedish textbook of infectious diseases does not even mention smallpox.

To those who have forgotten, we might add that the term "vaccination" itself is derived from Jenner's cowpox inoculation: *vacca* means cow in Latin, and the term was introduced by Louis Pasteur to honor Jenner.[2]

Andreas Aly, M.D., Ph.D.
Sophia Aly
Ersta Hospital
S-116 91 Stockholm, Sweden

1. Jenner E. The origin of the vaccine inoculation. London: D.N. Shury, 1801.
2. Fenner F, Henderson DA, Arita I, Ježek Z, Ladnyi ID. Smallpox and its eradication. Geneva: World Health Organization, 1988.

To the Editor: It seems unlikely that the image of smallpox appeared in the *Journal* by chance during the very week that the bicentenary of the first smallpox vaccination was commemorated. Thus, it seems perverse that the originator of vaccination, Edward Jenner, was not mentioned by name. It was on May 14, 1796, that Dr. Jenner, a country doctor from Berkeley, Gloucestershire, England, extracted the contents of a pustule from the arm of a cowpox-infected milkmaid, Sarah Nelmes, and injected it into the arm of eight-year-old James Phipps, thereby inaugurating vaccination, which has proved so successful in controlling not only smallpox but many other life-threatening infectious diseases in the subsequent 200 years. This contribution to medical science seems to me worthy of at least a passing reference.

Andrew J. Larner, M.R.C.P.
National Hospital for Neurology and Neurosurgery
London WC1N 3BG, United Kingdom

Dr. Herron replies:

To the Editor: It is possible that the generalized disease shown in my photographs is vaccinia rather than variola, but it is not very likely. The patient had been exposed to an unvaccinated person, known to have smallpox, before the onset of her rash and before her vaccination. The period between exposure and the onset of the rash

Correspondence Continued

was appropriate for an incubation period. The source case was the penultimate in a chain of transmission of well-documented smallpox cases among unvaccinated persons over a two-month period.[1]

Although the transmission of smallpox to unvaccinated contacts occurred at rates of 60 to 90 percent,[2] generalized vaccinia due to vaccination is extremely rare. Two large surveys documented attack rates of only 20.8 cases[3] and 23.4 cases[4] per million persons who had undergone primary vaccinations. These contrasting probabilities definitely favor variola over vaccinia as the diagnosis in the patient I described.

Dr. Maher's comments imply that extra-vigorous vaccination (two scarification strokes rather than one, and the initiation of bleeding at the vaccination site) led to high rates of generalized vaccinia in vaccine recipients, with secondary transmission to contacts, resulting in an incidence rate of about 40 percent in his village sample. Dixon, however, in discussing the incidence of generalized vaccinia, concluded that it "does not appear to be related to more vigorous technique" and "is exceedingly rare" regardless of the technique used.[5] The data he cites indicate that the syndrome occurs at a rate of about 48 cases per million persons of all ages who have undergone primary vaccination. He does note a "more common" occurrence after subcutaneous, rather than intradermal, introduction of vaccinia virus, but the rate cited was only 3 cases per 10,000, with the numerator probably including cases of isolated metastatic lesions, as well as generalized disease. Generalized vaccinia acquired from another person's vaccination is also rare, with only 2 cases reported by Lane et al. among contacts of 5,594,000 vaccine recipients.[4]

The apparent attack rate in Dr. Maher's village sample is unbelievably high for generalized vaccinia. This high rate, along with the report of six fatal cases in the first wave of illness, suggests that the disease he found among the Montagnards is much more likely to have been smallpox than vaccinia, so the similarity to my photograph is not at all surprising.

Charles A. Herron, M.D.
10014 Edgewater Dr.
Cleveland, OH 44102

1. Ogden HG. CDC and the smallpox crusade. Washington, D.C.: Government Printing Office, 1987:69-70. (HHS publication no. (CDC) 87-8400.)
2. DeQuadros CC, Morris L, DaCosta EA, Arnt N, Tigre CH. Epidemiology of variola minor in Brazil based on a study of 33 outbreaks. Bull World Health Org 1972;46:165-71.
3. Neff JM, Lane JM, Pert JH, Moore R, Millar JD, Henderson DA. Complications of smallpox vaccination. I. National survey in the United States, 1963. N Engl J Med 1967;276:125-32.
4. Lane JM, Ruben FL, Neff JM, Millar JD. Complications of smallpox vaccination, 1968: national surveillance in the United States. N Engl J Med 1969;281:1201-8.
5. Dixon CW. Smallpox. London: J&A Churchill, 1962:150-1, 356.

Dr. Kassirer replies: Some of our readers are exceptionally observant. Two years ago, readers noticed that we published an Image in Clinical Medicine on primary syphilis on page 1492, a number corresponding to the year Columbus came to the New World.[1] (It was only a coincidence.)

In today's Correspondence, Larner and Aly and Aly note that when we published the image of smallpox on May 16, we missed the 200th anniversary of Jenner's cowpox inoculation by a mere two days. It may seem a little spooky, but it is just another coincidence.

Jerome P. Kassirer, M.D.

1. Syphilis and coincidence. N Engl J Med 1995;332:1175-6.

Owl's-Eye Cells

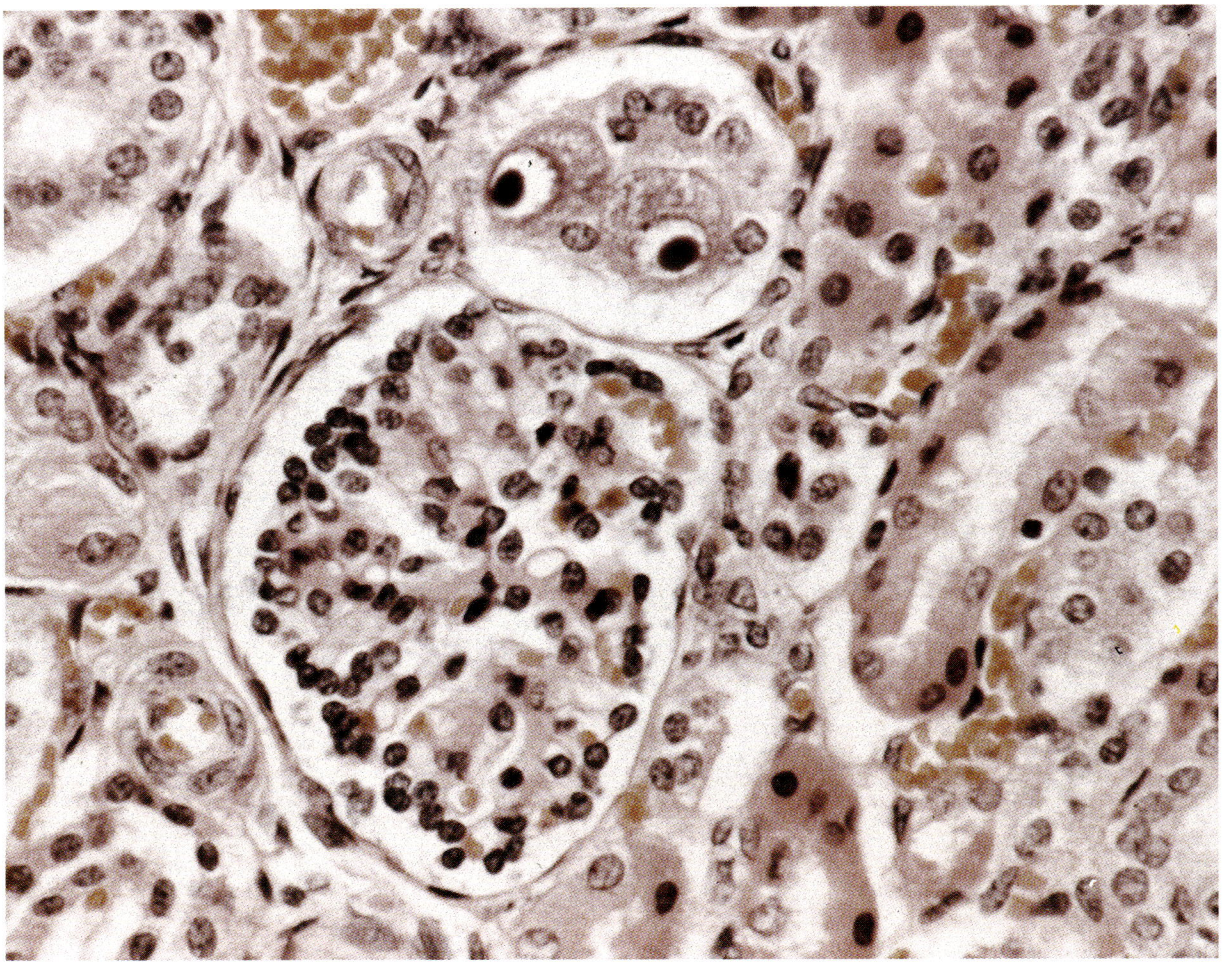

The photomicrograph shows a section of kidney taken at autopsy from a three-month-old boy who died of disseminated cytomegalovirus infection contracted in utero. A single periglomerular renal tubule contains large, intranuclear viral inclusion bodies typical of those found in cells infected with cytomegalovirus. Such inclusion bodies are commonly seen at autopsy or in biopsy specimens from the kidneys, lungs, and other organs in cases of congenital or acquired cytomegalovirus infection. (Hematoxylin and eosin, ×1920).

Richard Herriot, M.R.C.P., M.R.C.Path.
Elizabeth S. Gray, F.R.C.Path.

Aberdeen Royal Infirmary
Aberdeen AB9 2ZD, United Kingdom

September 8, 1994

Tropheryma whippelii

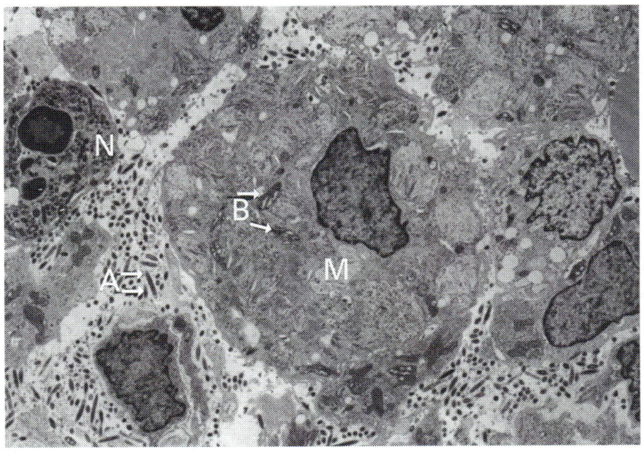

A

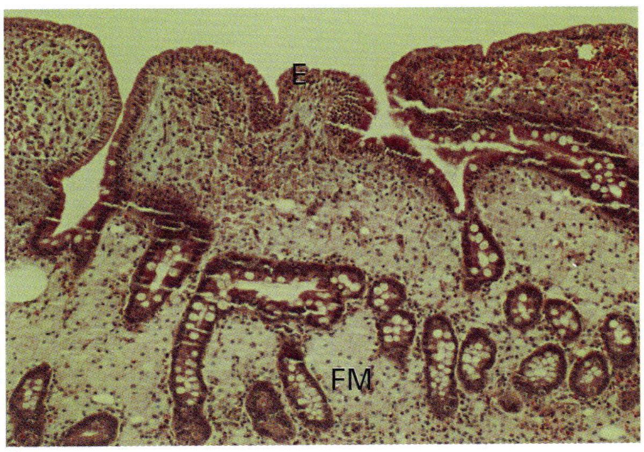

B

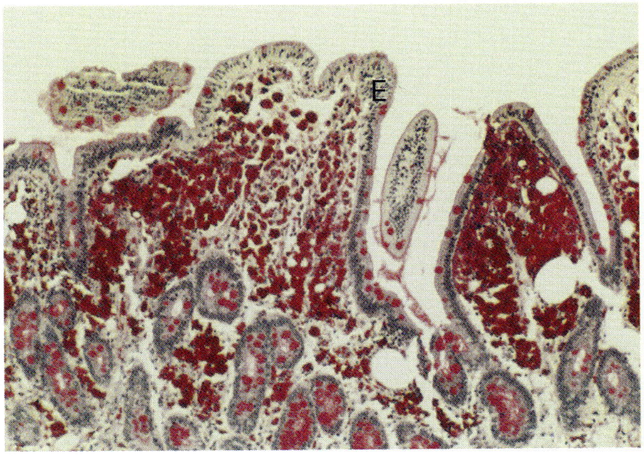

C

A 46-year-old man presented with a 50-lb (23-kg) weight loss and diarrhea. An electron micrograph (Panel A, ×6913) of tissue from the small bowel showed numerous extracellular bacilli (*Tropheryma whippelii;* A), a phagosome containing bacilli (B) within a macrophage (M), and a neutrophil (N). Staining of the tissue with hematoxylin and eosin (Panel B, ×10) revealed clubbed epithelial villi (E) and foamy macrophages (FM). Periodic acid–Schiff staining (Panel C, ×40) showed clubbed villi, lipid droplets, and lamina propria packed with positive-staining macrophages.

Whipple's disease was diagnosed, and the patient was treated with a two-week course of penicillin G (1.2 million units per day intramuscularly) and streptomycin (1 g intramuscularly per day), followed by one tablet of trimethoprim–sulfamethoxazole (Bactrim DS) given twice a day for one year. Twenty-four months after the diagnosis, the patient remained asymptomatic and had regained the weight lost during his illness. In this patient, electron microscopy was necessary to make the definitive diagnosis because a positive periodic acid–Schiff reaction was not diagnostic. The definitive diagnosis can now be made by the polymerase chain reaction.

Edward J. Fricker, M.D.

South Georgia Medical Center
Valdosta, GA 31602

Thomas J. McDonald, Jr., M.D.

Robert Packer Hospital
Sayre, PA 18840

July 4, 1996

Ehrlichiosis

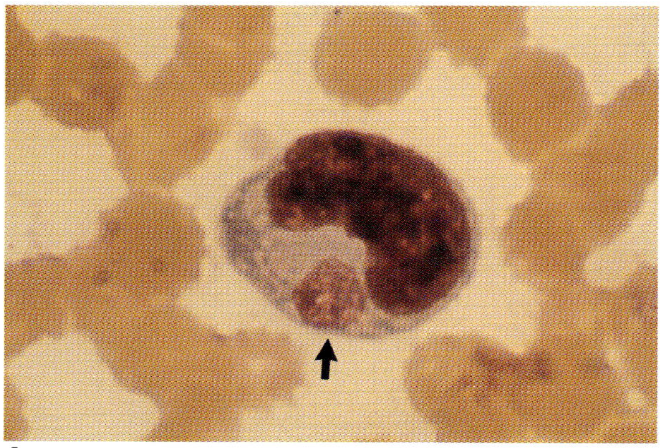

A

Intraleukocytic inclusion bodies of ehrlichia species are visible in buffy-coat smears from a 13-year-old girl with fever, encephalitis, neutropenia, and disseminated intravascular coagulation (×1000). The arrows in Panels A and B show the classic mulberry-like structures, or morulae; the arrow in Panel C shows an immature inclusion body. The patient had been bitten by ticks on a recent trip to Arkansas. The diagnosis of ehrlichiosis was made on the basis of these smears and later confirmed by serologic studies.

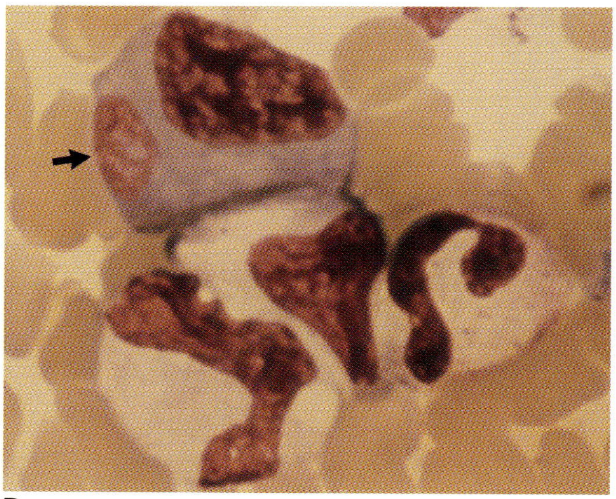

B

Carol Glaser, D.V.M., M.D.

University of California, San Francisco
San Francisco, CA 94105

Eileen Johnson, D.V.M., Ph.D.

University of California, Davis
Davis, CA 94116

May 25, 1995

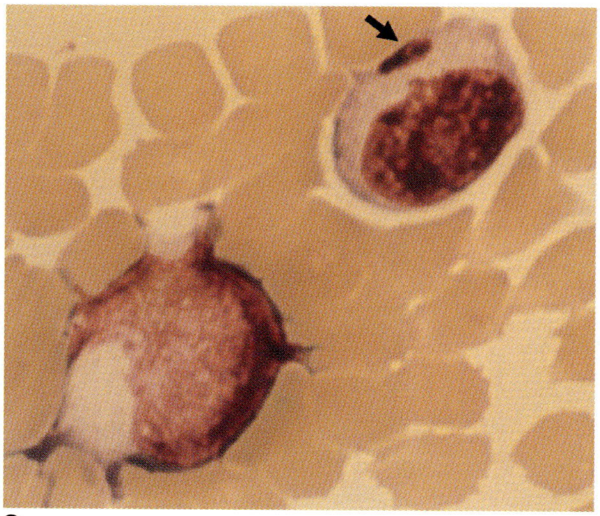

C

Rhinocerebral Mucormycosis

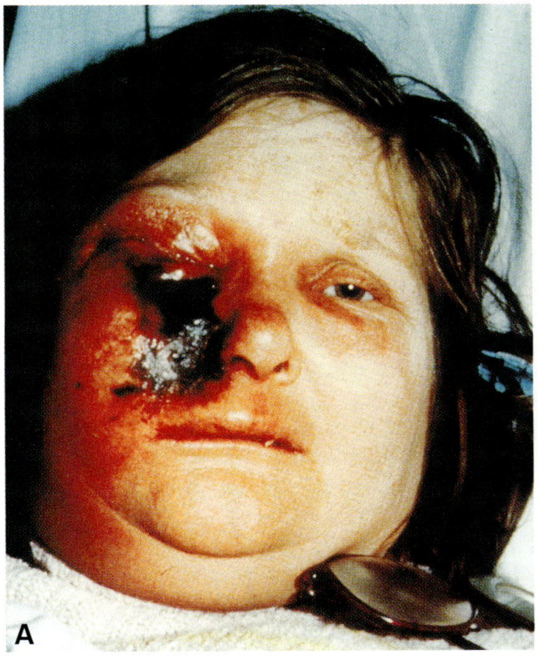

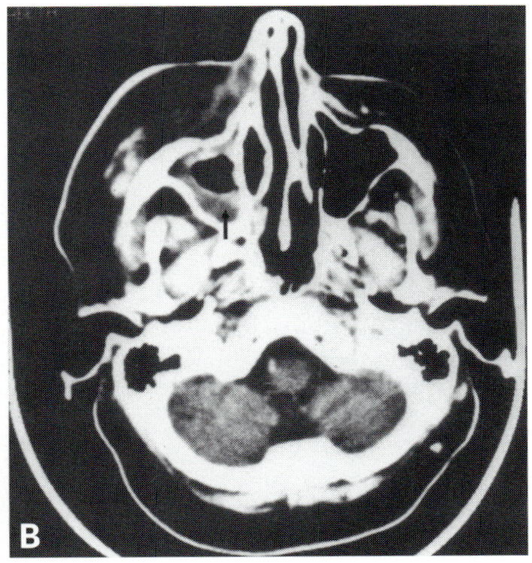

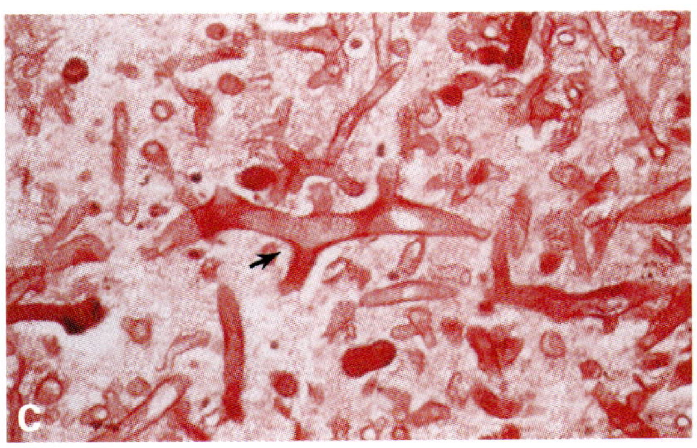

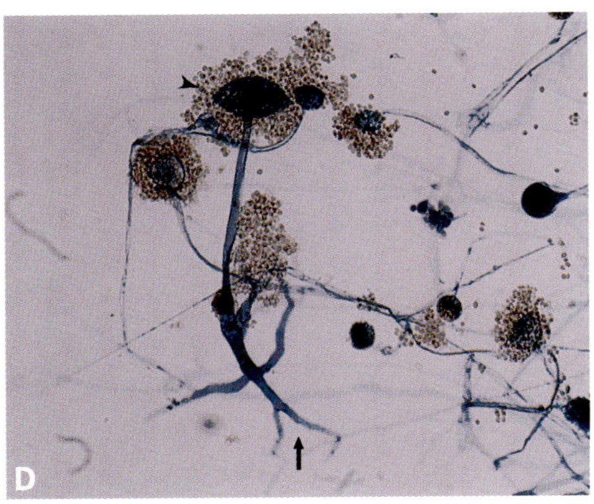

A 45-year-old woman with poorly controlled insulin-dependent diabetes mellitus had facial and periorbital swelling for three to four days. On the day of admission she was unable to open her right eye (Panel A). On admission she had a white-cell count of 22,000 per cubic millimeter, with 84 percent neutrophils and bands and a moderate degree of metabolic acidosis (blood pH, 7.22; plasma bicarbonate concentration, 8 mmol per liter). A computed tomographic scan of the head (Panel B) showed involvement of the paranasal sinuses (arrow) and periorbital soft tissues. Material from the periorbital tissue (Panel C), stained with periodic acid–Schiff stain (×560), demonstrated typical irregularly shaped broad hyphae with right-angle branching (arrow). In Panel D, the characteristic sporangia (arrowhead) and rhizoids (arrow) of the pathogen, rhizopus species, are apparent on staining with lactophenol blue (×130).

The patient was treated with amphotericin B (total dose, 2800 mg) for 35 days and surgical débridement, which included enucleation of the right eye and resection of the right paranasal sinuses. The patient is now undergoing reconstructive surgery.

Mark E. Rupp, M.D.

University of Nebraska Medical Center
Omaha, NE 68198

August 31, 1995

Fungus Ball

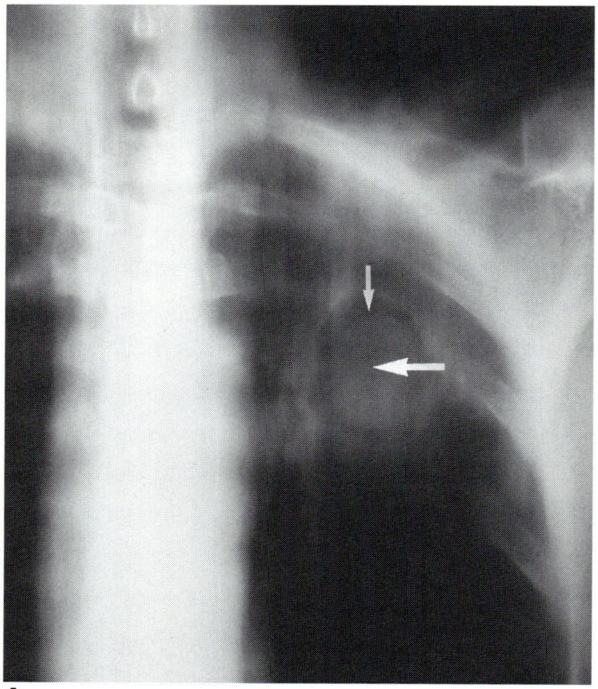

A

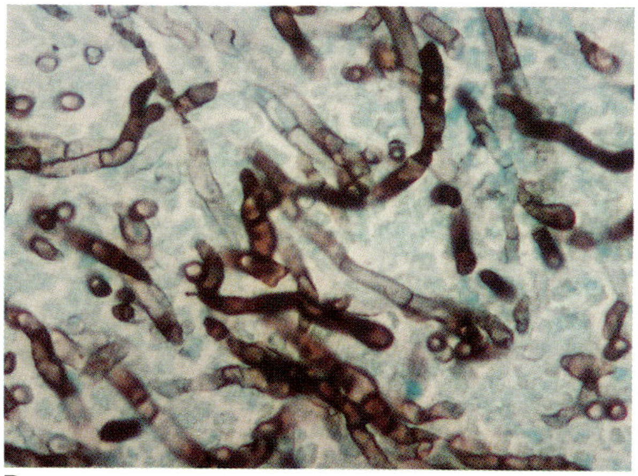

B

A 67-year-old man, adequately treated for tuberculosis 15 years previously, had a three-week history of hemoptysis that was not accompanied by fever, chills, malaise, night sweats, weight loss, or other systemic symptoms. He also had no chest pain, sputum production, or other pulmonary symptoms. He was not immunosuppressed. Linear tomography of the chest (Panel A) showed a cavity in the left upper lobe containing a round mass (large arrow) that was separated from the cavity wall by an air space (small arrow). Bronchoscopy performed preoperatively revealed no endobronchial lesion or tumor. Lobectomy was carried out for severe hemoptysis, and the presumptive diagnosis of fungus ball was confirmed. A tissue section obtained during lobectomy (Panel B) showed septate, dichotomously branching hyphae of aspergillus species (Gomori's methenamine silver, ×450).

Rao S. Mikkilineni, M.D.
David Flores, M.D.

Jersey City Medical Center
Jersey City, NJ 07304

January 12, 1995

Coccidioides immitis

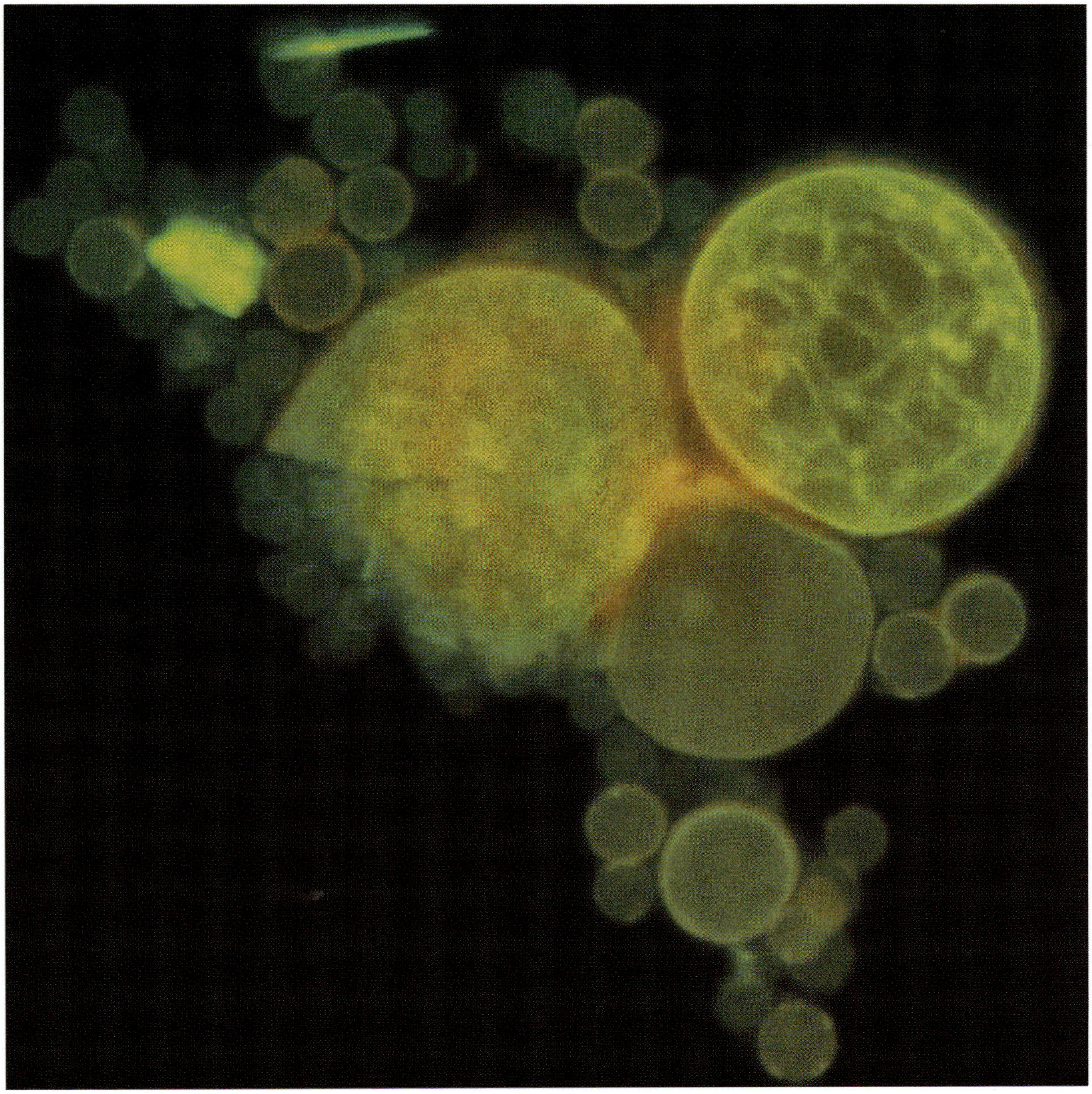

A specimen of bronchoalveolar-lavage fluid was obtained from a 33-year-old patient with the acquired immunodeficiency syndrome who had been admitted to the hospital with anorexia, weakness, dyspnea, cough, and fever. A chest film showed bilateral pulmonary infiltrates. The specimen was stained with Calcofluor white and photographed with a fluorescence microscope (×200). An intact spherule of *Coccidioides immitis* can be seen in the upper right portion of the image, and a ruptured spherule surrounded by released endospores in the left portion.

Luis M. de la Maza, M.D., Ph.D.

University of California, Irvine
Irvine, CA 92717

December 23, 1993

Pneumocystic Abscesses of the Spleen

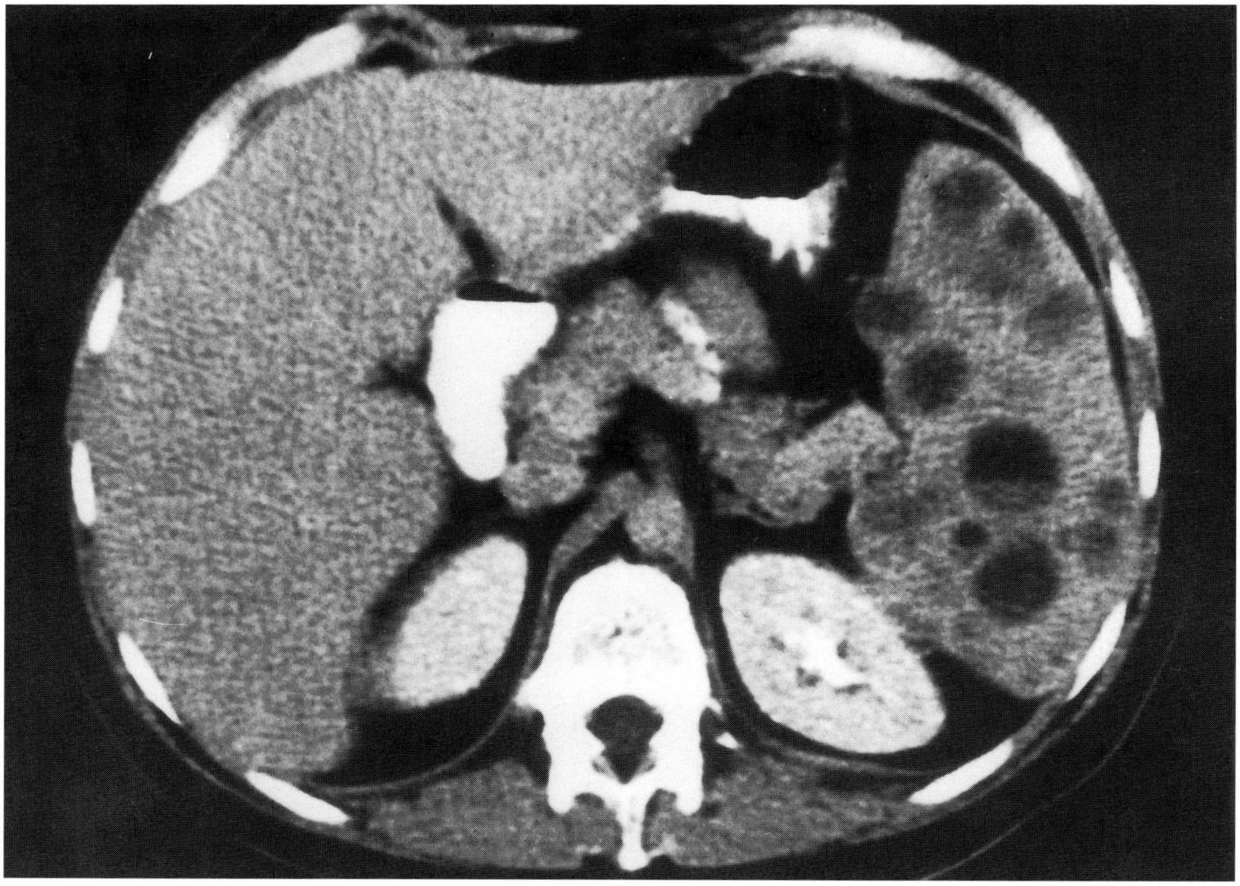

A computed tomographic scan of the spleen in an adult infected with the human immunodeficiency virus, who had a recurrence of *Pneumocystis carinii* pneumonia despite secondary prophylaxis with aerosolized pentamidine, shows abscesses characteristic of extrapulmonary pneumocystosis. Any type of pyogenic or parasitic abscess can have a similar appearance. Ultrasound-guided needle aspiration of the spleen demonstrated cysts of *P. carinii*. A second scan, obtained after several months of daily therapy with trimethoprim–sulfamethoxazole, showed marked diminution of the cysts.

Michael Landor, M.D.

Albert Einstein College of Medicine
Bronx, NY 10461

May 27, 1993

Streptococcus pneumoniae

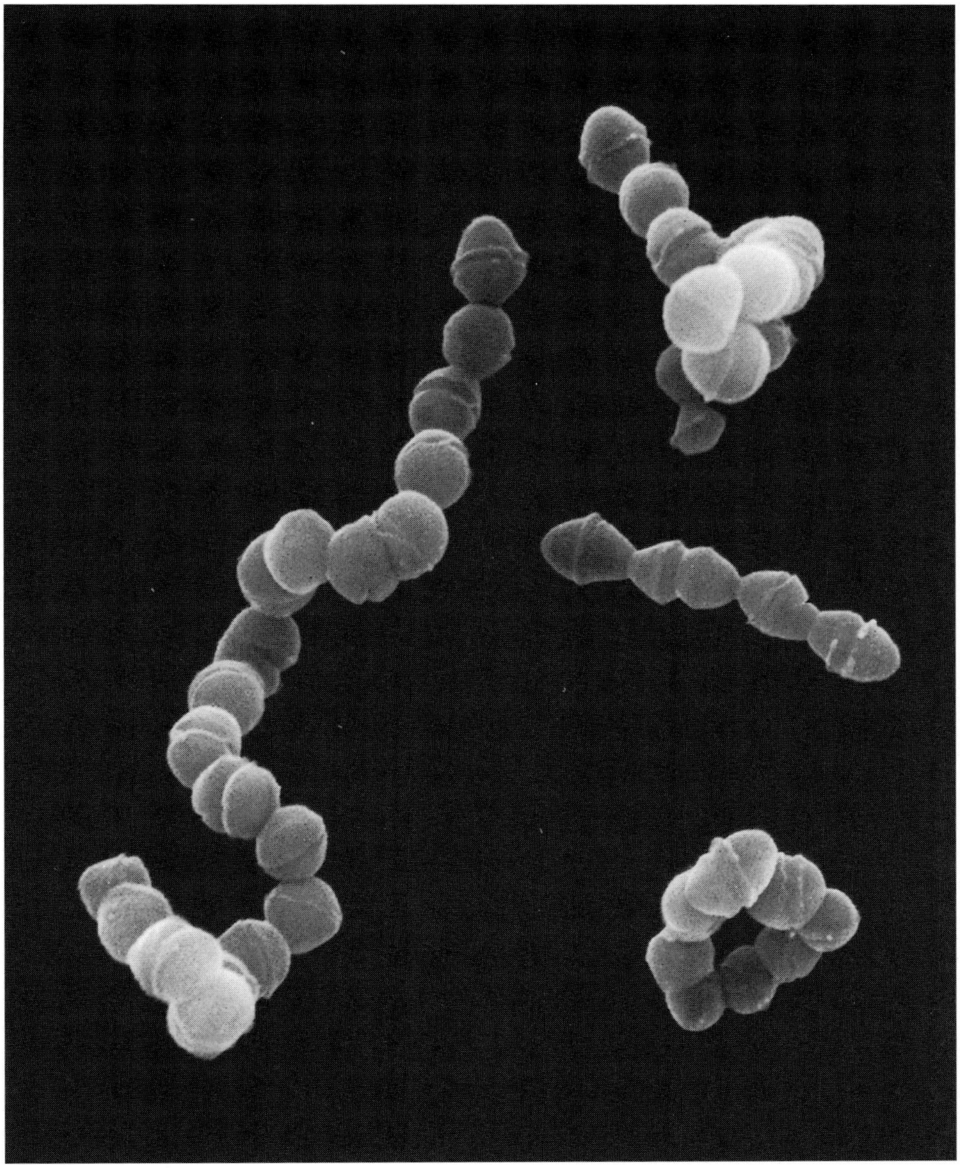

A ubiquitous gram-positive pathogen, *Streptococcus pneumoniae* often appears in a diplococcal form (×14,520).

David M. Phillips, Ph.D.

Population Council
New York, NY 10021

August 12, 1993

Enterococcus faecalis

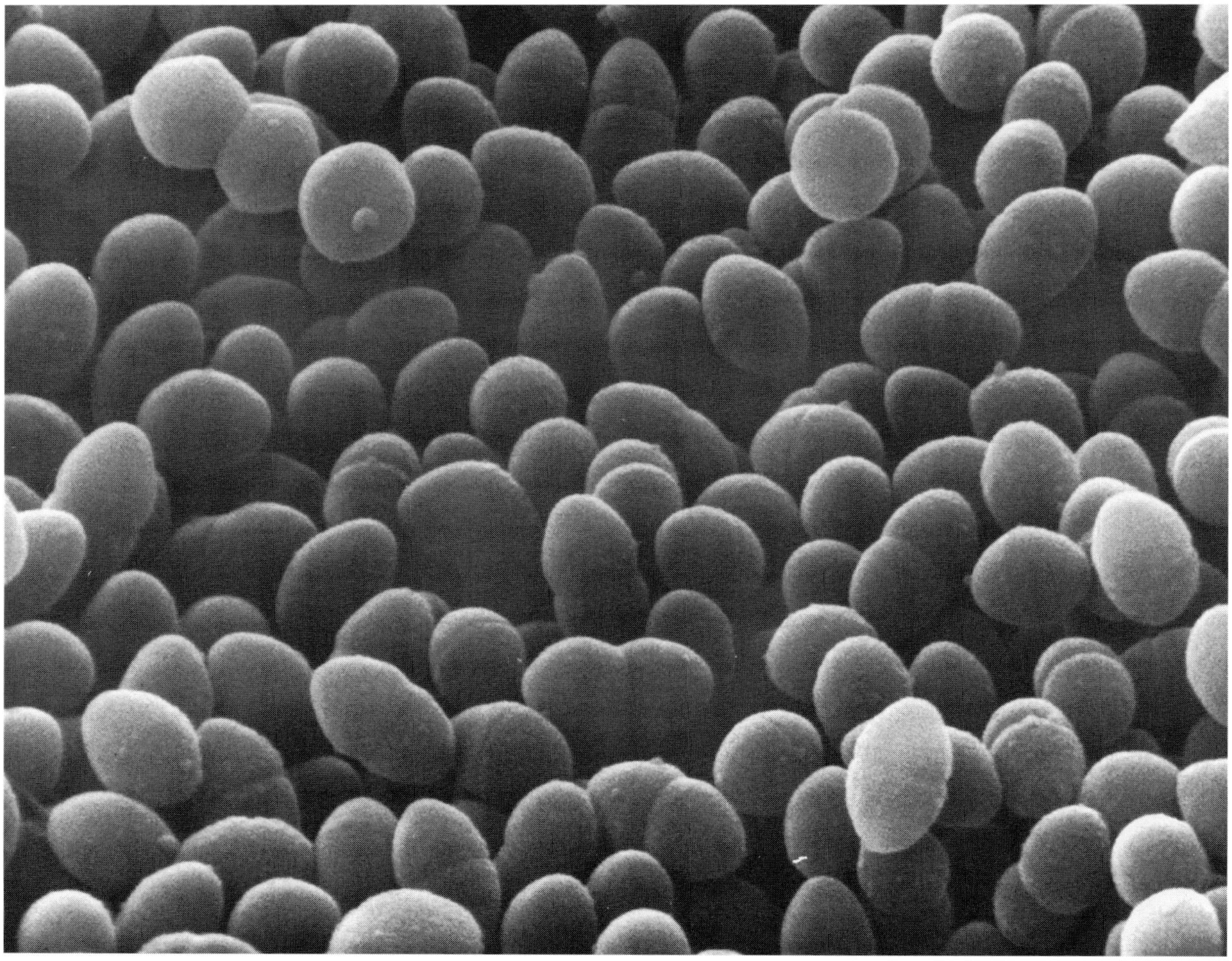

Although *Enterococcus faecalis* was once regarded as nonpathogenic, this opportunistic gram-positive coccus now ranks among the most troublesome hospital pathogens. It has intrinsic resistance to many antibiotics and a remarkable capacity for developing resistance to others (×17,160).

David M. Phillips, Ph.D.

Population Council
New York, NY 10021

January 5, 1995

Clostridium difficile

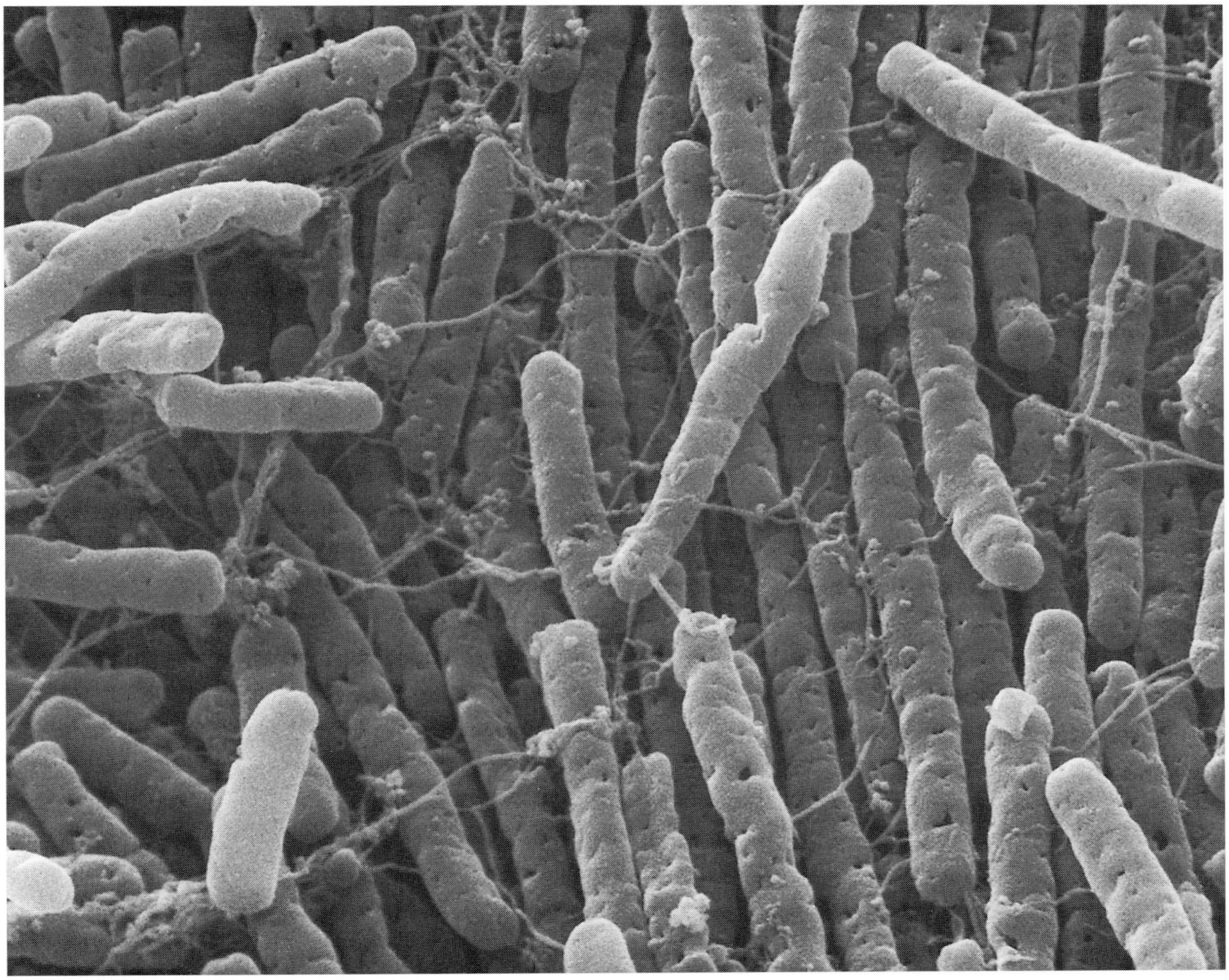

The use of antibiotics may allow *Clostridium difficile,* an anaerobic bacterium sometimes isolated as part of the normal fecal flora, to overgrow in the gut; the toxins it produces may cause pseudomembranous colitis. (Cultured in reinforced clostridium medium; source: American Type Culture Collection, Rockville, Md.; ×14,520.)

David M. Phillips, Ph.D.

Population Council
New York, NY 10021

January 27, 1994

Mycoplasma pneumoniae

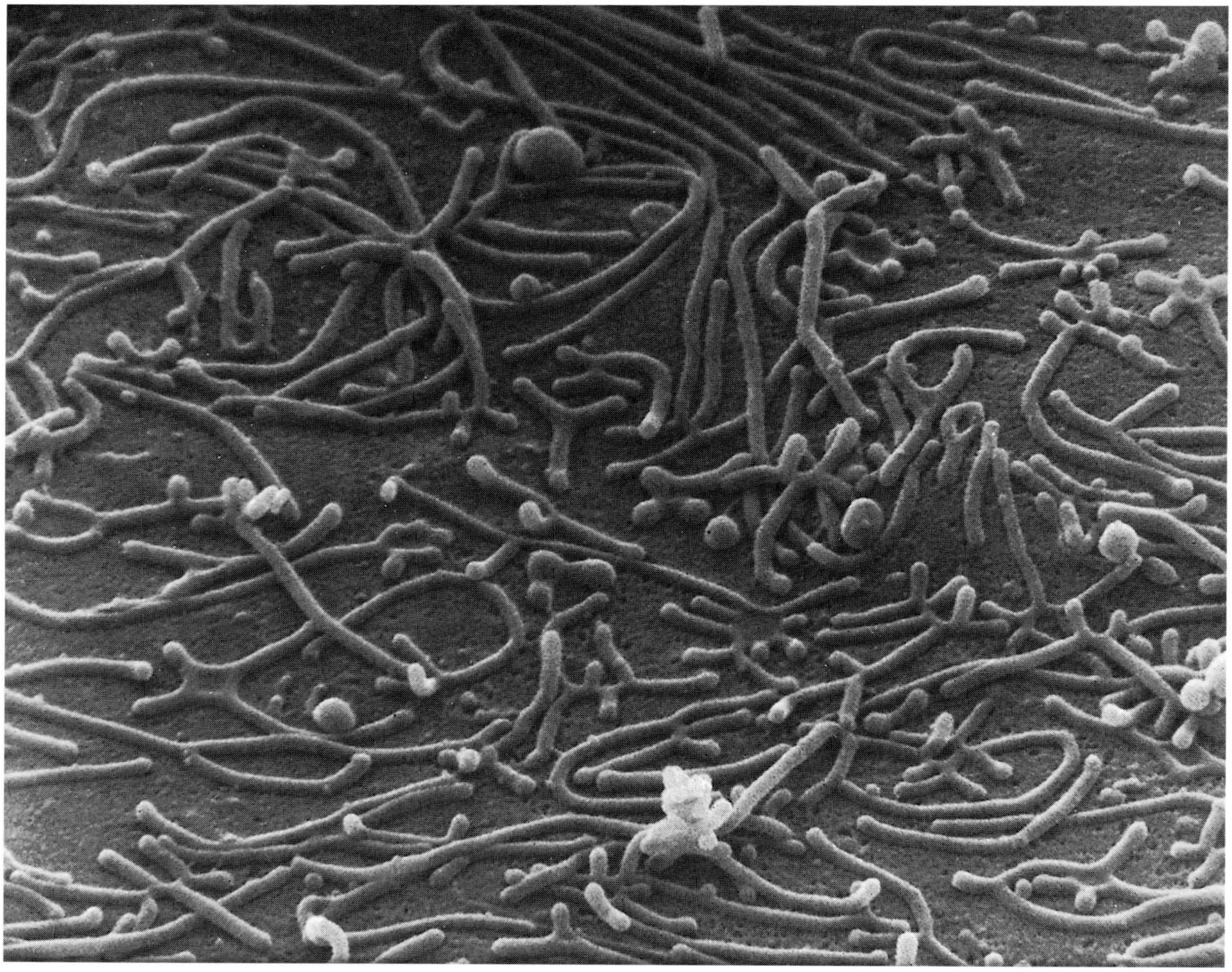

Probably the most common cause of community-acquired pneumonia, the commensal pathogen *Mycoplasma pneumoniae* is one of a group of cell-associated organisms that are the bane of tissue culturists (scanning electron micrograph, ×20,460).

David M. Phillips, Ph.D.

Population Council
New York, NY 10021

November 24, 1994

Correspondence

Mycoplasma Pneumoniae

May 11, 1995

To the Editor: In the November 24 issue of the *Journal,*[1] the legend below the elegant scanning electron micrograph of *Mycoplasma pneumoniae* states that the organism is "probably the most common cause of community-acquired pneumonia." This statement, which has important therapeutic implications, is incorrect. In a review article published in 1994, Marrie[2] concluded that the cause of the majority of cases of community-acquired pneumonia is unproved. Although outpatients seem to have a higher incidence of *M. pneumoniae* infection than inpatients, the chief threat remains *Streptococcus pneumoniae* in both groups, and treatment options must be weighed with this in mind.

Stephen Gordon, M.D.
University of Sheffield
Sheffield S10 2JF, United Kingdom

1. Phillips MD. *Mycoplasma pneumoniae.* N Engl J Med 1994;331:1421.
2. Marrie TJ. Community-acquired pneumonia. Clin Infect Dis 1994;18:501-15.

Human Immunodeficiency Virus

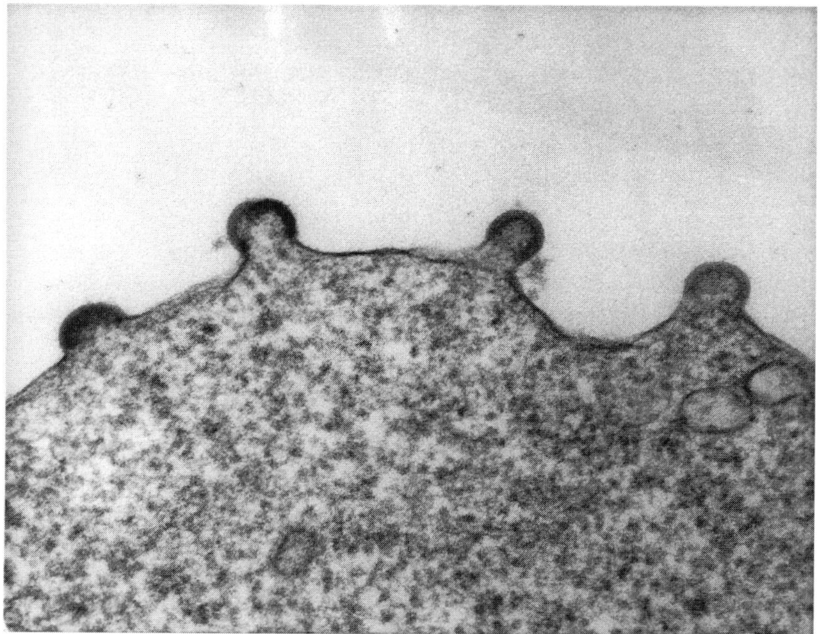

A

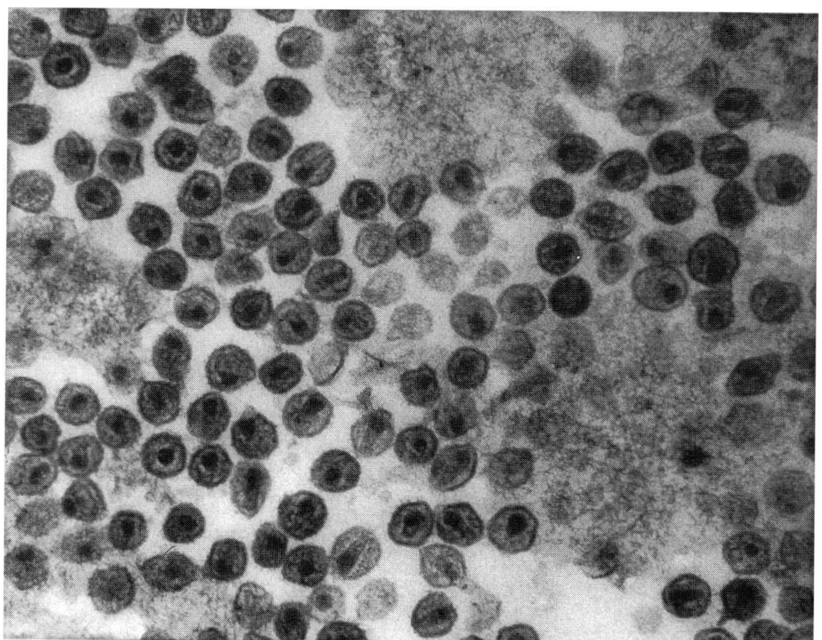

B

Transmission electron microphotographs of the human immunodeficiency virus (HIV) are shown. In Panel A, four viruses are shown budding from the surface of a cultured human lymphoma cell (×63,000). Like other enveloped viruses, HIV is unable to make lipids. The virus uses the lipid component of the membrane of the host cell as part of its envelope. During assembly at the cell surface, the viral envelope incorporates viral glycoprotein into the cell membrane. The membrane proteins of the cell are left behind when the virus buds off. Mature viruses are shown in Panel B (×50,000). The central dark spot in each virion is a cone-shaped core containing the RNA genome, reverse transcriptase, and core proteins.

David M. Phillips, Ph.D.

Population Council
New York, NY 10021

January 26, 1995

Correspondence

Human Immunodeficiency Virus

June 22, 1995

To the Editor: The caption to the transmission electron microphotograph of the human immunodeficiency virus (HIV) that shows HIV-1 budding from a cell (Jan. 26 issue)[1] states that during the budding process, "The membrane proteins of the cell are left behind when the virus buds off." We have recently shown that cellular proteins (HLA class I and class II proteins) are incorporated into the intact virus.[2] In fact, the concentrations of these cellular proteins may be even higher than those of the viral-envelope glycoproteins. Orentas and Hildreth,[3] using solid-phase capture techniques, have identified several other virus-associated cellular proteins, including CD71, CD63, CD43, CD8, LFA-1 (CD11A/CD18), and CD44. Also, we have shown that macaques immunized with purified HLA-DR are protected when they are challenged with the simian immunodeficiency virus grown in human cells.[4] Therefore, these virus-associated cellular proteins are not only present on the virus, but may play an important part in the design of an AIDS vaccine.

Larry O. Arthur, Ph.D.
Louis E. Henderson, Ph.D.
Raoul E. Benveniste, Ph.D., M.D.
National Cancer Institute–Frederick
Cancer Research and Development Center
Frederick, MD 21702

1. Phillips DM. Human immunodeficiency virus. N Engl J Med 1995;332:233.
2. Arthur LO, Bess JW Jr, Sowder RC II, et al. Cellular proteins bound to immunodeficiency viruses: implications for pathogenesis and vaccines. Science 1992;258:1935-8.
3. Orentas RJ, Hildreth JE. Association of host cell surface adhesion receptors and other membrane proteins with HIV and SIV. AIDS Res Hum Retroviruses 1993;9:1157-65.
4. Arthur LO, Bess JW, Urban RG, et al. Macaques immunized with HLA-DR are protected from simian immunodeficiency virus challenge. J Virol 1995;69:3117-24.

Dr. Phillips replies:

To the Editor: In the caption to my transmission electron microphotograph of HIV budding from the surface of a cultured human T cell, I noted that the viral envelope incorporates viral glycoproteins, a well-established observation. I added that the cell proteins are left behind. This point of view is also well accepted, although it may be true that people have not looked hard for cellular proteins in the viral envelope. The provocative experiments of Arthur et al. remind us that we should not be complacent about such apparent truisms. I appreciate their reminding me that some of the viral membrane protein may indeed include selected cellular proteins.

David M. Phillips, Ph.D.
Population Council
New York, NY 10021

Influenza A Virus

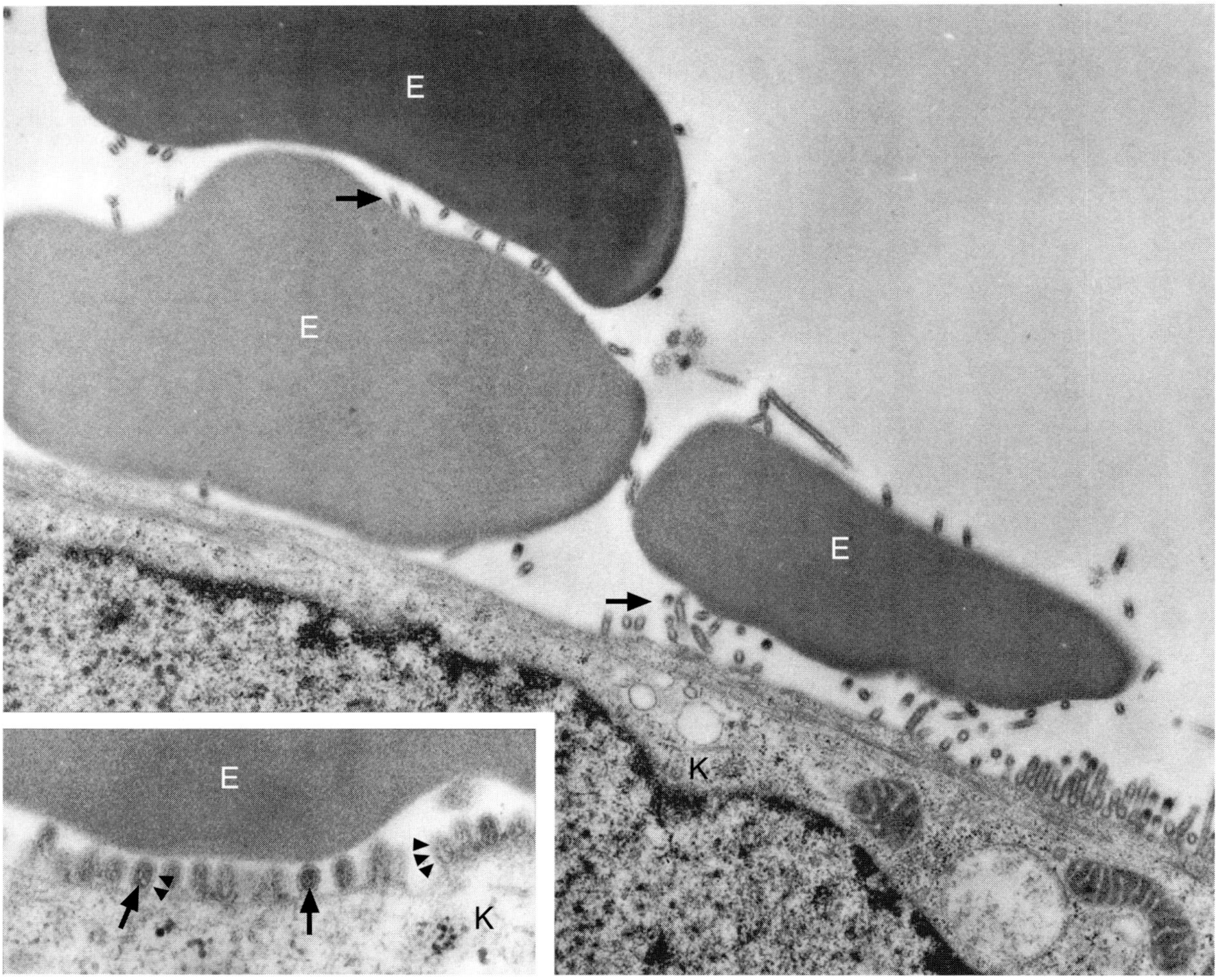

Virions of influenza A virus (arrows) are seen budding from the surface of kidney cells (K) from rhesus monkeys. In the inset, the dense nucleoprotein core of the virus (arrows) can be distinguished from the lighter fringe of individual hemagglutinin and neuraminidase spikes (arrowheads). The surface hemagglutinin is responsible for two important biologic phenomena. Hemadsorption of guinea-pig erythrocytes (E) onto the surface of the cellular monolayer (K) is an important tool for documenting the presence of virus in cell cultures. Hemagglutination is the aggregation by viral hemagglutinin of adjacent erythrocytes. The aggregates enlarge to form a lattice that becomes visible to the naked eye, providing the primary tool for epidemiologic typing of influenza isolates and the detection of serum antibodies after infection. Antigenic changes in the surface structures, especially the hemagglutinin molecule, render antibodies to viral strains prevalent in previous years less effective. Minor changes (antigenic drift) and especially major changes (antigenic shift) place a population at increased risk of infection. The hemagglutinin also has a critical role in the infectious process itself, because this exposed surface molecule mediates attachment of the virus to respiratory cells, the essential first step in human infection. (×24,000; inset, ×63,000.)

Washington C. Winn, Jr., M.D.
Fred W. Westenfeld, M.T.(A.S.C.P.), S.M.

University of Vermont College of Medicine
Burlington, VT 05405

October 5, 1995

Cryptococcal Meningitis

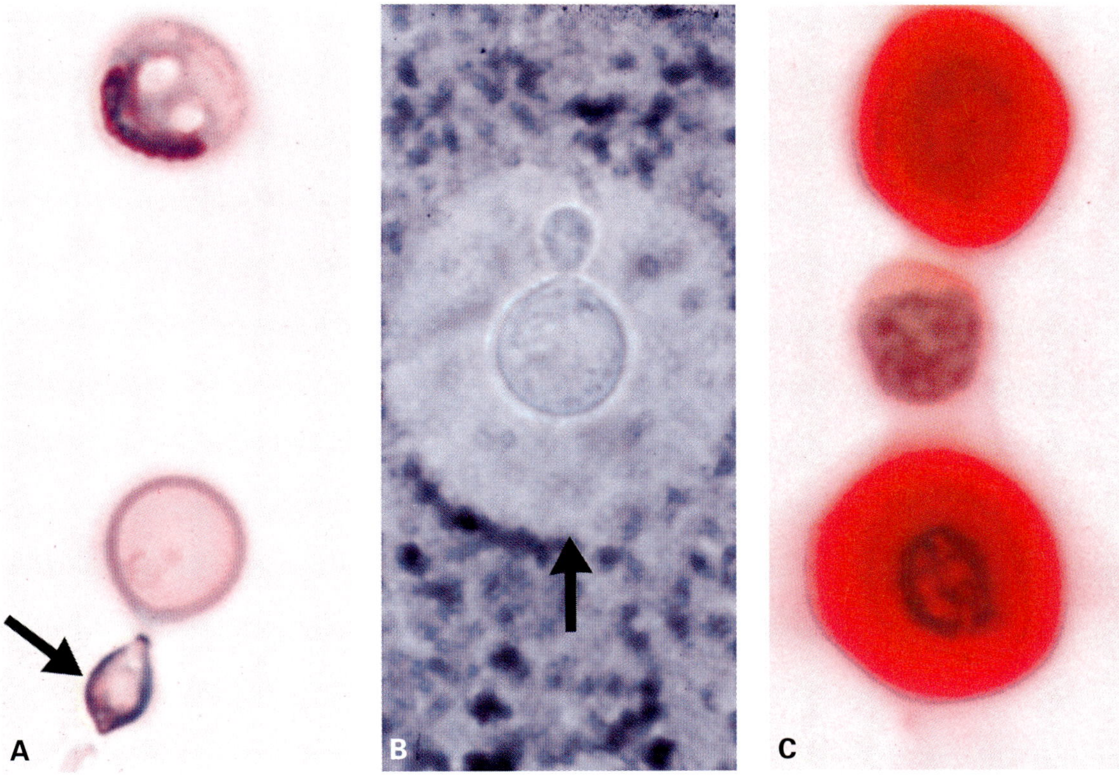

A 69-year-old white man had progressively more severe headaches for five weeks, and sudden persistent hearing loss developed four days before admission to the hospital. He had been healthy and had no history suggesting immune compromise or exposure to infectious agents. He was fully alert and oriented and had no neurologic abnormalities on examination, but he had severe bilateral sensorineural hearing loss and papilledema. A test for human immunodeficiency virus antibody was nonreactive. The results of magnetic resonance imaging of the brain and meninges with contrast agent were normal.

On lumbar puncture the opening pressure was 52 cm of water. Examination of the cerebrospinal fluid revealed a white-cell count of 34 per cubic millimeter (all mononuclear cells), a protein level of 59 mg per deciliter, and a glucose level of 26 mg per deciliter. A latex-agglutination test of the cerebrospinal fluid was positive for cryptococcal antigen at a dilution of 1:2048. In a cytologic preparation of cerebrospinal fluid (Panel A), numerous fungal elements were observed as narrowly budding (arrow) yeasts characteristic of cryptococcus (Papanicolaou's stain, ×1000). An India-ink preparation of the fresh cerebrospinal fluid (Panel B) showed the mucinous capsule of cryptococcus as a translucent halo (arrow) surrounding the budding yeast (×1000). The mucinous capsule appeared bright red on mucicarmine staining (Panel C, ×1000). Taken together, these findings were consistent only with infection by a cryptococcal species.

Fungal cultures of the cerebrospinal fluid subsequently grew *Cryptococcus neoformans,* as did blood cultures obtained at the same time, confirming the diagnosis of cryptococcal meningitis. We do not know how the patient acquired the infection. After the initiation of aggressive therapy with intravenously administered amphotericin B the patient had slowly progressive confusion and lethargy and renal insufficiency. He died on the 22nd hospital day. Permission for a postmortem examination was not granted.

J. Howard Jaster, M.D.
Mark J. Malecha, M.D.

University of Tennessee
Memphis, TN 38163

December 26, 1996

Candida albicans

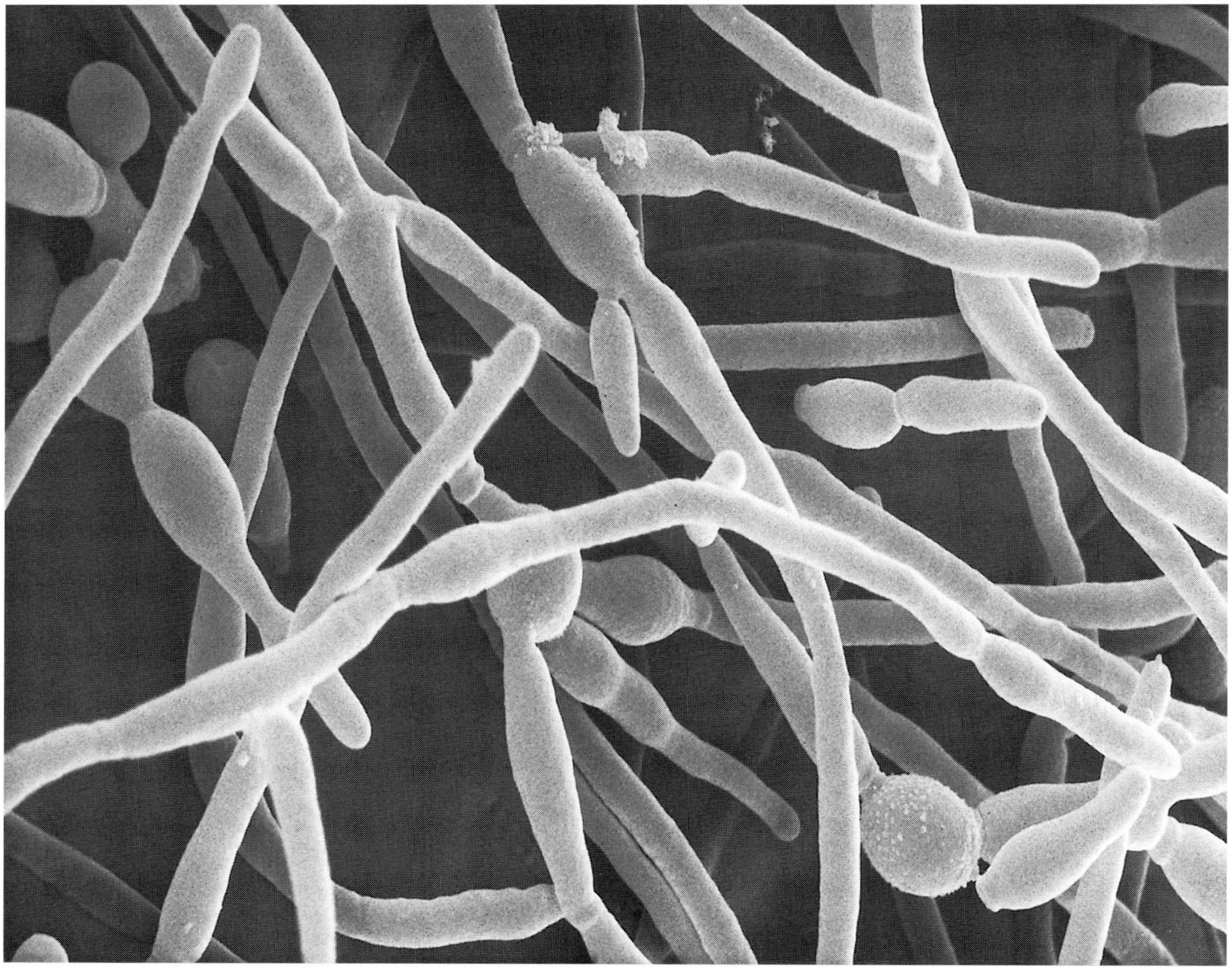

A scanning electron micrograph shows a pure culture of *Candida albicans* (×6030).

David M. Phillips, Ph.D.

Center for Biomedical Research
New York, NY 10021

May 6, 1993

Cardiology

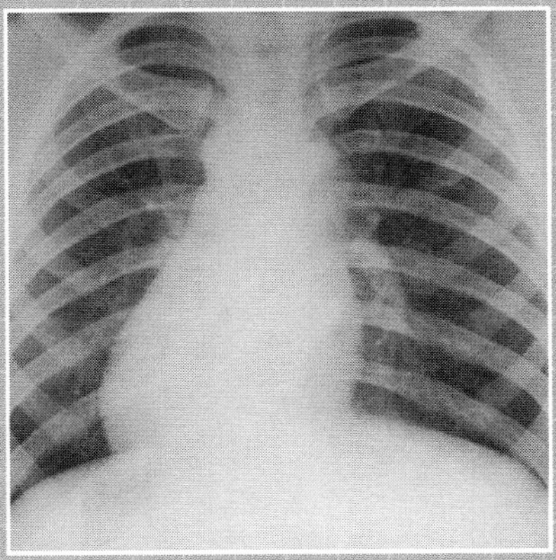

Situs Inversus

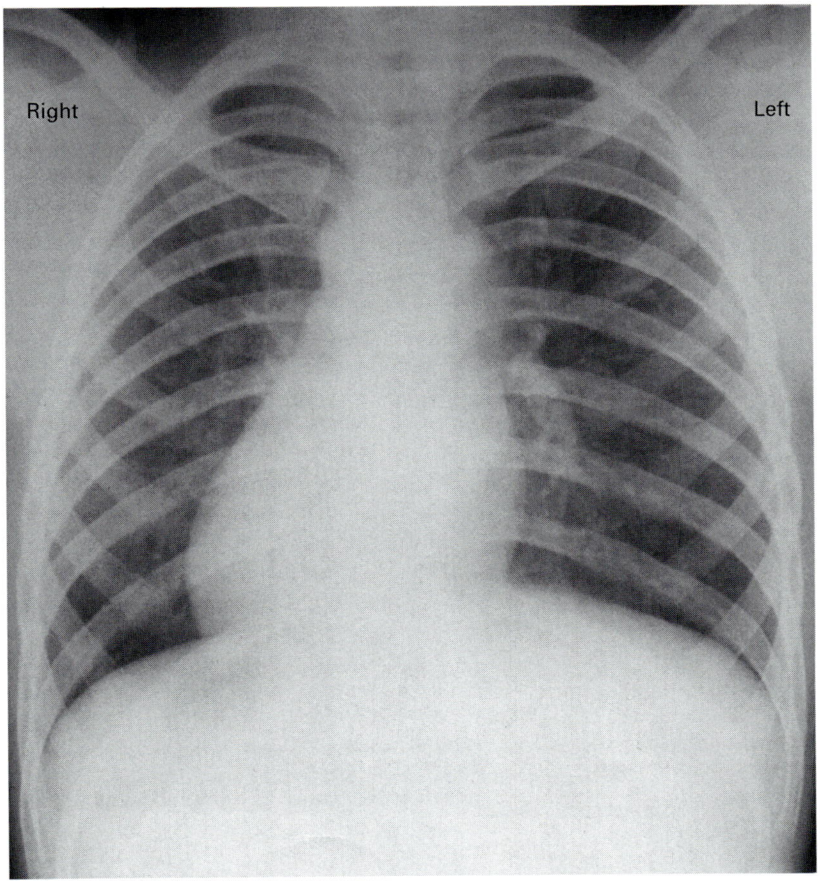

A chest film was obtained in an 11-year-old girl who presented with pain and tenderness of the left iliac fossa. Chest auscultation revealed right-sided heart sounds. The position of the heart suggested situs inversus totalis. The left iliac fossa was incised to remove an acutely inflamed appendix. Other causes of left-sided appendicitis include situs inversus indeterminus (only the abdominal contents are transposed), a mobile cecum, and a very long appendix.

Allan D. Spigelman, F.R.A.C.S.

St. Mary's Hospital Medical School
London W2, United Kingdom

March 3, 1994

Acute Myocardial Infarction and Coronary Spasm

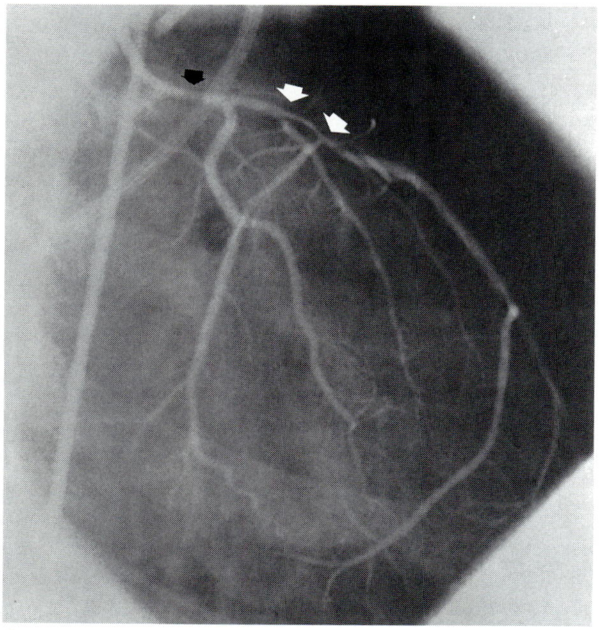

A

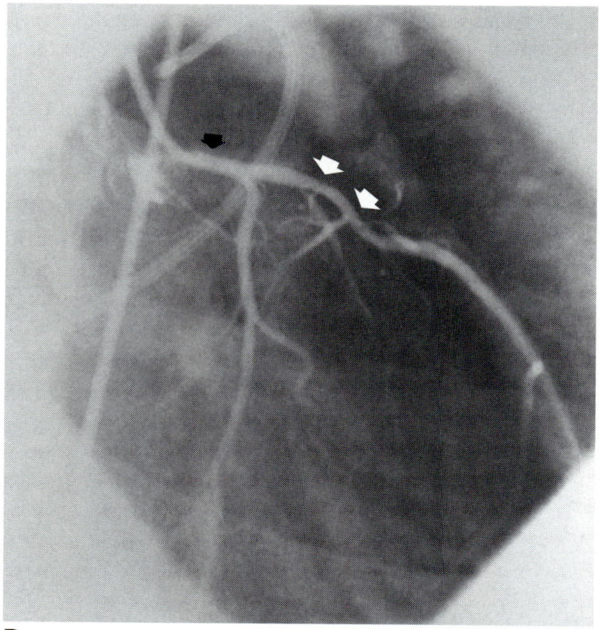

B

A 41-year-old woman with a history of hypertension and cigarette smoking was admitted to the emergency department with chest pain. Electrocardiography revealed changes consistent with acute anterior myocardial infarction. Recurrent ventricular fibrillation required several electric cardioversions. At coronary angiography, spontaneous spasm of the proximal left anterior descending artery (white arrows) was evident (Panel A), as was mild catheter-induced spasm of a portion of the left main coronary artery (black arrow). Intracoronary nitroglycerin reversed the coronary spasm (Panel B). The patient was treated with nitrates and a calcium-channel blocker. Two weeks after admission she died suddenly.

Ik-Kyung Jang, M.D., Ph.D.

Massachusetts General Hospital
Boston, MA 02114

May 19, 1994

Negative U Waves as an Indicator of Stress-Induced Myocardial Ischemia

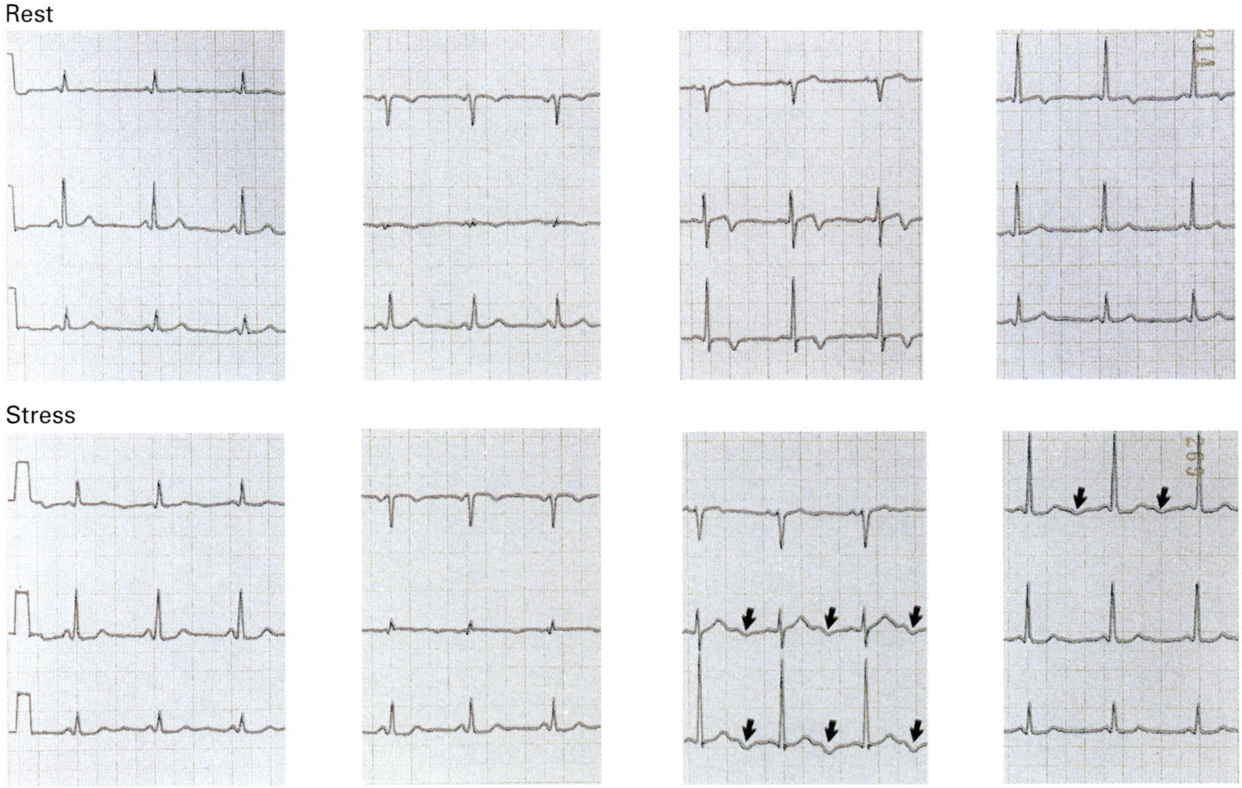

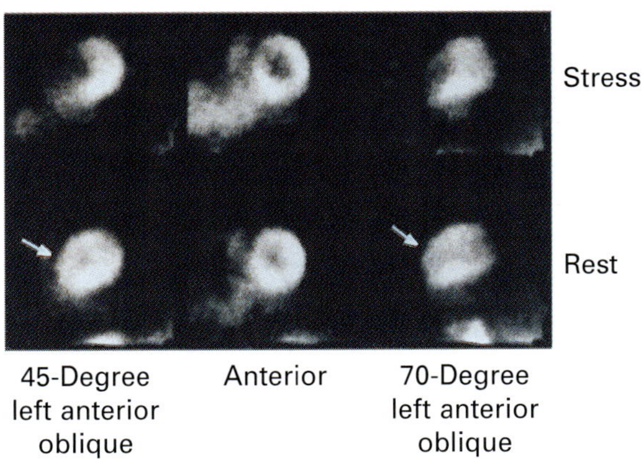

Chest discomfort and negative U waves in precordial leads V_2, V_3, and V_4 of the electrocardiogram (black arrows) with T-wave inversion occurred after the infusion of dipyridamole in a patient with severe stenosis of the proximal left anterior descending coronary artery. These findings occurred concomitantly with severe myocardial hypoperfusion in the anteroseptal region during a thallium stress test. The area of hypoperfusion subsequently filled in (white arrows). Among the electrocardiographic signs of transient myocardial ischemia, negative U waves in the precordial leads have been reported to be very specific for coronary artery disease, especially stenosis or spasm of the anterior descending coronary artery.

Michele Galli, M.D.
PierLuigi Temporelli, M.D.

Fondazione Clinica del Lavoro
28010 Veruno, Italy

June 23, 1994

Emergency Coronary-Artery Angioplasty for Cardiogenic Shock Complicating Acute Myocardial Infarction

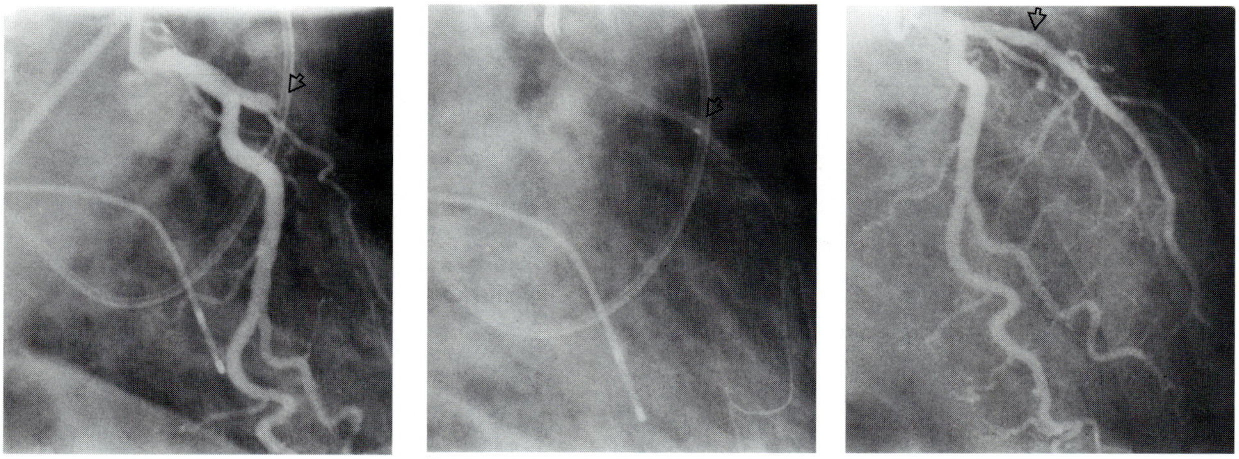

A B C

Coronary-artery angioplasty was performed in a 45-year-old man who presented with two hours of crushing retrosternal chest pain and hypotension (blood pressure, 90/60 mm Hg). Electrocardiography revealed evidence of an acute anterior-wall myocardial infarction. Coronary arteriography (Panel A) showed a left anterior descending artery that was totally occluded in its proximal portion (indicated by the arrow in each panel), with normal right and circumflex coronary arteries. Emergency coronary-artery angioplasty (Panel B) resulted in rapid antegrade flow without residual stenosis at the site of the occlusion (Panel C). The patient's hemodynamic status stabilized, and the rest of his hospital course was unremarkable. An echocardiogram obtained the day after catheterization and angioplasty showed an akinetic anterior wall and an ejection fraction of 20 percent. An exercise test before discharge from the hospital was negative for signs of residual myocardial ischemia. Six weeks after discharge, echocardiography demonstrated an estimated ejection fraction of 50 percent, and a maximal exercise test was negative.

Harry Feld, M.D.

Maimonides Medical Center
Brooklyn, NY 11219

March 11, 1993

Coronary Atherectomy

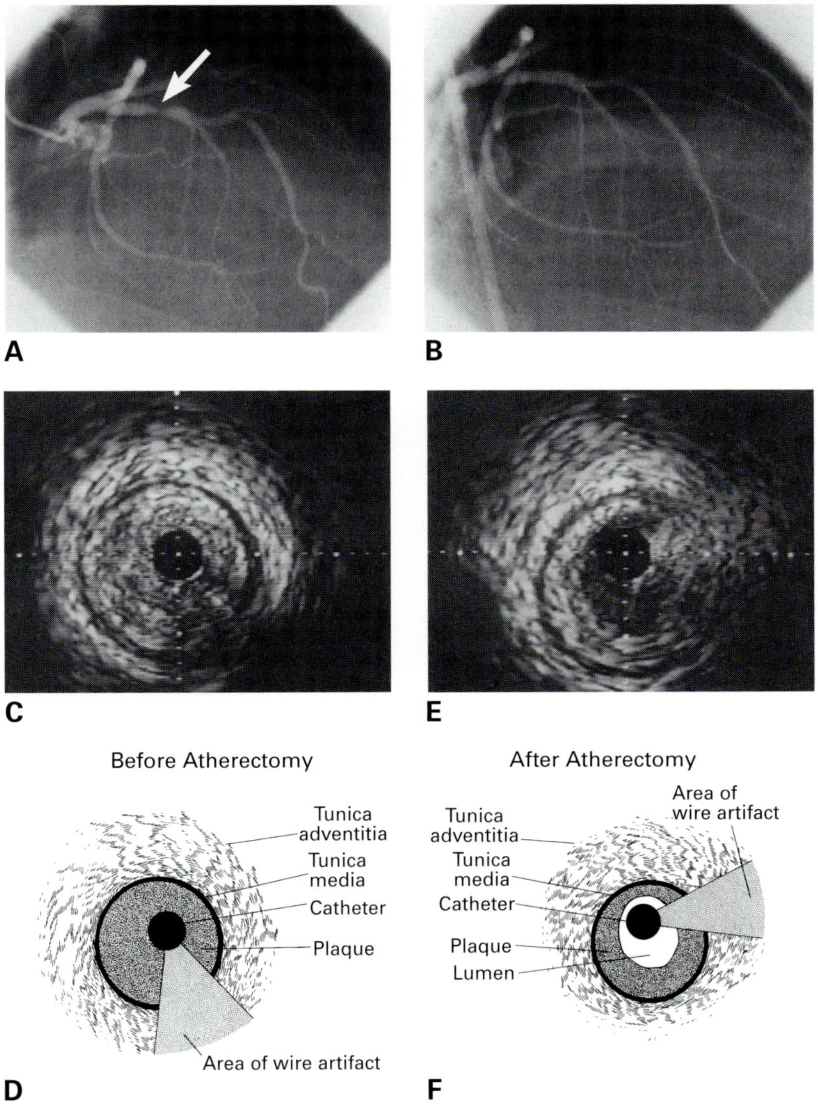

A proximal stenosis of the left anterior descending coronary artery (arrow in Panel A) was found in a 41-year-old man during coronary arteriography for unstable angina. The stenosis improved after atherectomy (Panel B). Intravascular ultrasonography was performed before and after atherectomy. Before atherectomy a plaque occupies the entire artery and closely surrounds the ultrasound catheter (Panels C and D). After atherectomy the size of the lumen has increased and the area of the plaque has decreased (Panels E and F). Although the intervention appears to have resulted in a normal vessel with no evidence of stenosis on angiography, the intravascular ultrasound images reveal a substantial amount of residual plaque.

Neil J. Weissman, M.D.
Arthur E. Weyman, M.D.

Massachusetts General Hospital
Boston, MA 02114

February 24, 1994

Left Ventricular Aneurysm

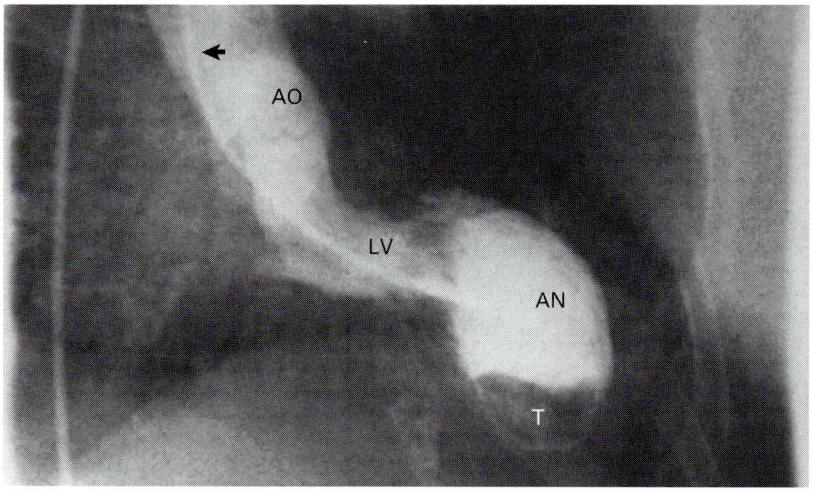

A

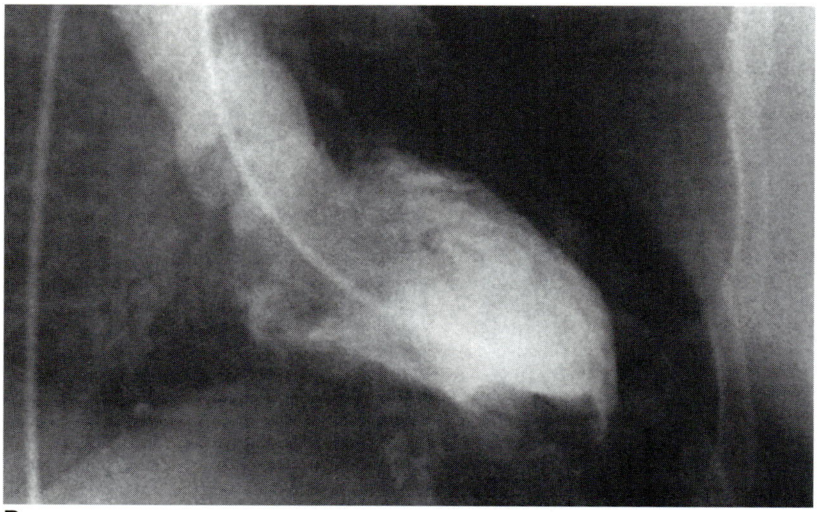

B

The images show the results of contrast left ventriculography in a 72-year-old woman who presented with progressive cardiac failure after myocardial infarction. Panel A is a right anterior oblique view showing the left ventricle during systole. The contrast medium was injected through an angiographic catheter (arrow) passed into the left ventricle in a retrograde fashion from the aorta (AO). A large ventricular aneurysm (AN) is located at the apex of the left ventricle. The stasis of blood in the aneurysm is revealed by the contrast density, which is greater in the aneurysm than in the left ventricle. The large filling defect inside the aneurysm is a mural thrombus (T). In the diastolic frame of the left ventriculogram (Panel B), the size of the uninfarcted left ventricular segments has increased, whereas that of the aneurysm remains unchanged.

Rajendra Patel, M.D.
Mohandas M. Shenoy, M.D.

Coney Island Hospital
Brooklyn, NY 11235

July 22, 1993

Coronary Arteriovenous Fistula on Coronary Angiography

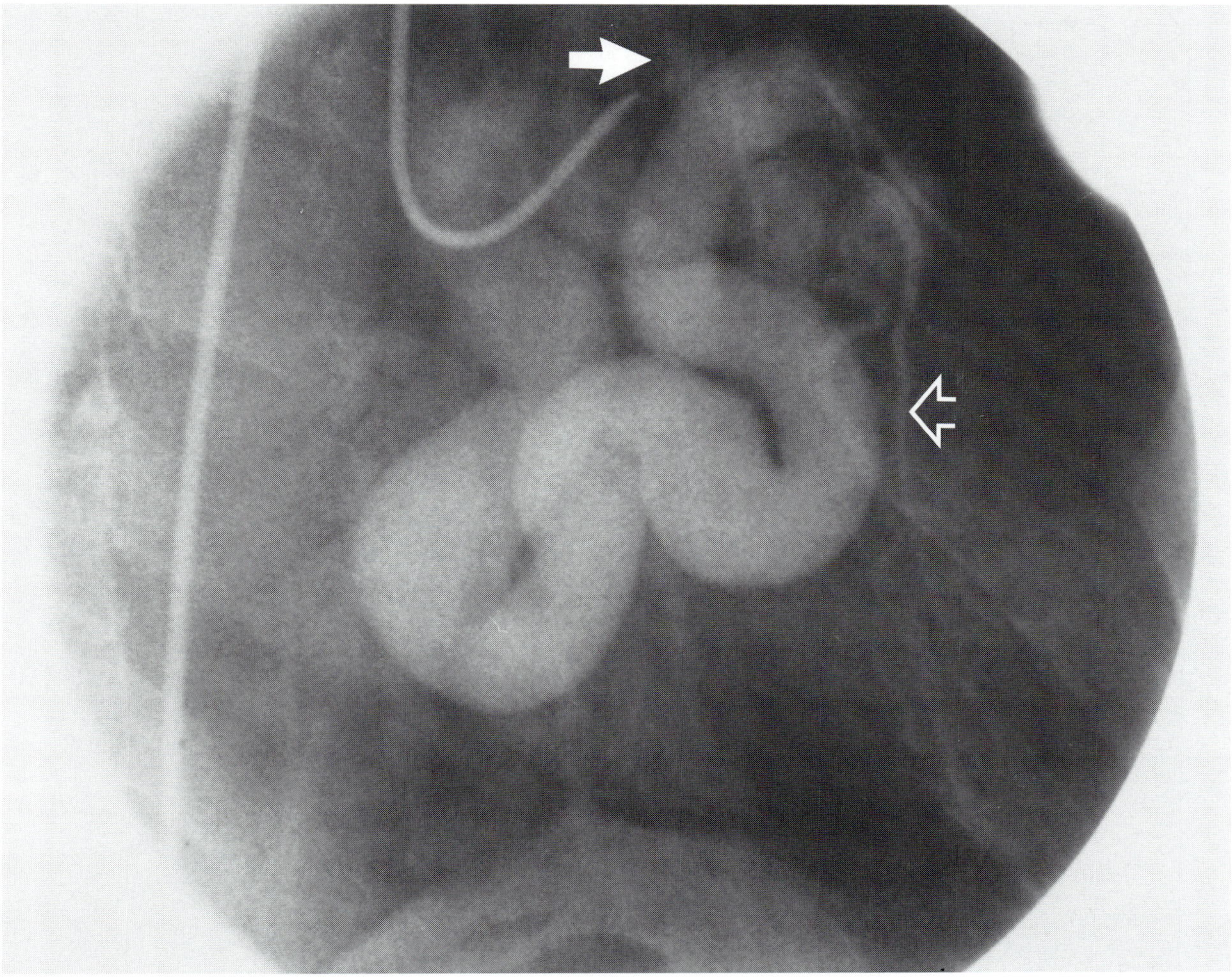

A large coronary arteriovenous fistula can be seen originating in the left coronary artery, coursing over the lateral and posterior walls of the left ventricle, and eventually emptying into the right atrium. The solid arrow indicates the origin of the fistula (not well visualized), and the open arrow indicates a normal-sized left anterior descending coronary artery, which is of much smaller caliber than the greatly dilated fistula. Patients with such fistulas often have loud continuous cardiac murmurs and may have congestive heart failure, myocardial ischemia (due to a coronary-artery "steal" phenomenon), and pulmonary hypertension. Coronary arteriovenous fistulas typically arise as congenital anomalies. With obliteration of the fistula by suturing, the prognosis is usually excellent.

Kenichi Fujise, M.D.

University of Texas Health
Science Center at Houston
Houston, TX 77030

Warren Sherman, M.D.

Beth Israel Medical Center
New York, NY 10003

November 10, 1994

Ostium Secundum Atrial Septal Defect

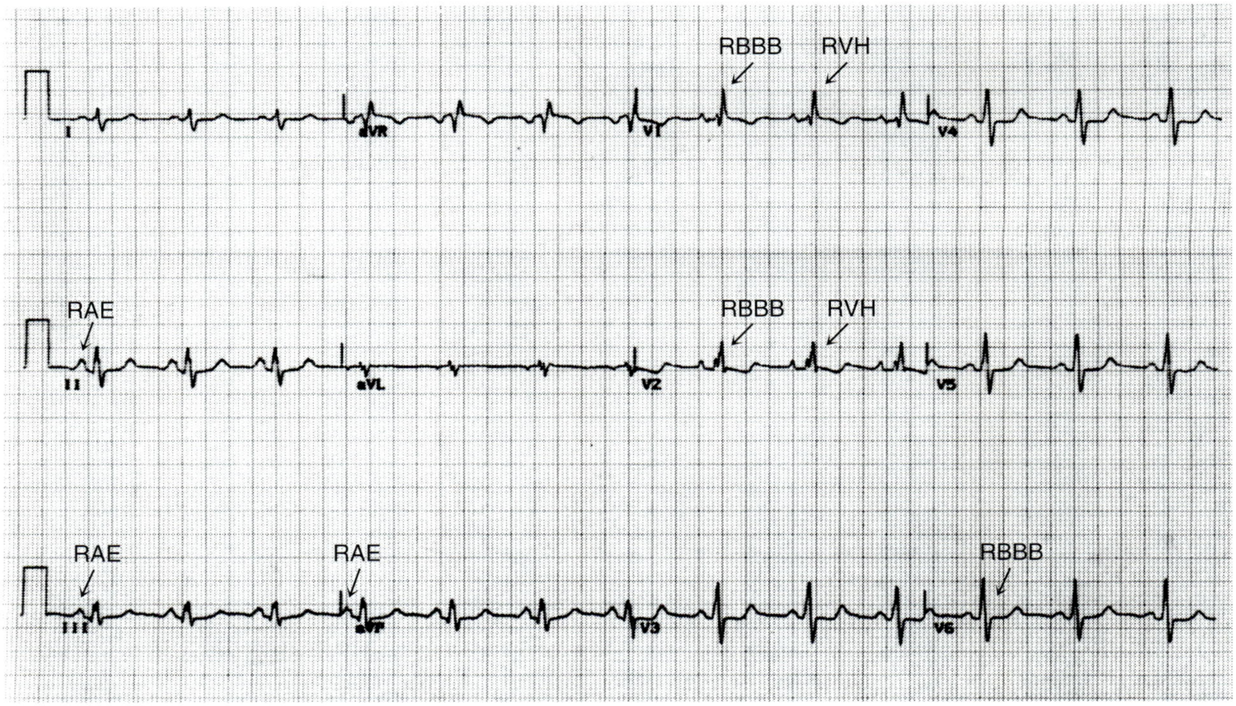

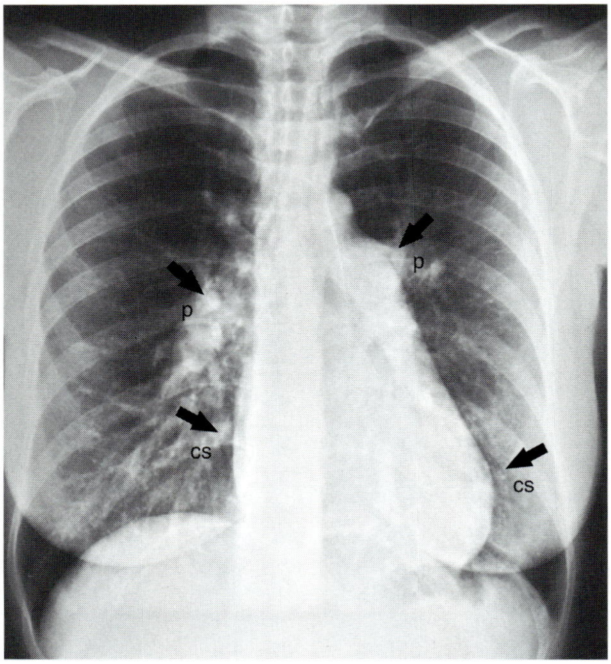

The electrocardiogram of a 42-year-old woman with the ostium secundum type of atrial septal defect shows normal sinus rhythm with incomplete right bundle-branch block (RBBB), indicated by the rSR′ pattern in leads V_1 and V_2 and the terminal S wave in V_6; right atrial enlargement (RAE), indicated by the tall P waves in leads II, III, and aVF; and right ventricular hypertrophy (RVH), indicated by the tall R waves in leads V_1 and V_2. The chest radiograph of the same patient shows a globular cardiac silhouette with prominent pulmonary arteries (p); cs denotes cardiac silhouette. Two-dimensional echocardiography confirmed the presence of an ostium secundum atrial septal defect.

Judy R. Mangion, M.D.

Baystate Medical Center
Springfield, MA 01199

May 18, 1995

Ostium Secundum Atrial Septal Defect

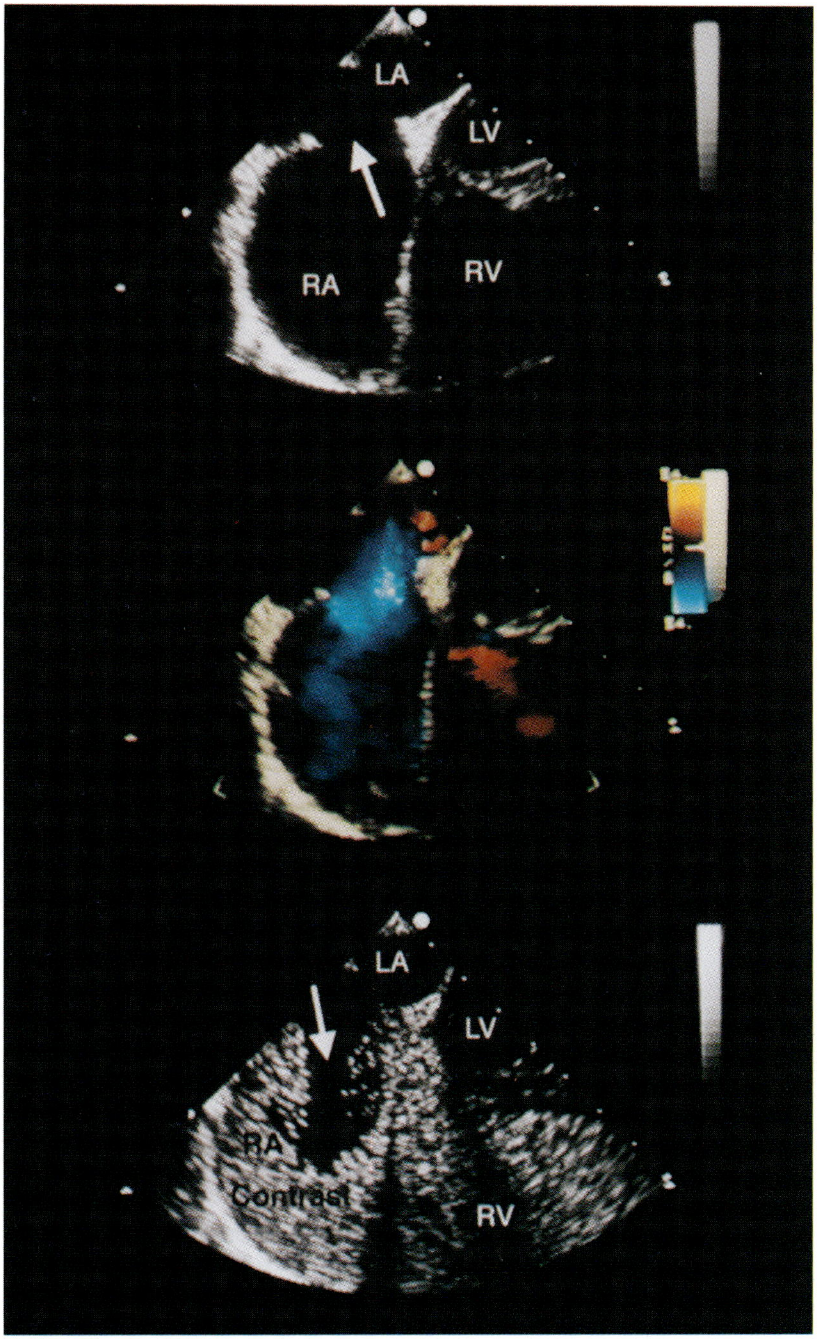

Transesophageal echocardiography was performed in a 23-year-old patient who presented with exertional dyspnea, fatigue, and palpitations. Cardiac auscultation revealed fixed splitting of the second heart sound and a short mid-diastolic murmur (grade 1/4) in the fourth left intercostal space parasternally. An rSR′ pattern was present in precordial lead V_1 on the electrocardiogram. Doppler studies showed a pulmonary–systemic flow ratio (QP/QS) of 2.3:1. The patient underwent successful surgical closure of the atrial septal defect.

A four-chamber transesophageal echocardiogram (top) shows a large defect in the interatrial septum (arrow). In the middle, a color-flow image shows left-to-right flow in blue (away from the transducer), through the defect in the interatrial septum. In a contrast echocardiogram (bottom) obtained after the injection of agitated saline into the antecubital vein, a "negative contrast effect" (arrow) is apparent, caused by left-to-right flow across the interatrial septum. LA denotes left atrium, LV left ventricle, RA right atrium, and RV right ventricle.

Roberto M. Lang, M.D.
Richard H. Marcus, M.D.

University of Chicago
Chicago, IL 60637

May 18, 1995

Percutaneous Mitral Balloon Valvotomy

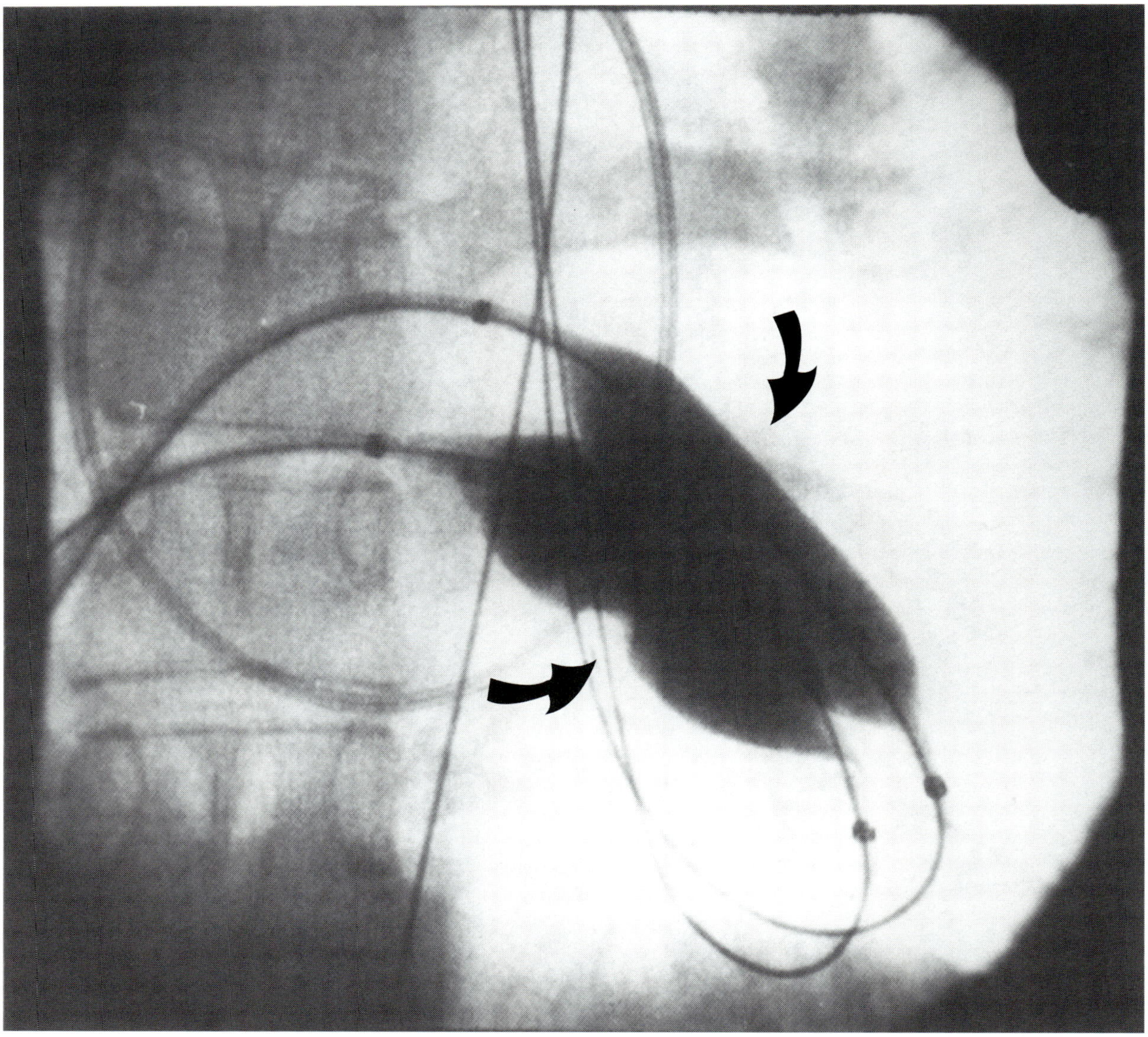

Percutaneous mitral balloon valvotomy by means of the double-balloon technique.

The inflation of 18-mm (above) and 20-mm (below) dilating balloons can be seen in a stenotic mitral valve. Note the "waist" produced by the stenotic valve (arrows) before full inflation causes commissural splitting. The balloons were placed in the mitral valve over two transfer wires passed through the right femoral vein, the interatrial septum (the transseptal route), and the mitral valve into the left ventricle, the aorta, and the descending aorta.

Peter C. Block, M.D.

March 19, 1992

"Floppy Mitral Valve"

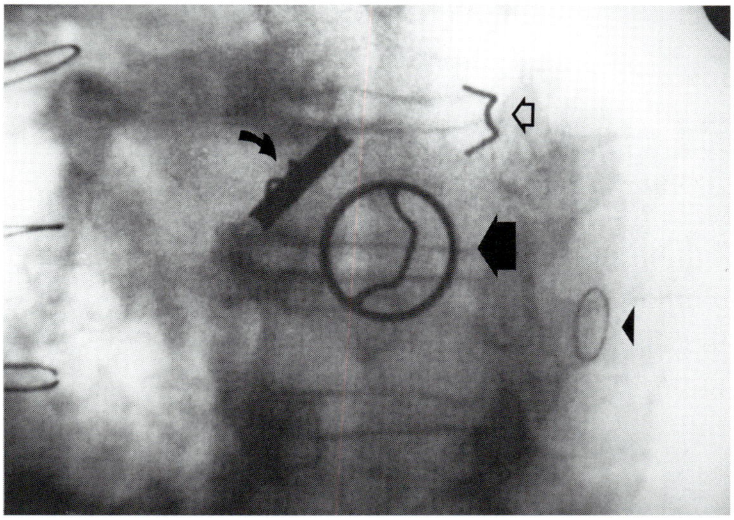

A

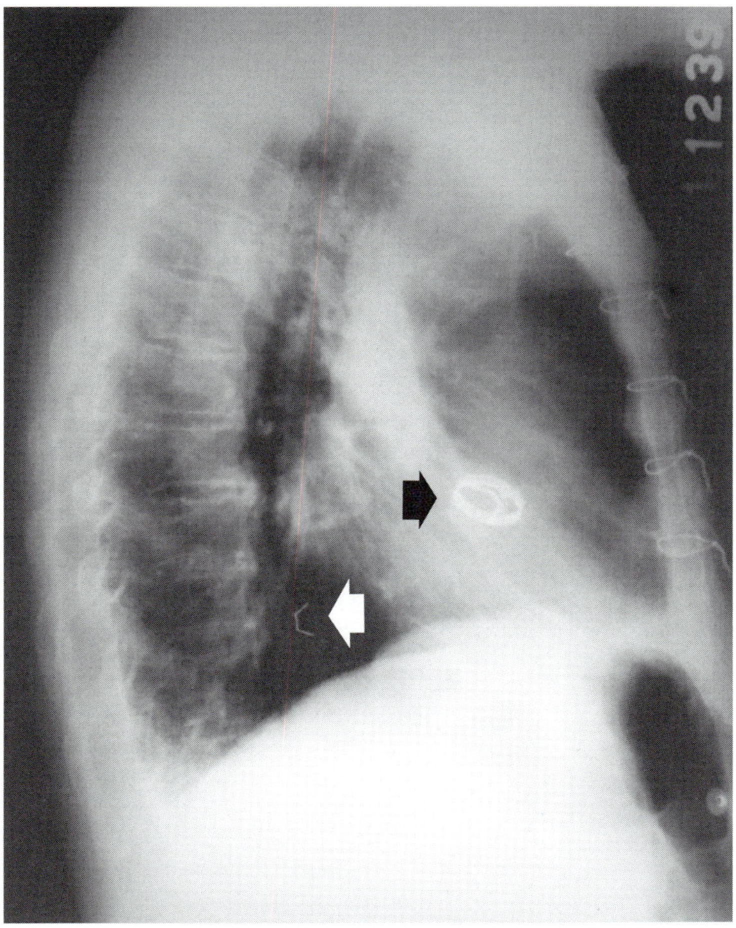

B

A 71-year-old man presented with acute pulmonary edema and cardiogenic shock nine years after his mitral and aortic valves had been replaced by Bjork–Shiley prostheses. Cinefluoroscopy showed that the minor strut of the mitral-valve prosthesis had broken off, and the disk was flopping wildly in the left ventricle. A frame from the cinefluoroscopy (Panel A) shows the severed minor strut (open arrow), the free-floating disk (arrowhead), the defective mitral-valve prosthesis (solid arrow), and the intact aortic-valve prosthesis (curved arrow). Echocardiography revealed wide-open mitral regurgitation.

The disk was removed from the left ventricle, and the defective valve was removed and replaced with a St. Jude prosthesis, but the broken strut could not be located. A lateral chest film (Panel B) taken one week after surgery shows the strut in a pulmonary vein (white arrow) and the intact aortic-valve prosthesis (black arrow). The patient made a gradual, uneventful recovery; the broken strut remained in place in the pulmonary vein.

Wolf F.C. Duvernoy, M.D.
Delano R. Small, M.D.

Providence Hospital
Southfield, MI 48075

August 18, 1994

Long-QT Syndrome

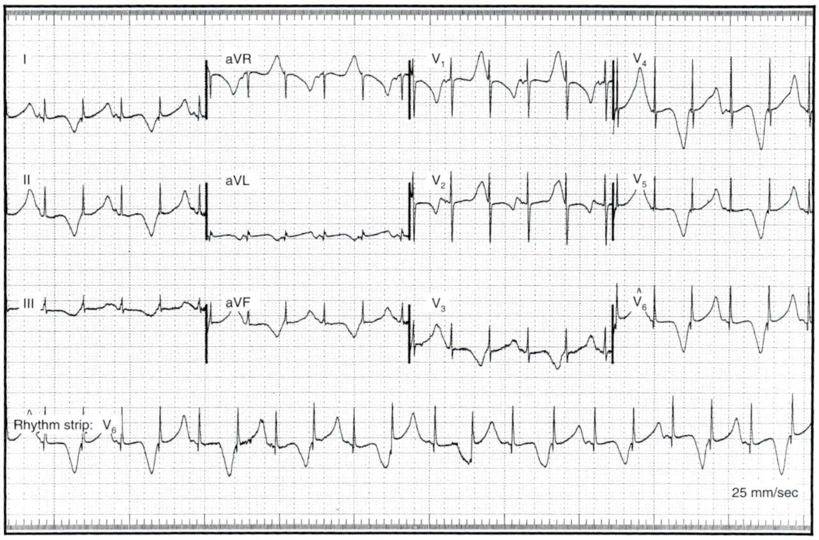

A

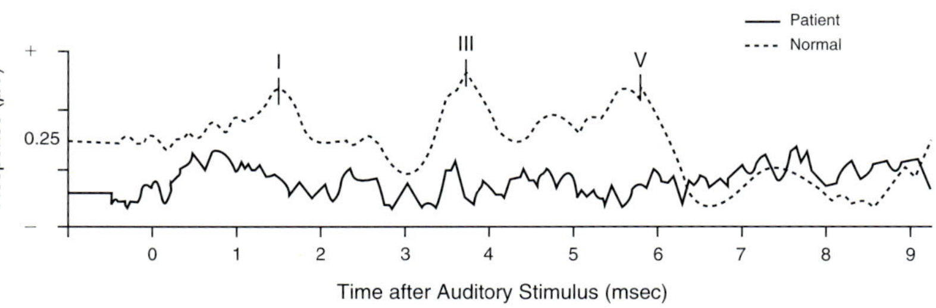

B

A two-year-old boy came to medical attention because he lost consciousness four times over a period of five months. Three of the episodes occurred when the child became upset. These episodes had previously been diagnosed as "breath-holding spells." He was also found to have severe sensorineural hearing loss. The child was taking no medication. There was no family history of sudden cardiac death.

Panel A is a 12-lead electrocardiogram, showing marked prolongation of the QT interval (QT corrected for heart rate, 0.75 sec) with T-wave alternans. Panel B compares the flattened and diminished auditory evoked responses of this patient (an indication of severe sensorineural hearing loss) with the responses of a subject with normal hearing. A single auditory stimulus (a click) was presented at time 0, and the electroencephalogram was recorded continuously. Peaks I, III, and V represent recordings of activity in the acoustic nerve, the pons, and the midbrain, respectively.

These findings are consistent with the autosomal recessive form of the congenital long-QT syndrome (called the Jervell and Lange-Nielsen syndrome). This syndrome, along with the more common Romano–Ward form of the long-QT syndrome (autosomal dominant inheritance, normal hearing), is associated with sudden cardiac death. Syncopal episodes are probably due to nonsustained polymorphic ventricular tachycardia (torsade de pointes). The patient has been asymptomatic since being treated with a beta-blocker.

Wayne H. Franklin, M.D.
Robert W. Hickey, M.D.

Columbus Children's Hospital
Columbus, OH 43205

August 10, 1995

Post-Tachycardia T-Wave Syndrome

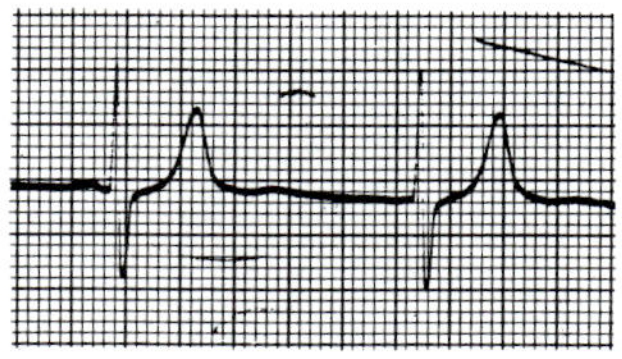

6/28/83

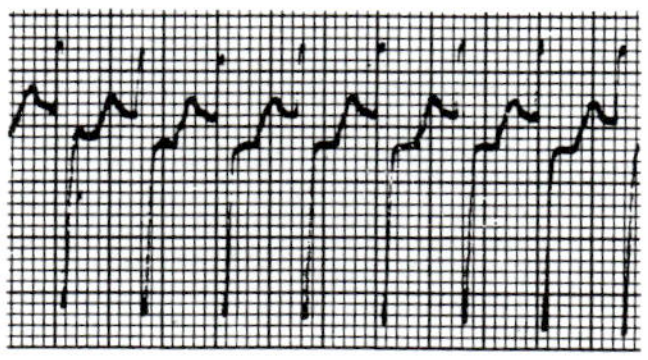

8/15/83

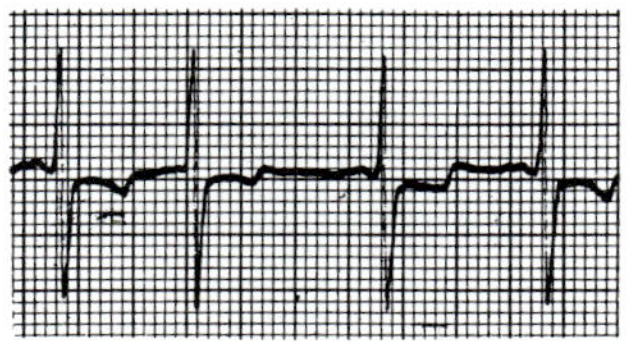

8/15/83

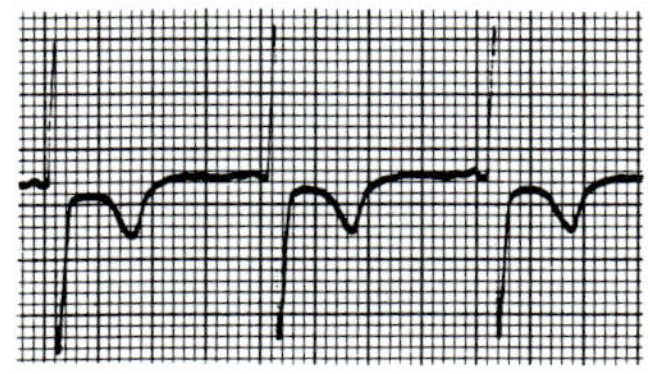

8/16/83

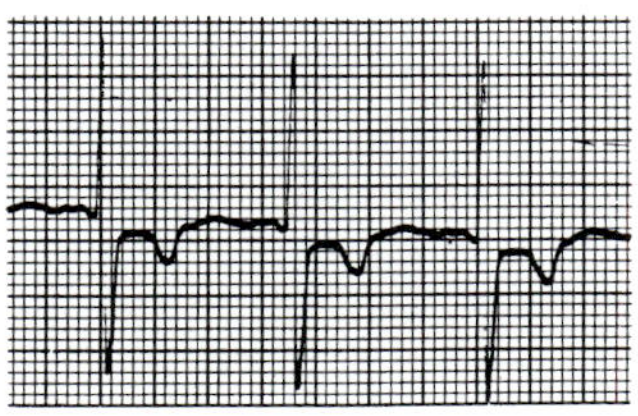

8/17/83

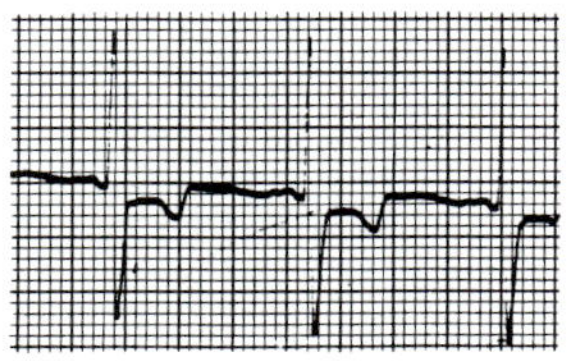

8/18/83

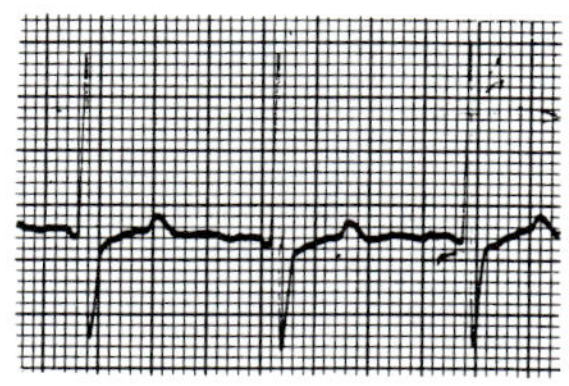

8/25/83

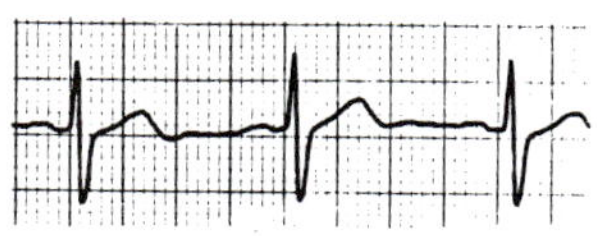

1987

Serial electrocardiograms (lead V_4) were obtained in a 67-year-old man taking digoxin for paroxysmal supraventricular tachycardia. An electrocardiogram obtained on June 28, 1983, showed no abnormalities. About six weeks later on August 15, while awaiting surgery for peripheral vascular disease, the patient had an episode of paroxysmal supraventricular tachycardia (first electrocardiogram in second row) that responded to carotid-sinus massage. An electrocardiogram obtained shortly after conversion to sinus rhythm showed atrial premature beats and minor T-wave inversions (second electrocardiogram in second row), which became deeper over the next 24 hours (third electrocardiogram in second row). The patient was given verapamil at a dose of 80 mg four times daily. Because of persistent T-wave inversions (recorded on August 17 and 18) he underwent cardiac catheterization and angiography, which revealed normal coronary arteries and normal left ventricular function. The T-wave abnormalities, which are those classically seen in the post-tachycardia syndrome, had decreased by August 25, and he underwent successful femoral-artery bypass surgery. Four years later, in 1987, his electrocardiogram had returned to normal.

Arnold M. Katz, M.D.

University of Connecticut
Health Center
School of Medicine
Farmington, CT 06030

January 19, 1995

Shock Delivered by an Implantable Cardioverter–Defibrillator in Response to Spontaneous Ventricular Fibrillation

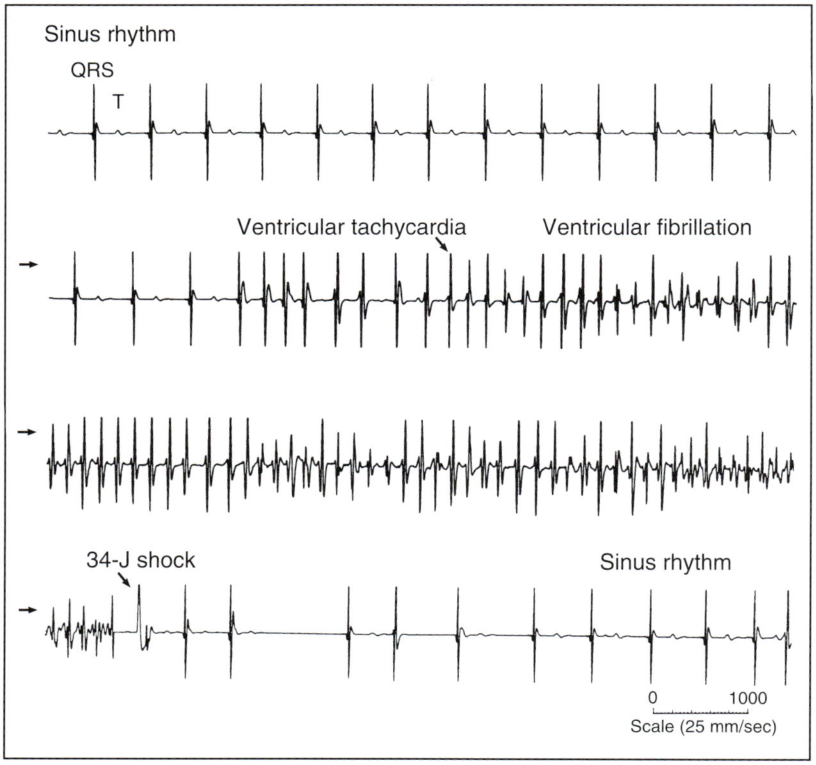

Stored bipolar intracardiac electrograms obtained from a 66-year-old man with an implantable cardioverter–defibrillator were retrieved during a routine office visit. The patient had reported a brief episode of lightheadedness followed by a sudden jolt in his chest. He remained conscious. The intracardiac electrograms are recorded from a right ventricular rate-sensing lead. The initial rhythm is sinus, with characteristic intracardiac recordings analogous to the QRS complex and the T wave. Rapid ventricular tachycardia developed spontaneously and degenerated into ventricular fibrillation. The rapid ventricular rate was detected by the cardioverter–defibrillator, which delivered a high-energy DC shock. Defibrillation restored sinus rhythm.

Marc Roelke, M.D.

Newark Beth Israel Medical Center
Newark, NJ 07112

Sean S. O'Nunain, M.B.

Massachusetts General Hospital
Boston, MA 02114

March 30, 1995

Radiofrequency Catheter Ablation of a Left Posterior Accessory Atrioventricular Connection in a Patient with the Wolff–Parkinson–White Syndrome

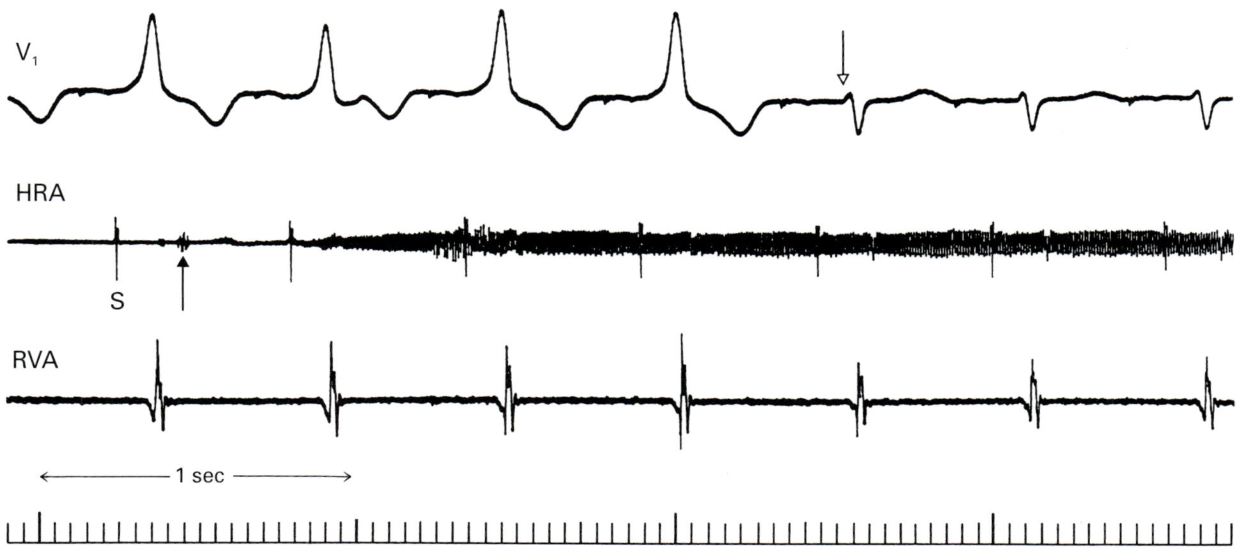

From top to bottom the tracings represent the surface electrocardiogram (Lead V_1) and bipolar intracardiac electrograms recorded from the high right atrium (HRA) and right ventricular apex (RVA) during right atrial pacing (S denotes a stimulus artifact of the right atrial pacer). Radiofrequency current (55 V for 30 seconds) was applied through the distal electrode of an exploring catheter positioned on the ventricular side of the mitral annulus close to the ventricular insertion of the accessory atrioventricular connection. Within three beats after the application of radiofrequency current (solid arrow), conduction over the accessory pathway was eliminated and ventricular preexcitation disappeared, as evidenced by normalization of the QRS complex (open arrow).

Jeremy N. Ruskin, M.D.
Hasan Garan, M.D.

Massachusetts General Hospital
Boston, MA 02114

August 27, 1992

Large Left Atrial Thrombus

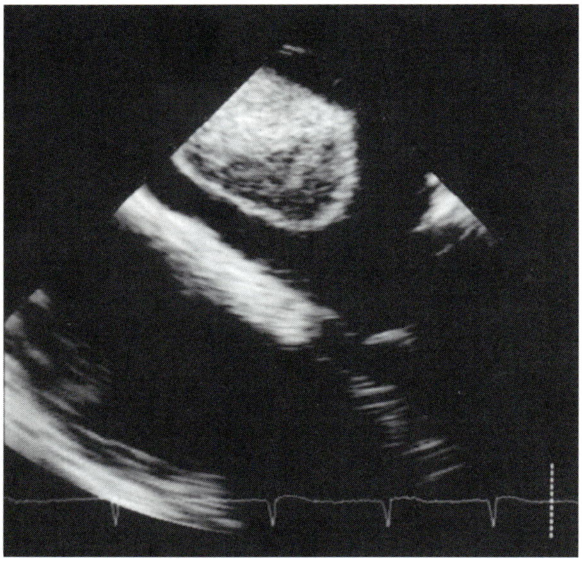

A

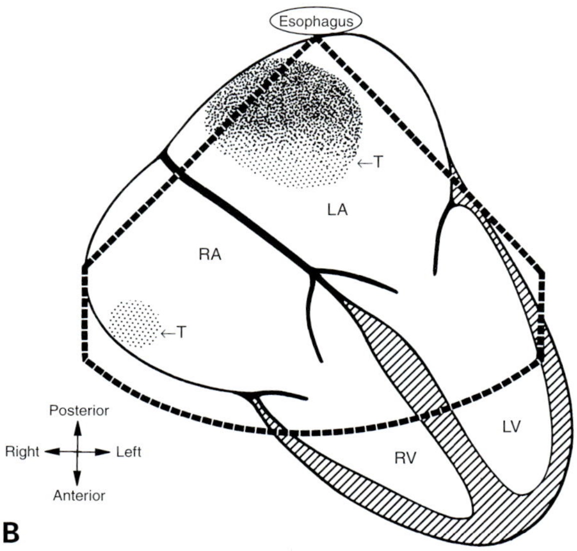

B

This four-chamber view of the heart (Panel A) was obtained by transesophageal echocardiography in a 75-year-old man with longstanding nonvalvular atrial fibrillation who had recently had a transient ischemic attack. A large, immobile thrombus (T in the schematic drawing in Panel B) is attached to the posterior wall of the left atrium (LA). A smaller thrombus (T) is attached to the lateral wall of the right atrium (RA). A third thrombus was present in the left atrial appendage (not shown). The large left atrial mass is unlikely to be a myxoma because of the absence of a pedicle and the lack of attachment to the atrial septum in the area of the fossa ovalis. In addition, the presence of a mass in the left atrial appendage and the spontaneous echo contrast in the right atrium (not shown) are most consistent with the presence of multiple atrial thrombi. After this echocardiogram was obtained, the patient received anticoagulation. Transesophageal echocardiography performed three weeks later revealed a reduction in the size of both left atrial thrombi. RV denotes right ventricle, and LV left ventricle.

Bibiana Cujec, M.D., F.R.C.P.C.
Marc Baltzan, M.D., F.R.C.P.C.

Department of Medicine
University of Saskatchewan
Saskatoon, SK S7N 0X0, Canada

March 18, 1993

Fracture of a Retention Wire in an Atrial J Pacemaker Lead

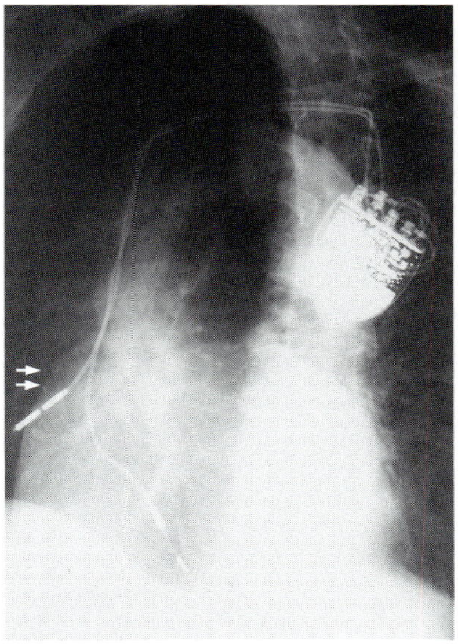

A

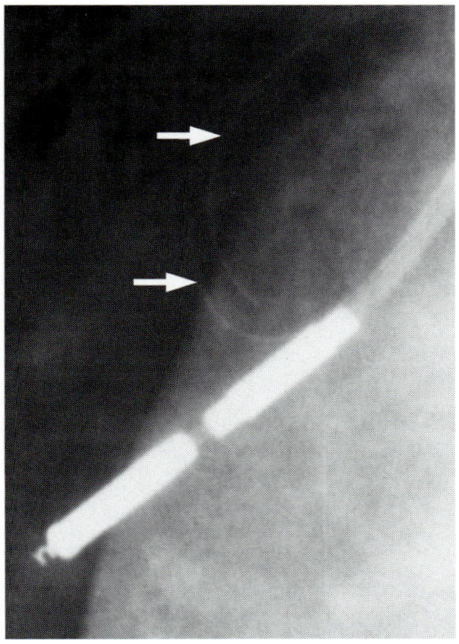

B

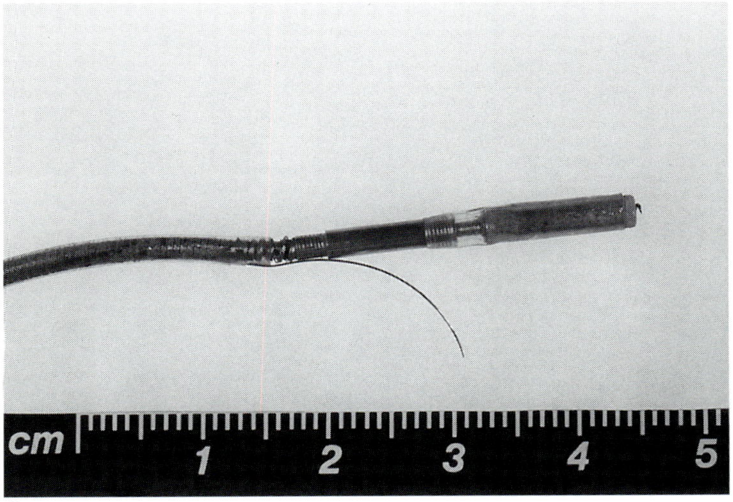

C

A fracture of a retention wire in an atrial J pacemaker lead (model 330-801, Telectronics, Englewood, Colo.) was detected by chest radiography. The wire, which maintains the J shape of the lead, had fractured, and the distal fragment had migrated from the lead body. Both fragments, visible on the initial chest x-ray film taken at an oblique angle (Panel A, arrows), became more apparent when the image was enlarged (Panel B, arrows).

The patient was asymptomatic, and the lead was functioning properly. Nearly 42,000 such leads have been implanted worldwide, and the rate of fracture is approximately 17 percent. Patients with retention wires that protrude from the lead body or in whom a wire fragment has protruded and migrated from the lead body (as in this patient) are considered at high risk for laceration and cardiac tamponade. In the vast majority of cases, however, the retention wire is not protruding and thus not life threatening, and removal of the lead is generally not indicated. Panel C shows the lead body in this case after extraction, with the retention-wire fragment protruding conspicuously. The detached wire segment that had migrated remained embedded in the atrial wall.

Marc Roelke, M.D.
Victor Parsonnet, M.D.

Newark Beth Israel Medical Center
Newark, NJ 07112

January 11, 1996

Neurocardiogenic (Vasodepressor) Syncope

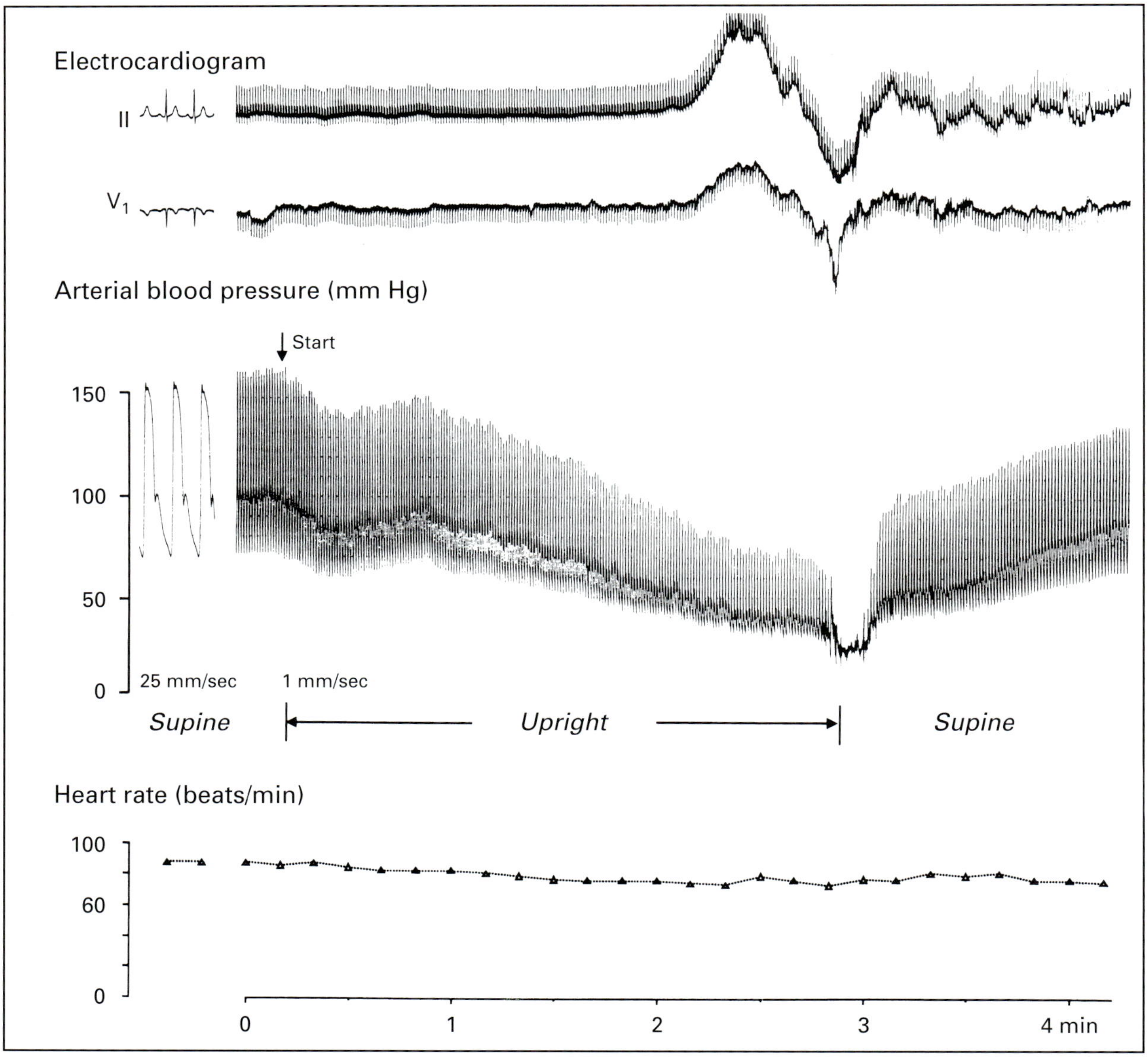

A 72-year-old woman with breast cancer that had metastasized to the glossopharyngeal region had recurrent episodes of sudden lightheadedness, diaphoresis, and syncope. A dual-chamber pacemaker was implanted, but syncope recurred, always preceded by severe neck pain. During the tilt-table test with the pacemaker inactivated, the results of which are shown here, the patient's usual symptoms developed. She lost consciousness and had a seizure, but regained consciousness immediately after she was returned to the supine position. The study shows a profound vasodepressor reaction with minimal slowing of the sinus rhythm. Treatment with disopyramide (150 mg three times a day) eliminated the syncopal episodes over five months of follow-up.

Stefan Osswald, M.D.
Thomas G. Trouton, M.D.

Massachusetts General Hospital
Boston, MA 02114

July 1, 1993

Correspondence

Neurocardiogenic Syncope

December 23, 1993

To the Editor: The Images in Clinical Medicine in the July 1 issue[1] intrigued me. I am uncertain whether the hemodynamic reaction shown represents syncope mediated by the neurocardiogenic (Bezold–Jarisch) reflex or carotid-sinus hypersensitivity with only a vasodepressor component. Generally, bradycardia is expected in neurocardiogenic syncope, which is thought to be mediated by vagal afferent and efferent fibers.[2,3] Conversely, carotid-sinus hypersensitivity mediated by glossopharyngeal afferent fibers occurs without bradycardia in a pure vasodepressor reaction.[4] Given the patient's history of metastatic cancer of the neck, carotid-sinus hypersensitivity seems to be a strong candidate for having produced the illustrated hemodynamic reaction. I am interested in the results of carotid-massage testing in this patient and the authors' interpretation of the reflex arcs involved in the patient's syncopal episode.

Stephen E. Piwinski, M.D.
John Peter Smith Hospital, Fort Worth, TX 76104

1. Osswald S, Trouton TG. Neurocardiogenic (vasodepressor) syncope. N Engl J Med 1993;329:30.
2. Sra JS, Jazayeri MR, Avitall B, et al. Comparison of cardiac pacing with drug therapy in the treatment of neurocardiogenic (vasovagal) syncope with bradycardia or asystole. N Engl J Med 1993; 328:1085-90.
3. Linzer M. Syncope: 1991. Am J Med 1991;90:1-5.
4. Taylor AA, Mitchell JR. Laboratory evaluation of autonomic nervous system function. In: Laragh, JH, Brenner BM, eds. Hypertension: pathophysiology, diagnosis, and management. Vol. 2. New York: Raven Press, 1990:1461-78.

The authors reply:

To the Editor: Dr. Piwinski has made a reasonable suggestion that glossopharyngeal-nerve involvement and carotid-sinus hypersensitivity might have had a role in triggering clinical syncope in our patient.[1] Furthermore, the patient was initially treated with carbamazepine, which relieved her neuralgia but did not prevent recurrent syncope. However, there are several features that are not adequately explained by the occurrence of classic carotid hypersensitivity alone. First, palpation of the patient's neck did not induce syncope, whereas head-up tilt testing in the absence of carotid-sinus irritation did reproducibly induce her syncope. Second, her frequent syncopal episodes were completely abolished by treatment with disopyramide, a drug that is thought to inhibit cardiac mechanoreceptors (C fibers) in neurocardiogenic syncope by means of its negative inotropic properties.[2] This property of disopyramide in unlikely to be effective in the management of carotid hypersensitivity.

On the basis of the current understanding,[3] the afferent limb of the reflex arc in neurocardiogenic syncope may be quite variable, whereas the uniformity of the efferent response suggests the involvement of a final common pathway.[4,5] This concept is supported by the clinical observation that multiple stimuli, such as pain, fear, psychological stress, use of vasodilators, inferior myocardial ischemia, and gastrointestinal hemorrhage, have the potential to trigger a uniform vasodepressor response.[4,5] This suggests that mechanisms in addition to abnormal afferent parasympathetic activity, such as lowering of the central nervous system threshold for activation of the efferent autonomic response, may have a pivotal role in people susceptible to neurocardiogenic syncope.

Stefan Osswald, M.D., Thomas G. Trouton, M.D., Brian A. McGovern, M.D.
Massachusetts General Hospital, Boston, MA 02114

1. Wallin BG, Westerberg CE, Sundlof G. Syncope induced by glossopharyngeal neuralgia: sympathetic outflow of muscle. Neurology 1984;34:522-4.
2. Milstein S, Buetikofer J, Dunningan A, Benditt DG, Gornick C, Reyes WJ. Usefulness of disopyramide for prevention of upright tilt-induced hypotension-bradycardia. Am J Cardiol 1990;65:1339-44.
3. Abboud FM. Neurocardiogenic syncope. N Engl J Med 1993;328:1117-20.
4. Benditt DG, Remole S, Bailin S, Dunnigan A, Asso A, Milstein S. Tilt table testing for evaluation of neurally-mediated (cardioneurogenic) syncope: rationale and proposed protocols. PACE Pacing Clin Electrophysiol 1991;14:1528-37.
5. Rea RF, Thames MD. Neural control mechanism and vasovagal syncope. J Cardiovasc Electrophysiol 1993;4:587-95.

Pressure Tracings in Obstructive Cardiomyopathy

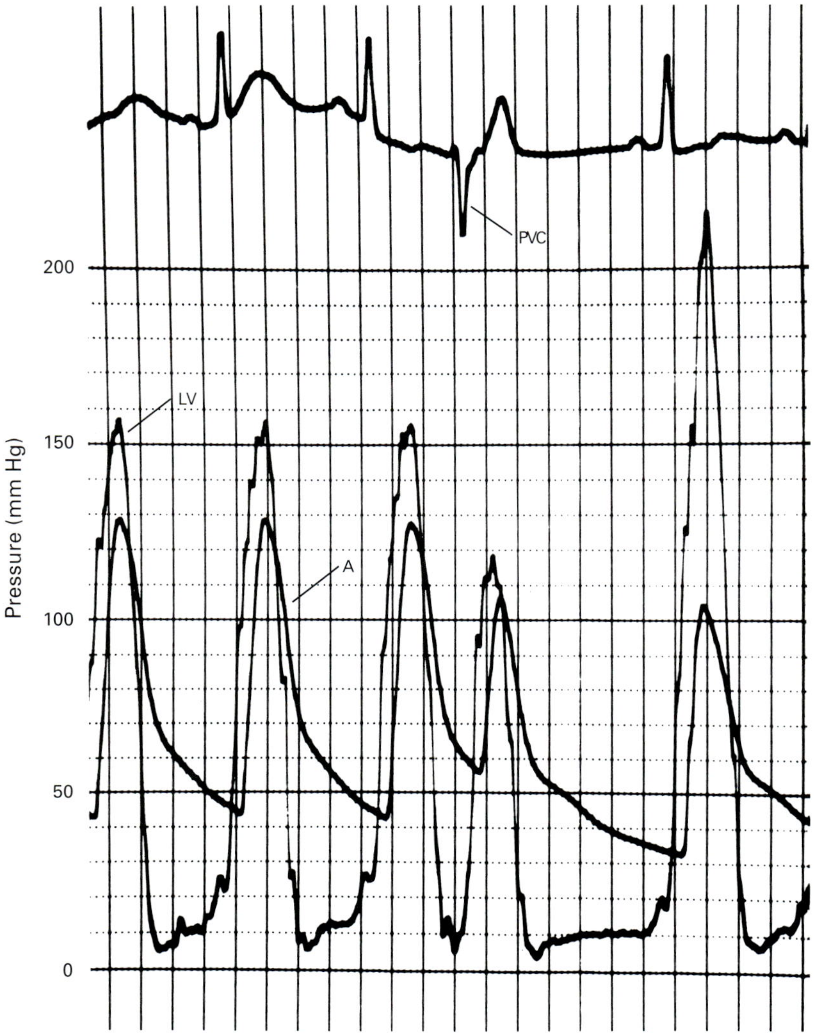

Simultaneous arterial (A) and left ventricular (LV) pressures were recorded in a patient with hypertrophic obstructive cardiomyopathy. The first three beats show a peak systolic gradient of 25 mm Hg. On the first sinus beat after a premature ventricular contraction (PVC), the peak-systolic gradient increases to over 100 mm Hg, but the pulse pressure (arterial systolic pressure minus diastolic pressure) decreases. This characteristic pattern is known as the Brockenbrough–Braunwald sign. The decrease in pulse pressure after a premature ventricular contraction is due to reduced stroke volume caused by increased dynamic obstruction, which is due, in turn, to post-extrasystolic potentiation.

Stewart G. Pollock, M.D.

Harrisonburg Medical Associates
Harrisonburg, VA 22801

July 28, 1994

Correspondence

The Brockenbrough–Braunwald–Morrow Sign

December 8, 1994

To the Editor: With regard to the clinical image depicting the "Brockenbrough–Braunwald sign" (July 28 issue),[1] the authors of the 1961 article that initially described the diminished pulse pressure in the post-extrasystolic beat were Brockenbrough, Braunwald, and Morrow.[2] The late Andrew G. Morrow was a prolific investigator of hypertrophic cardiomyopathy and deserves equal recognition. The criterion for a positive post-extrasystolic response was later modified by the authors to include instances in which the pulse pressure fails to increase.[3] It was also later found that this sign is not unique to hypertrophic cardiomyopathy but has frequently been observed in discrete forms of aortic stenosis.[4] Figure 1 depicts this response in patients with valvular and discrete subvalvular aortic stenosis.

It has also been found that the ventricle in hypertrophic cardiomyopathy actually empties more rapidly and completely in situations in which the gradient is augmented,[5,6] including post-extrasystolic and inotropic stimulation. These observations belie the explanation offered for the diminished pulse pressure — namely, a "reduced stroke volume caused by increased dynamic obstruction."

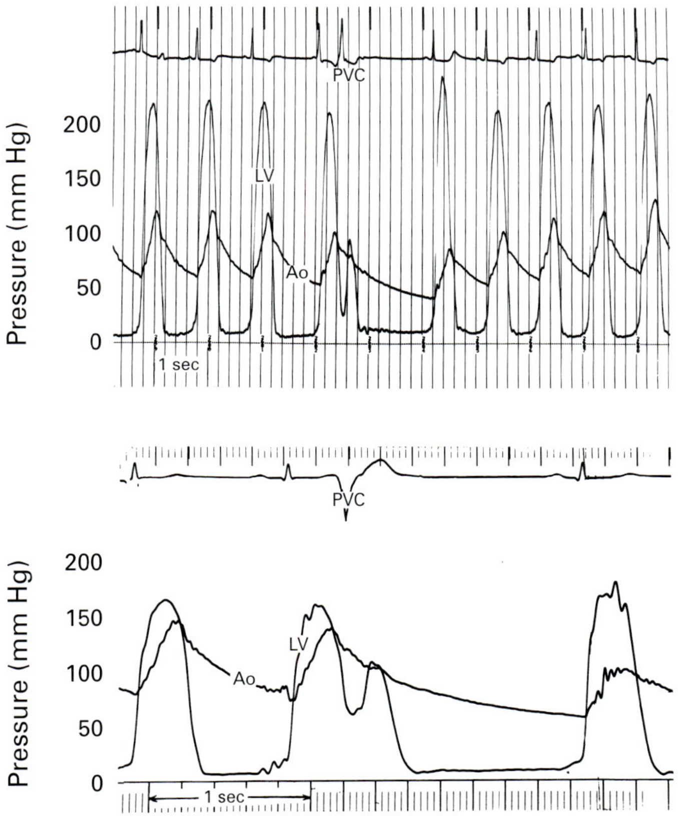

Figure 1. Brockenbrough–Braunwald–Morrow Sign in Aortic Stenosis.
Left ventricular (LV) pressure and central aortic (Ao) pressure were recorded simultaneously in a patient with calcific valvular aortic stenosis (upper panel) and a patient with discrete subvalvular aortic stenosis (lower panel). Both patients had a diminished aortic upstroke rate, which is typical of fixed obstruction; post-extrasystolic potentiation of the left ventricular pressure and pressure gradient after the premature ventricular contraction (PVC); and a fall in the aortic pulse pressure.

Since it is unlikely that the severity of obstruction in aortic stenosis increases during the post-extrasystolic beat, other mechanisms should be considered to explain this fall in pulse pressure. The prolonged diastolic aortic runoff time decreases the aortic impedance, and an increase in mitral regurgitation driven by the higher left ventricular pressure may lower the forward stroke volume. Either or both of these explanations may also apply to hypertrophic cardiomyopathy.

John Michael Criley, M.D.
Steven L. Goldberg, M.D.
William J. French, M.D.
Harbor–UCLA Medical Center
Torrance, CA 90502

1. Pollock SG. Pressure tracings in obstructive cardiomyopathy. N Engl J Med 1994;331:238.
2. Brockenbrough EC, Braunwald E, Morrow AG. A hemodynamic technic for the detection of hypertrophic subaortic stenosis. Circulation 1961;23:189-94.
3. Braunwald E, Lambrew CT, Morrow AG, Pierce GE, Rockoff SD, Ross J Jr. Idiopathic hypertrophic subaortic stenosis. Circulation 1964;30:Suppl IV:IV-1–IV-213.
4. Kramer DS, French WJ, Criley JM. The postextrasystolic murmur response to gradient in hypertrophic cardiomyopathy. Ann Intern Med 1986;104:772-6.

Correspondence Continued

5. Wilson WS, Criley JM, Ross RS. Dynamics of left ventricular emptying in hypertrophic subaortic stenosis: a cineangiographic and hemodynamic study. Am Heart J 1967;73:4-16.
6. Siegel RJ, Criley JM. Comparison of ventricular emptying with and without a pressure gradient in patients with hypertrophic cardiomyopathy. Br Heart J 1985;53:283-91.

Dr. Pollock replies:

To the Editor: Criley et al. correctly point out that Dr. Morrow contributed to the first description of the post-extrasystolic fall in pulse pressure seen in idiopathic hypertrophic subaortic stenosis (as the disorder was then called). They also question my explanation of the mechanism of this hemodynamic finding.

I used the term "Brockenbrough–Braunwald sign," excluding Dr. Morrow's name, because it is the name commonly used for this sign.[1] Although it is technically incorrect to omit one of the investigators' names, such terms are often abbreviated for convenience. For instance, the preoperative assessment is guided by the "Goldman class," a term that would be cumbersome if it included the names of all 13 authors.[2]

I explained the post-extrasystolic fall in blood pressure as a reduction in stroke volume due to an increase in dynamic obstruction, which is the usual explanation for this finding but may, like the sign's name, be incorrect.[1,3] Criley et al. argue this point by presenting a pressure tracing from a patient with fixed valvular stenosis. The tracing purports to show the Brockenbrough–Braunwald–Morrow sign. The pulse pressure, however, is reduced not just for one beat after the premature ventricular contraction but for four beats. Furthermore, the pulse pressure is reduced even before the premature ventricular contraction. This is not an example of the Brockenbrough–Braunwald–Morrow sign. Although the tracing does not rule out a role for dynamic obstruction in causing the Brockenbrough–Braunwald–Morrow sign, the suggestion that enhanced mitral regurgitation or arterial compliance contributes to the physiologic process is intriguing. The second tracing, from a patient with discrete subvalvular aortic stenosis, supports this idea.

Stewart G. Pollock, M.D.
Harrisonburg Medical Associates
Harrisonburg, VA 22801-7500

1. Grossman W. Profiles in dilated (congestive) and hypertrophic cardiomyopathies. In: Grossman W, ed. Cardiac catheterization and angiography. Philadelphia: Lea & Febiger, 1986:420-1.
2. Goldman L, Caldera DL, Nussbaum SR, et al. Multifactorial index of cardiac risk in noncardiac surgical procedures. N Engl J Med 1977;297:845-50.
3. Wynne J, Braunwald E. The cardiomyopathies and myocarditides. In: Braunwald E, ed. Heart disease: a textbook of cardiovascular medicine. 3rd ed. Vol. 2. Philadelphia: W.B. Saunders, 1988:1428.

Pulsus Alternans

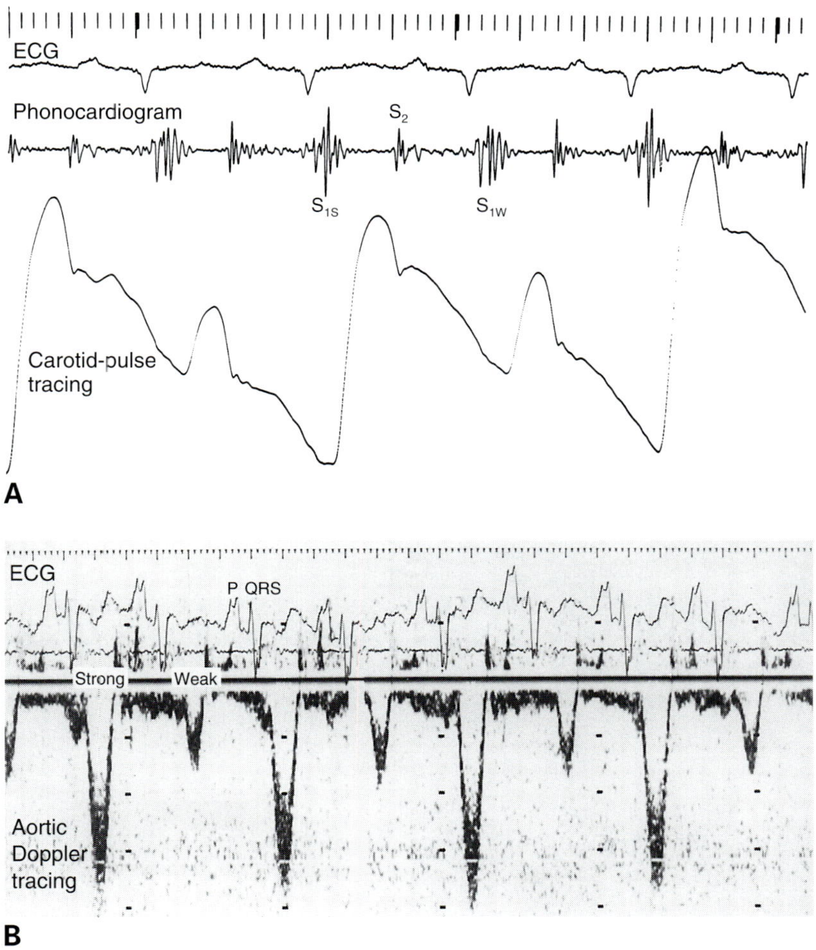

Physical examination of two patients with severe left ventricular failure revealed pulsus alternans in the radial pulse. Pulsus alternans is a physical finding characterized by a regular alternation of the force of the arterial pulse. It almost invariably indicates the presence of severe left ventricular systolic dysfunction.

Panel A shows a simultaneous electrocardiogram (ECG), phonocardiogram, and carotid-pulse tracing in a 64-year-old man with an ejection fraction of 15 percent due to dilated cardiomyopathy. Alternating strong and weak beats are seen in the carotid pulse tracing that corresponded to an alternation of approximately 40 mm Hg in the systolic blood pressure. There is also an alternation of the first heart sound on the phonocardiogram, characterized by a more pronounced sound with a strong contraction (S_{1S}) and a less pronounced sound with a weak beat (S_{1W}). This is due to a more rapid increase in left ventricular pressure with the stronger contraction.

Panel B shows a simultaneous ECG and Doppler tracing in a 29-year-old woman with cardiomyopathy related to the acquired immunodeficiency syndrome and an ejection fraction of 10 percent. Marked alternation in aortic flow is present, corresponding to a calculated alternation in the stroke volume of 2.2:1 between the strong and weak beats.

Karen Cha, B.S.
Rodney H. Falk, M.D.

Boston University Medical Center
Boston, MA 02118

March 28, 1996

Dissection of the Ascending Thoracic Aorta

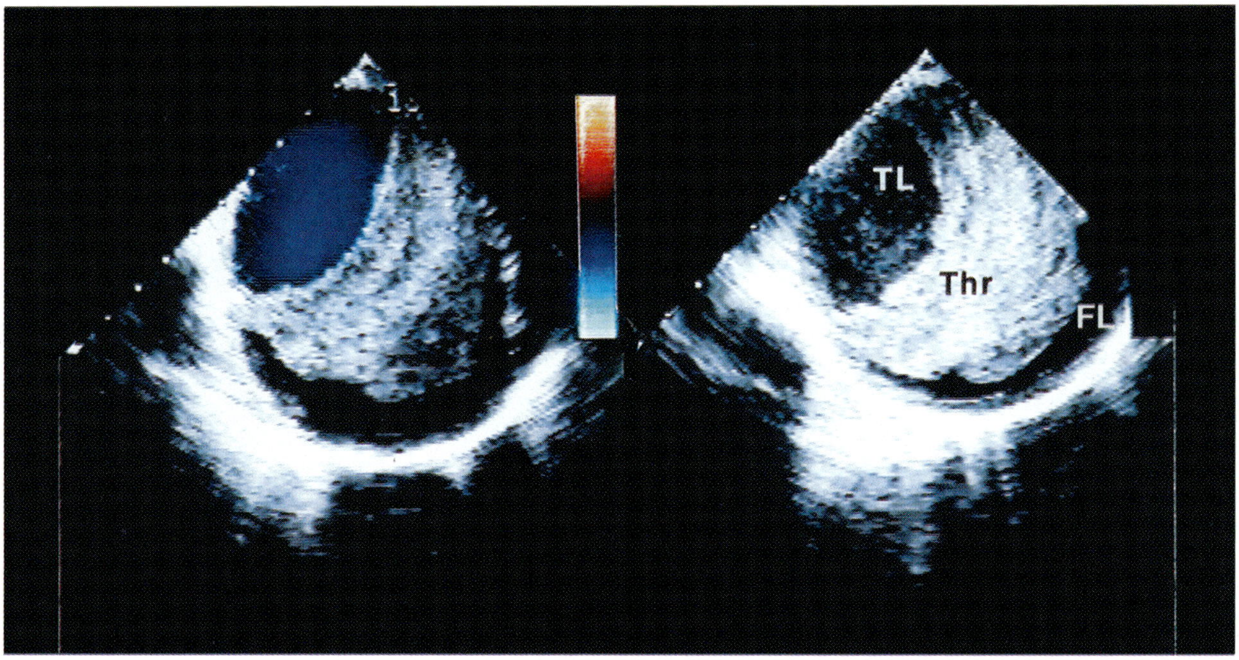

A dissecting aneurysm of the ascending segment of the thoracic aorta was diagnosed by two-dimensional transesophageal echocardiography. The horizontal imaging plane is approximately 3 cm above the aortic valve and shows a separation of the true lumen (TL) and the false lumen (FL) of the dissecting aneurysm. A color-coded flow signal in blue identifies flow away from the aortic valve in the true lumen. An echogenic crescent-shaped thrombus (Thr) almost completely fills the false lumen and leaves only a narrow unobstructed mural rim. Two images, taken at slightly different gray-scale gain settings, are shown side by side; the lower setting in the image on the left allows better visualization of the color-coded flow signal. Blue denotes flow away from and red or yellow flow toward the transducer.

Christoph A. Nienaber, M.D.

University Hospital Eppendorf
20246 Hamburg, Germany

May 12, 1994

Correspondence

Aortic Dissection

September 22, 1994

To the Editor: Nienaber (May 12 issue)[1] presented an image of an aortic dissection obtained by transesophageal echocardiography in a horizontal plane. He described the dissection as located in the ascending aorta, approximately 3 cm above the aortic valve. The absence of any visualized structure between the transesophageal echocardiographic probe and the aorta suggests that the probe was in immediate proximity to the aortic wall. Because the esophagus normally lies adjacent only to the descending aorta, we suspect that the segment of the aorta depicted corresponds to the descending rather than the ascending aorta.

Markus Jakob, M.D.
Donat R. Spahn, M.D.
Rolf Jenni, M.D., M.S.E.E.
University of Zurich
CH-8091 Zurich, Switzerland

1. Nienaber CA. Dissection of the ascending thoracic aorta. N Engl J Med 1994;330:1361.

The author replies:

To the Editor: We thank our colleagues for their vigilance and attentive comments. As they point out, the ultrasonographic image of an aortic dissection shows the descending aorta at the level described, rather than the ascending segment. Legends from various sets of ultrasonographic images were inadvertently intermixed.

Christoph A. Nienaber, M.D.
Dietmar Koschyk, M.D.
University Hospital Eppendorf
20246 Hamburg, Germany

Usefulness of MRI in Aortic Dissection

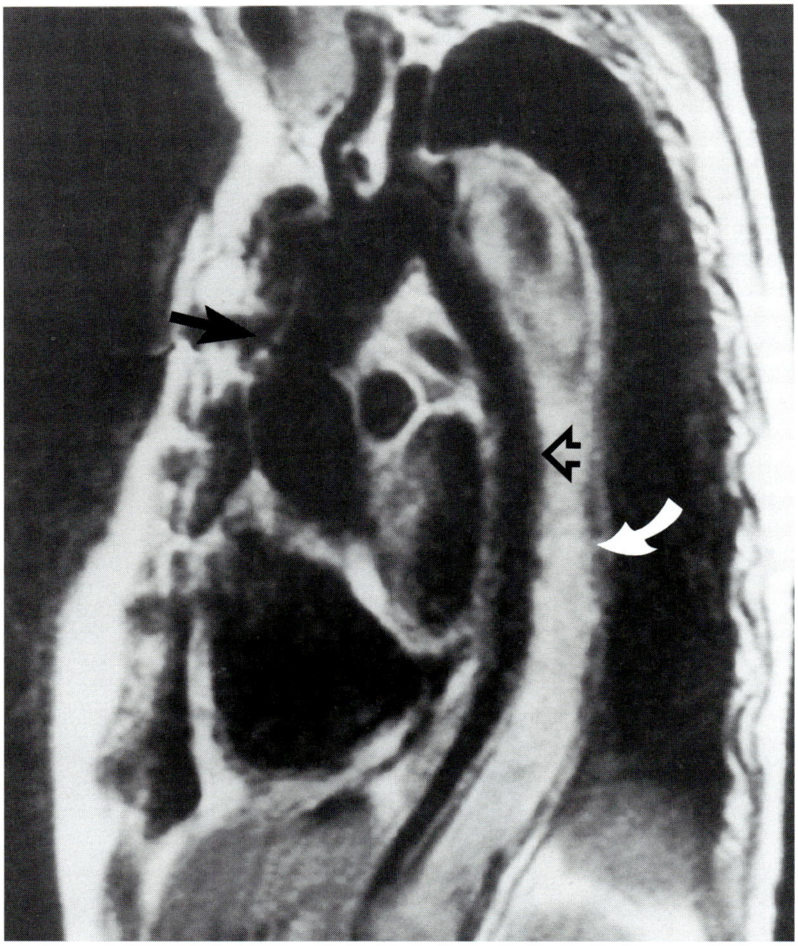

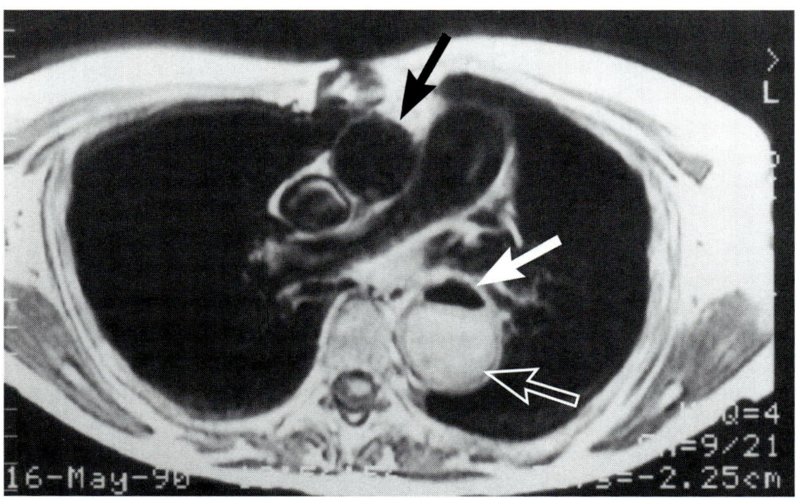

The top panel is an oblique sagittal magnetic resonance image (MRI) aligned to give a long-axis view of the thoracic aorta in a 55-year-old patient with Marfan's syndrome and aortic dissection. The intimal flap begins in the ascending aorta (solid black arrow) at the level of the distal anastomosis of a graft used in a previous repair of the aortic root. The left carotid and left subclavian arteries can be seen originating from the aortic arch. In the descending aorta a relatively high signal is returned by the blood in the false channel (white arrow), a result consistent with slow flow (or possibly thrombosis) in this area. The signal intensity in the true lumen (open black arrow) is low, indicating faster flow in this channel.

The bottom panel is a transverse image at the level of the right pulmonary artery. There is a signal void in the true lumen of the descending aorta (solid white arrow). Again, a high signal intensity is observed in the false channel (open white arrow). Reconstruction of the same data in a phase image (not shown) revealed a phase change in the false channel relative to the surrounding stationary tissue, indicating that this channel contains slowly flowing blood rather than a solid thrombus. The appearance of the graft in the ascending aorta (black arrow) is normal. Both images were obtained with a spin–echo technique (time to echo, 30 msec; y resolution, 160; field of view, 31 cm).

Godtfred Holmvang, M.D.

June 18, 1992

Tension Pneumopericardium

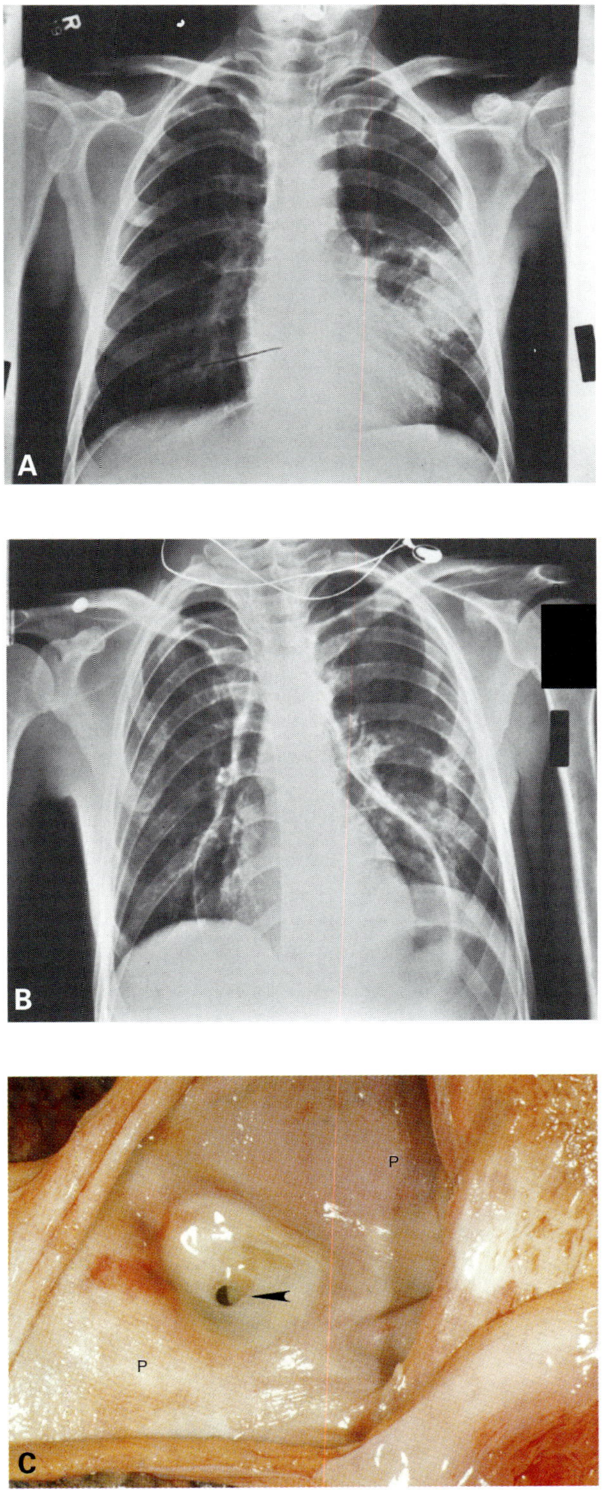

Tension pneumopericardium, a rare complication of pyogenic lung abscess, occurred in a 27-year-old white man with the acquired immunodeficiency syndrome. Cultures of specimens obtained through a bronchoscopic sheath catheter had yielded *Pseudomonas aeruginosa* and *Staphylococcus aureus.* Despite antibiotic treatment, the patient had spontaneous rupture of the abscess into the pericardial sac and died from a tension pneumopericardium and cardiac tamponade. The chest x-ray film in Panel A shows cavitating pneumonia in the left mid-lung field, adjacent to the cardiac silhouette. In Panel B, another chest film, air under pressure is evident in the pericardial sac, with the original abscess cavity now clear of fluid. In Panel C, a photograph taken at autopsy, showing the parietal pericardial surface, the fistula (arrowhead) connecting the pericardial sac (P) to the lung abscess can be seen.

Lawrence G. Smith, M.D.

Mount Sinai Medical Center
New York, NY 10029

Tasneem Naqvi, M.D.

State University of New York
at Stony Brook
Stony Brook, NY 11794

June 1, 1995

Löffler's Endocarditis

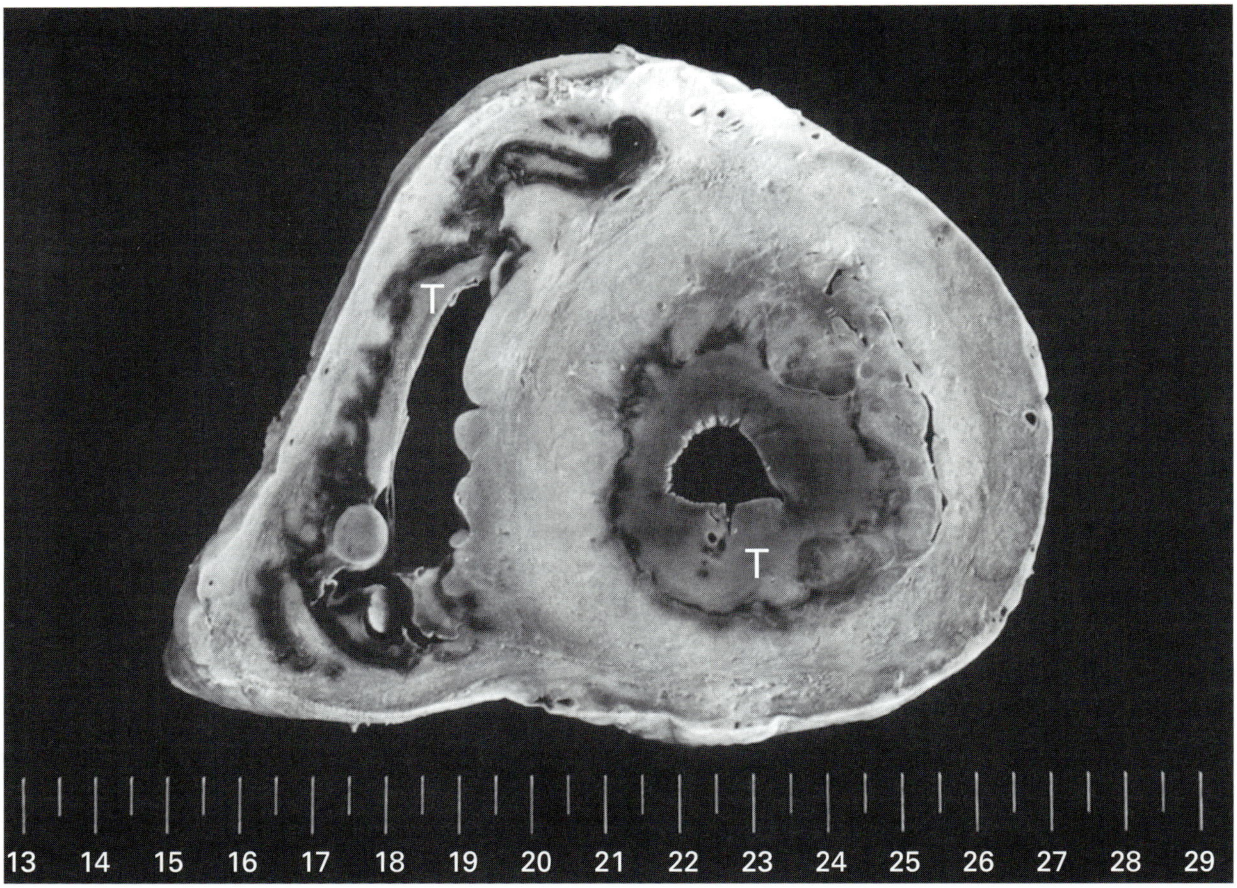

A transverse slice of the heart from a 65-year-old man with Löffler's endocarditis shows large mural thrombi (T) surrounding the thickened endocardium in both ventricles. Löffler's endocarditis is characterized by hypereosinophilia and endocardial thickening, which typically causes restrictive cardiomyopathy.

Tsutomu Imaizumi, M.D.
Keiji Aibara, M.D.

Kyushu University School of Medicine
Higashi-Ku, Fukuoka, Japan 812

July 7, 1994

Cardiac Amyloidosis

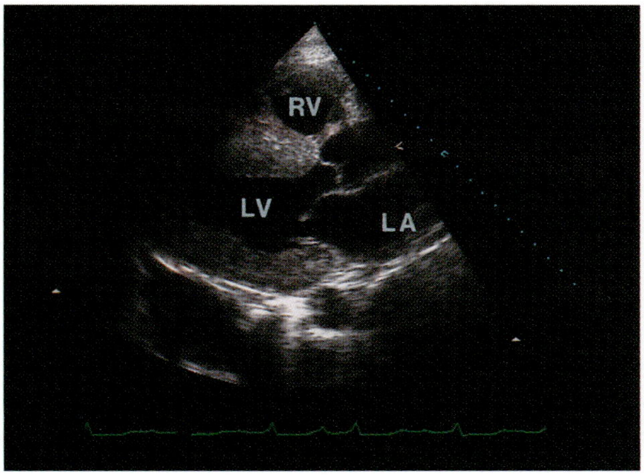

A

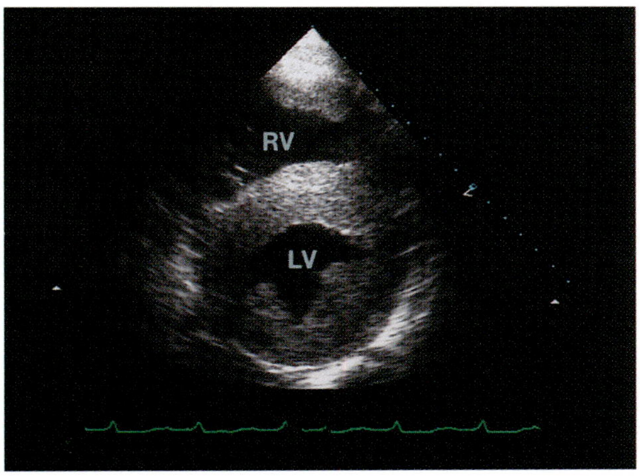

B

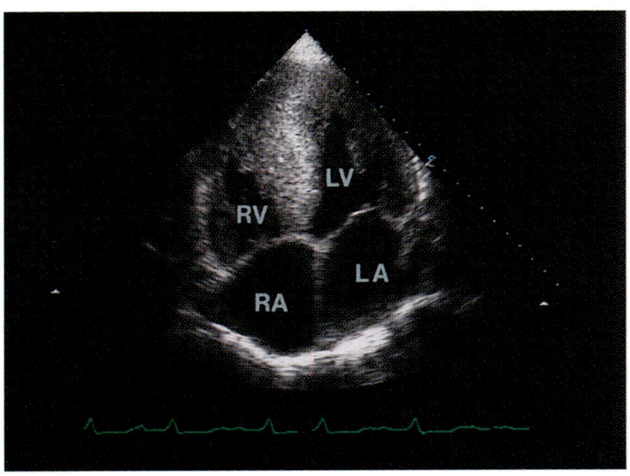

C

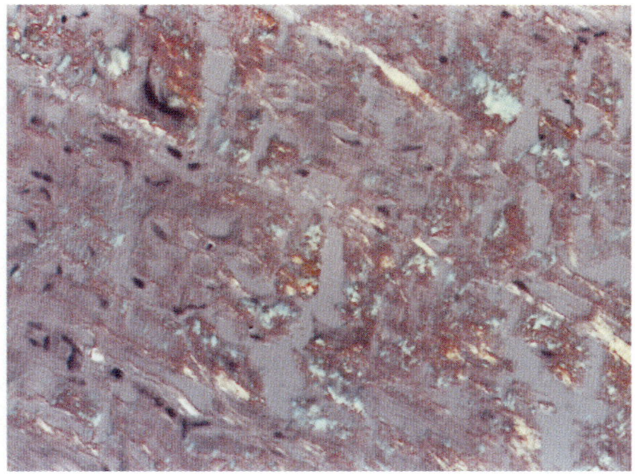

D

Both the two-dimensional echocardiogram (Panels A, B, and C) and the cardiac-biopsy specimen (Panel D) of a 68-year-old man with increasing symptoms of cardiac failure and a history of hypertensive heart disease demonstrate the presence of cardiac amyloidosis. In Panel A, a parasternal long-axis view shows marked concentric hypertrophy of the left ventricle (LV), with thickening of both the mitral and the aortic valves. In Panel B, a parasternal short-axis view of the left ventricle at the level of the papillary muscles shows concentric left ventricular hypertrophy as well as a prominent speckled pattern of the myocardium that is characteristic of infiltrative cardiomyopathy. In Panel C, an apical four-chamber view shows hypertrophy of the right ventricle (RV) as well as the left ventricle and thickening of both the mitral and the tricuspid valves and the interatrial septum. In the photomicrograph of a specimen obtained by percutaneous transvenous cardiac biopsy (Panel D), the specimen has been stained with Congo red and is viewed under polarized light; amyloid protein can be recognized by its apple-green birefringence (×3). LA denotes left atrium, and RA right atrium.

Pamela S. Douglas, M.D.
Sarah E. Katz

Beth Israel Hospital
Boston, MA 02215

November 26, 1992

Right Atrial Tumor

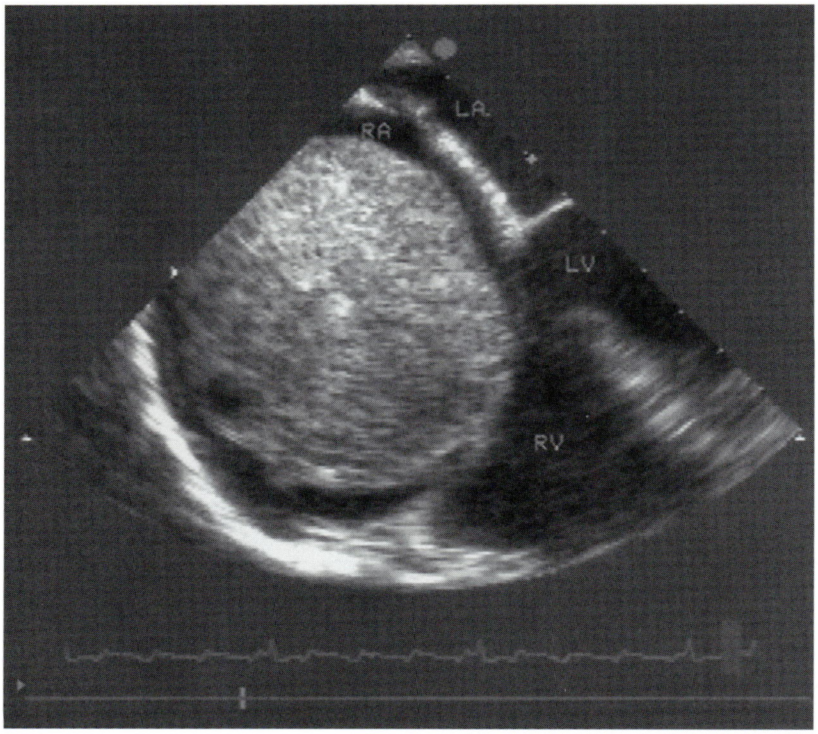

A

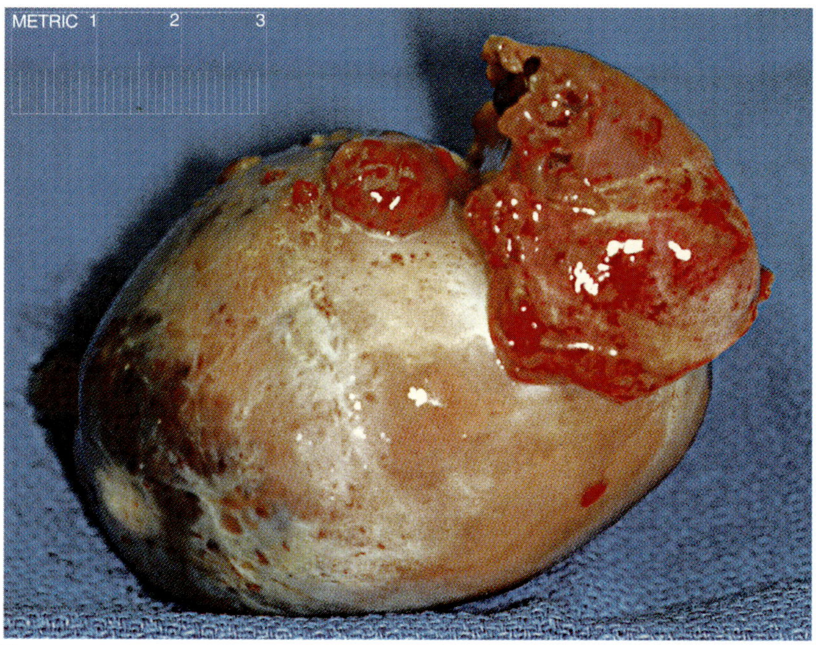

B

A right atrial mass was observed in a 42-year-old woman who presented with atrial fibrillation. A four-chamber view of the heart (Panel A) obtained intraoperatively by transesophageal echocardiography, demonstrated a mass in the right atrium (RA) obstructing the right ventricular inflow (RV). An encapsulated cystic rhabdomyoma (9 cm by 6 cm by 3 cm) and attached atrial stalk (Panel B) were excised during hypothermic circulatory arrest. A transesophageal echocardiogram obtained immediately thereafter showed a persistently enlarged right atrium. Two years after the excision of this rare tumor, the right atrial and ventricular dilatation had not resolved, tricuspid regurgitation persisted, and atrial fibrillation was still present. LA denotes left atrium, and LV left ventricle.

Joseph S. Savino, M.D.
Stuart J. Weiss, M.D., Ph.D.

University of Pennsylvania Medical School
Philadelphia, PA 19104

December 14, 1995

CT Scan Demonstrating Air in the Right Ventricle

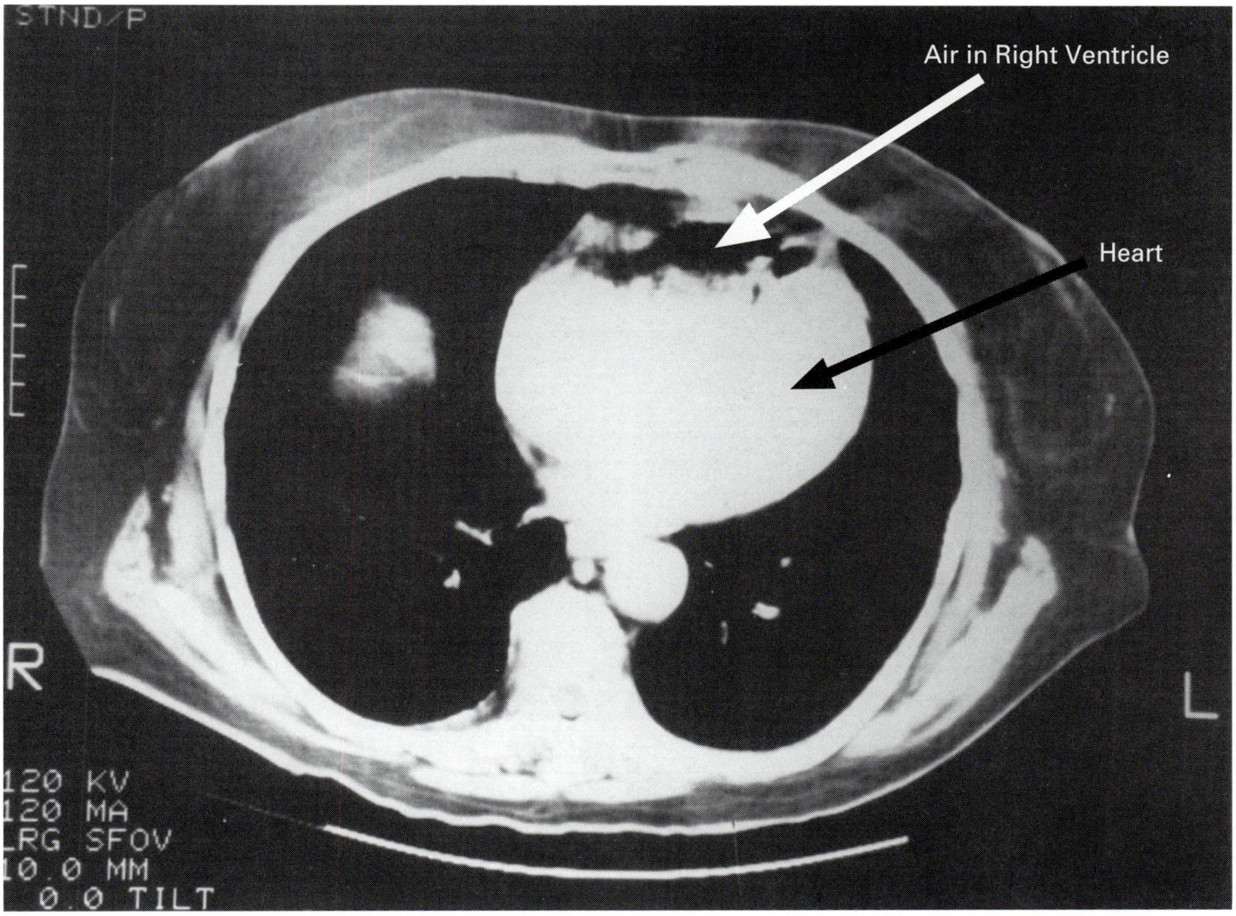

To increase the rate of infusion of an intravenous contrast agent, air was forced into a patient's intravenous bottle. Shortly afterward, the patient became dyspneic, diaphoretic, and hypotensive, and computed tomography demonstrated air in the right ventricle. The air was removed by aspiration through a Swan–Ganz catheter placed in the ventricle, and the patient's condition immediately improved. In the vast majority of instances, the amount of air is small and is not associated with symptoms.

Ralph G. Oriscello, M.D.
Michael E. Robertello, M.D.

Elizabeth General Medical Center
Elizabeth, NJ 07201

March 25, 1993

Digitalis purpurea *(Foxglove)*

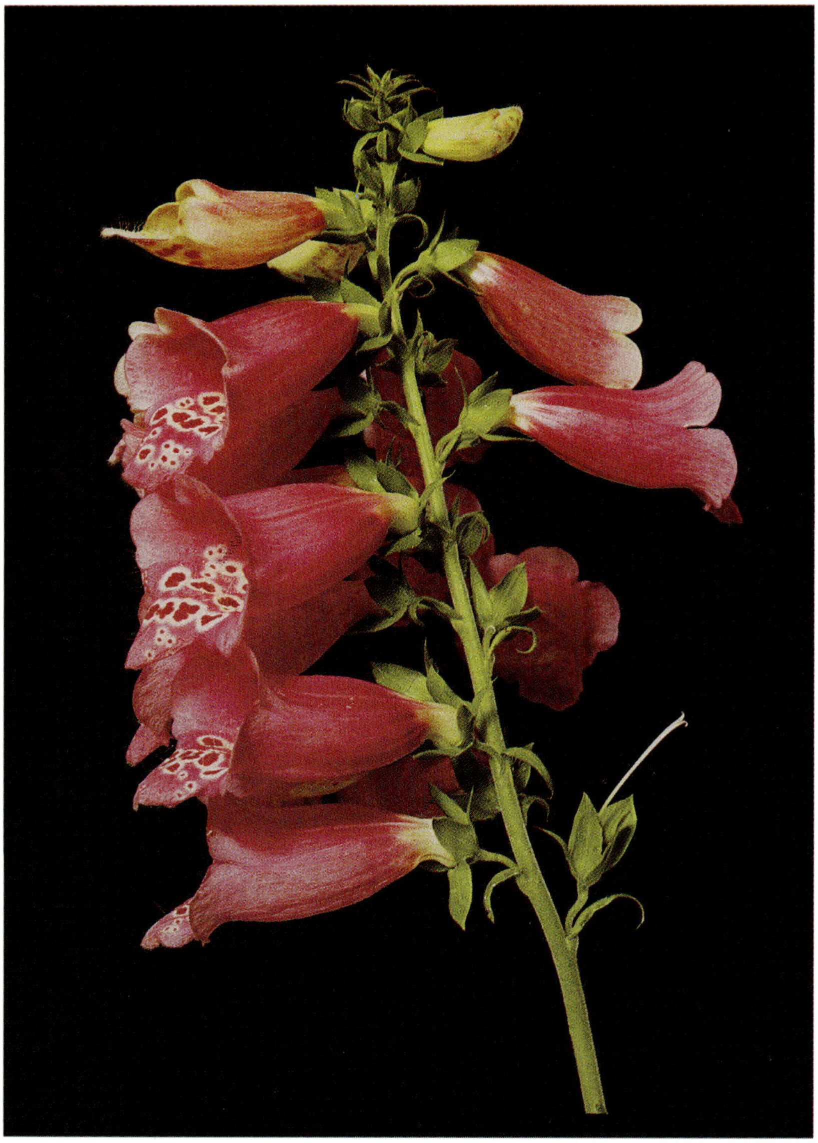

In 1775 William Withering demonstrated that the leaves of the foxglove plant alleviated certain forms of dropsy (edema), and in 1799 John Ferriar ascribed their beneficial effects to a primary action on the heart. All physicians have learned about digitalis, but few recognize its plant source. Digoxin, the preparation most commonly used in the United States, is derived from related plants, *Digitalis lanata* and *D. orientalis.*

J. Lawrence Naiman, M.D.

Stanford University
School of Medicine
Stanford, CA 94303

December 8, 1994

Correspondence

Foxglove

May 18, 1995

To the Editor: Naiman's magnificent photograph of *Digitalis purpurea* (Dec. 8 issue)[1] illustrates the derivation of its common name: because of its color and resemblance to fingers, it was called foxglove by the botanist Leonhard Fuchs in 1542. William Withering first used the foxglove in 1775, but his classic account was published 10 years later.[2]

Frank J. Lepreau, M.D.
74 River Rd.
Westport, MA 02790

1. Naiman JL. *Digitalis purpurea* (Foxglove). N Engl J Med 1994;331:1563.
2. Withering W. An account of the foxglove and some of its medical uses: with practical remarks on dropsy, and other diseases. London: G.G.J. and J. Robinson, 1785.

Thromboangiitis Obliterans

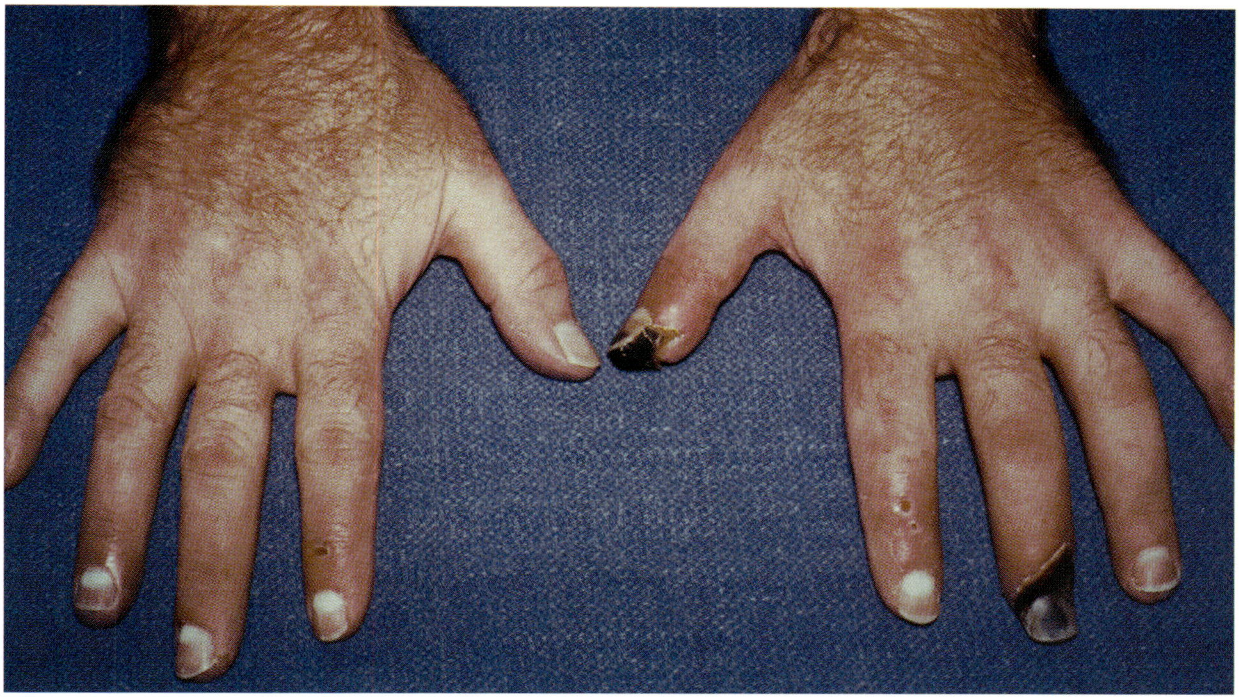

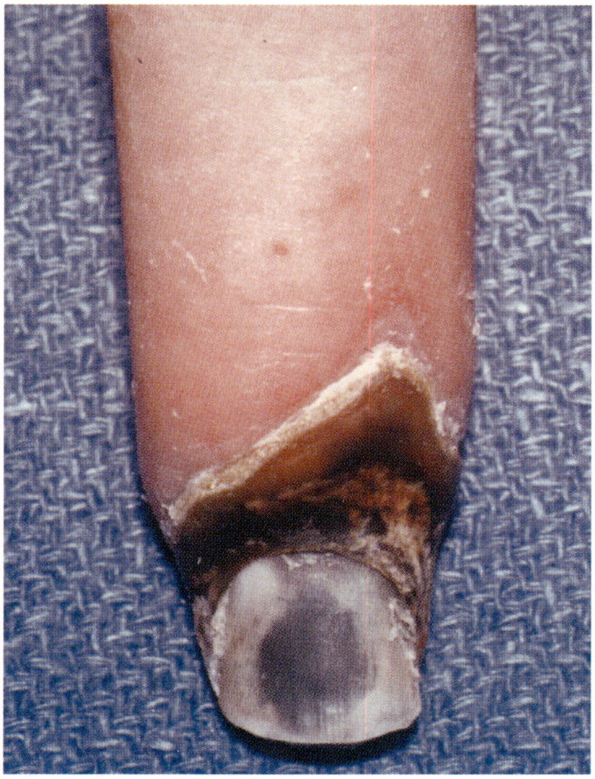

A 35-year-old man who had smoked two packs of cigarettes per day for 20 years presented with necrosis of the ends of the middle finger and the thumb of the left hand. These lesions had been preceded for three to four years by burning sensations and bluish discoloration of the fingers and toes on exposure to cold. Brachial pulses were only slightly diminished, but radial pulses were markedly diminished. The results of all laboratory studies were normal. The patient stopped smoking, and two months later, the fingers were better perfused, though he had lost the distal portions of the thumb and middle finger by autoamputation.

Greg Rosencrance, M.D.
Timothy Thistlewaite, M.D.

Robert C. Byrd Health Sciences Center of West Virginia University
Charleston, WV 25304

April 4, 1996

Hematology and Oncology

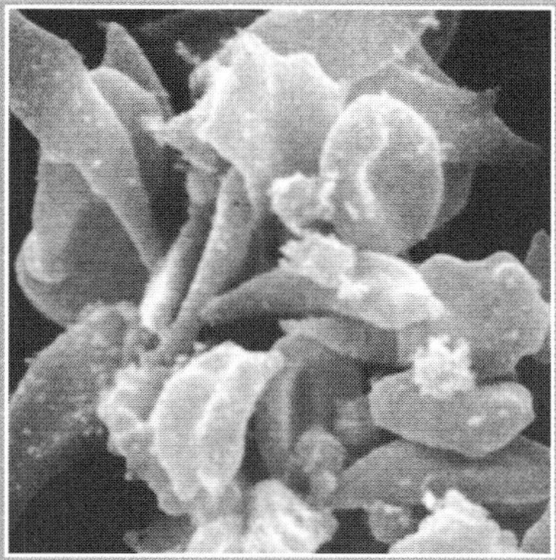

Spontaneous Human Erythrocyte Rosette

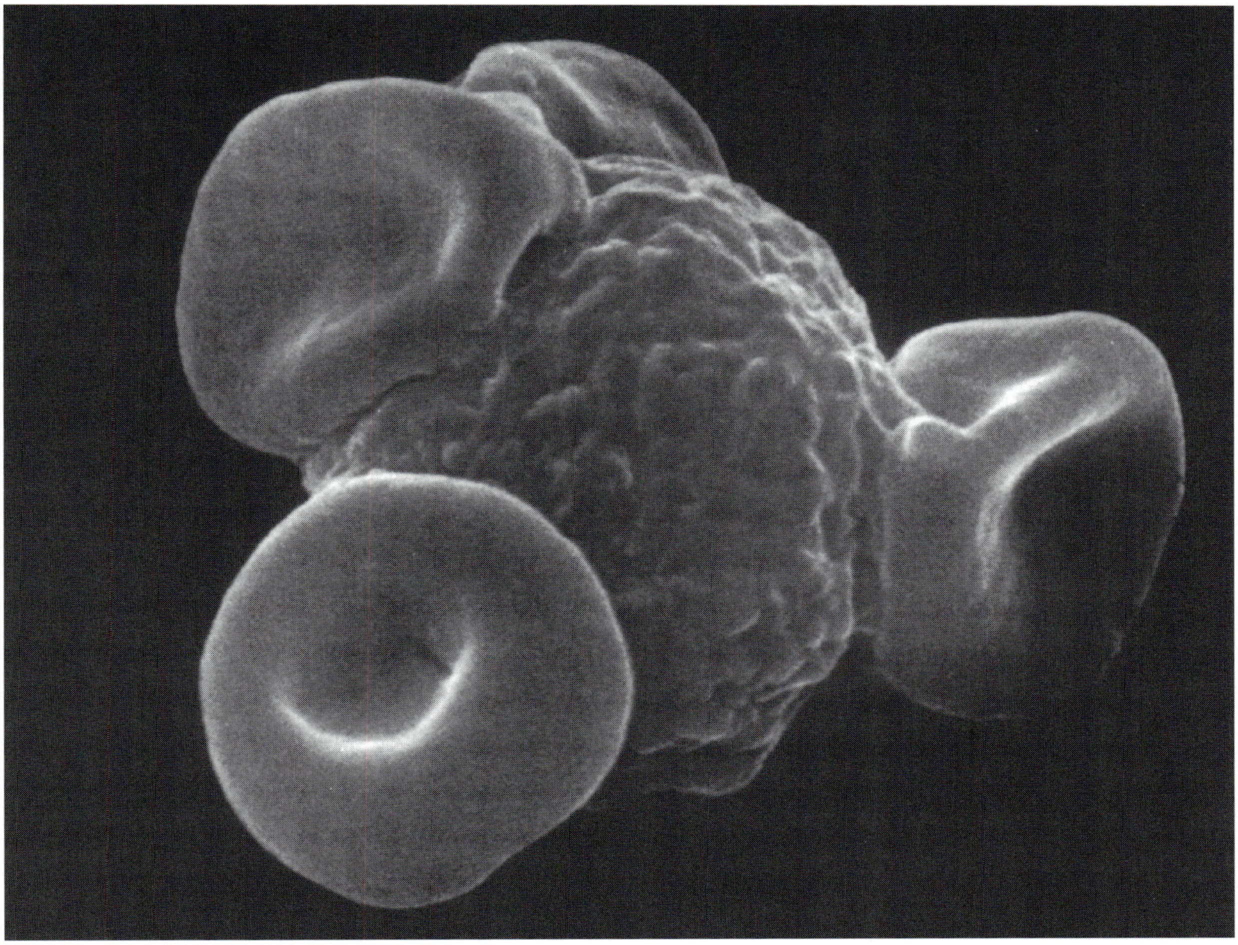

This scanning electron micrograph of a peripheral-blood lymphocyte from a patient with chronic T-cell lymphocytic leukemia shows red cells attached to the surface of the lymphocyte, forming a spontaneous rosette (×9800). Formation of such rosettes does not occur with normal T cells, but appears to be a property of an abnormal T-cell subpopulation.

Giorgio Lambertenghi-Deliliers, M.D.

University of Milan
20122 Milan, Italy

February 3, 1994

Spur Cells

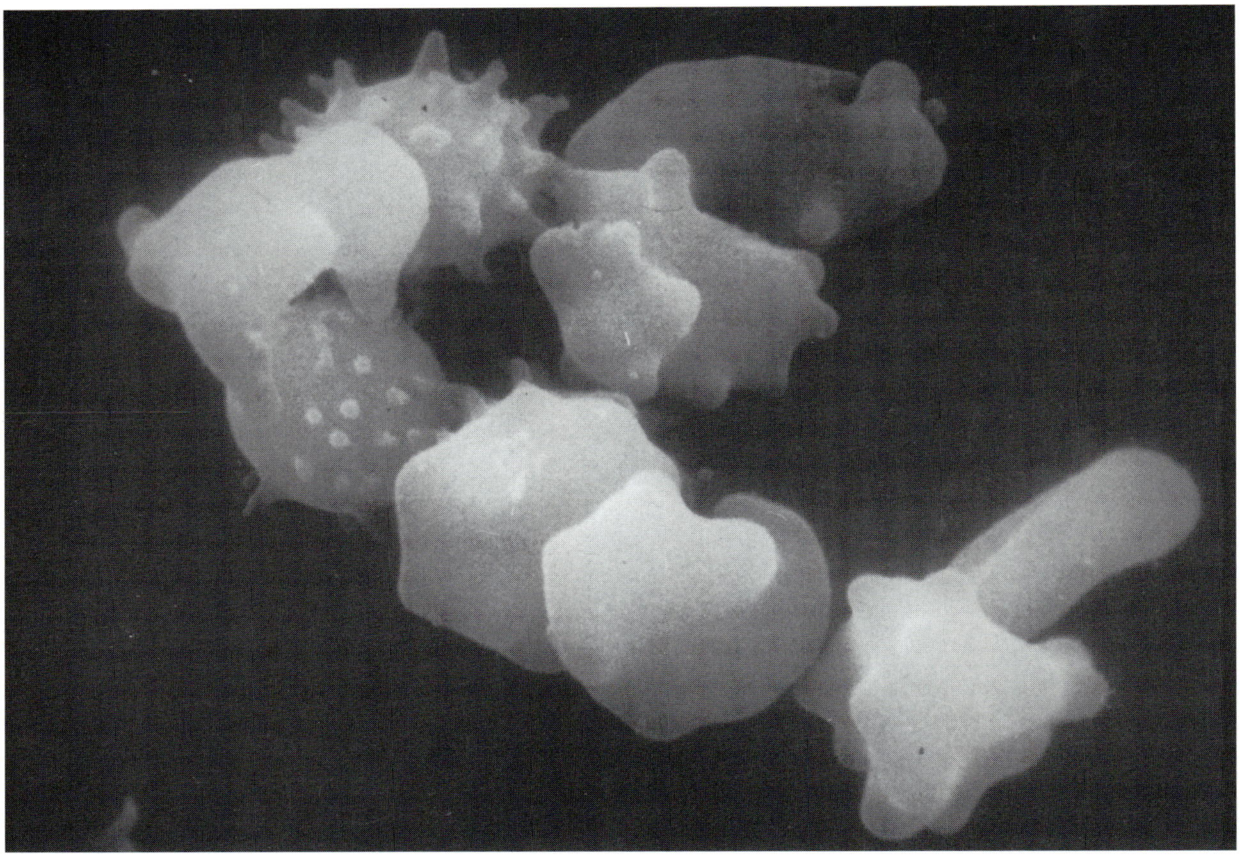

Scanning electron microscopy (×5000) reveals numerous acanthocytes diagnostic of spur-cell anemia in a peripheral-blood specimen from a jaundiced 43-year-old woman with alcoholic cirrhosis and anemia. Several putative factors, including an altered ratio of cholesterol to phospholipid in the erythrocyte membrane, stagnation of sterols on the red-cell membrane, retention of bile acids, and changes in plasma lecithin–cholesterol acyltransferase concentrations, may be involved in the pathogenesis of spur cells.

Donald C. Doll, M.D.

Harry S Truman Veterans Affairs Medical Center
Columbia, MO 65201

November 2, 1995

Sickle Cell Anemia

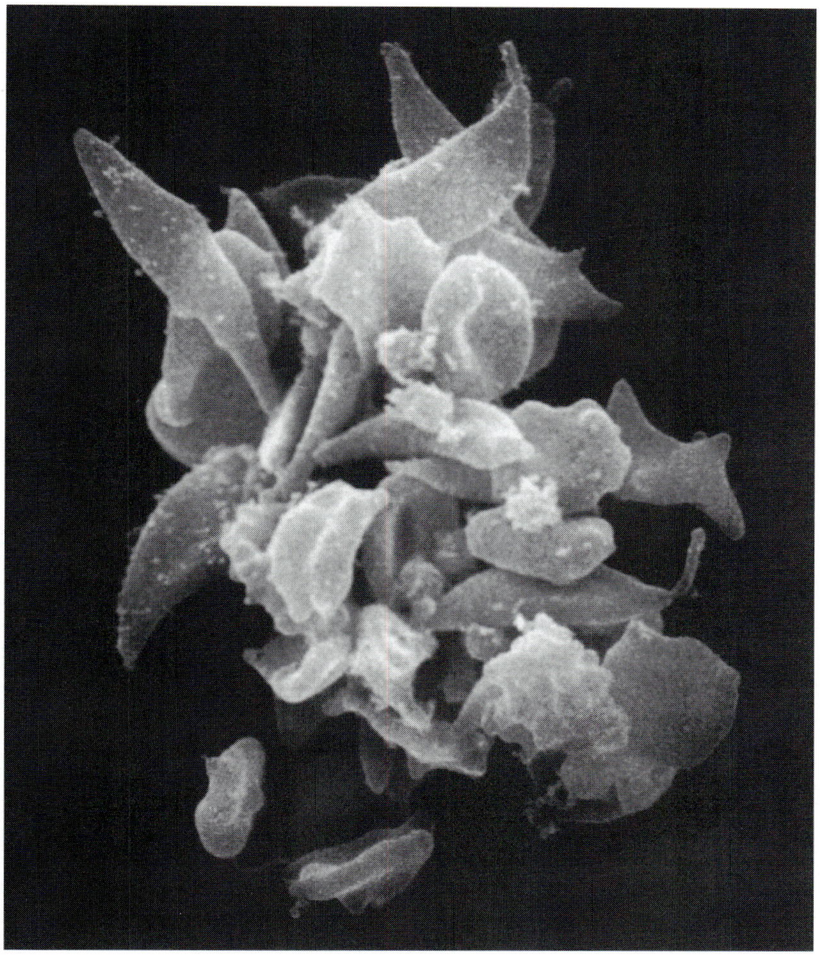

Scanning electron microscopy shows numerous sickled erythrocytes in a peripheral-blood specimen from a 21-year-old black woman with sickle cell anemia who was admitted to the hospital with acute chest and abdominal pain (×1380).

Donald C. Doll, M.D.

Harry S. Truman Memorial Veterans Hospital
Columbia, MO 65201

January 14, 1993

Vitamin B_{12} Deficiency

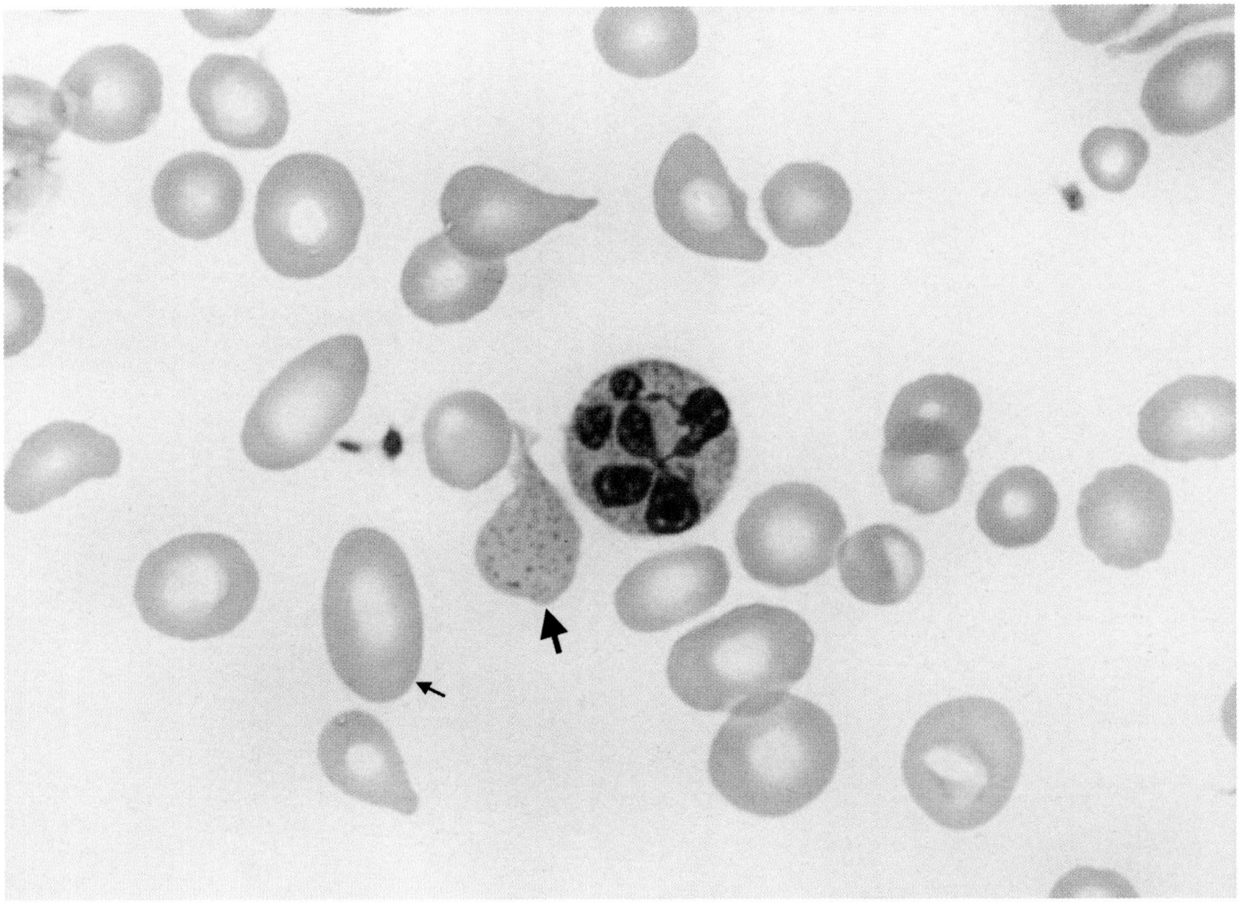

A 72-year-old man with a several-week history of fatigue, loss of appetite, and feeling feverish presented at the hospital with severe pallor and signs of left and right ventricular failure. Neurologic examination disclosed poor short-term memory and decreased sense of vibration in the legs.

An electrocardiogram showed changes consistent with the presence of cardiac ischemia. The hemoglobin level was 3.7 g per deciliter, with a mean corpuscular volume of 103 μm^3, a white-cell count of 3200 per cubic millimeter, and a platelet count of 57,000 per cubic millimeter. The peripheral-blood film showed the typical changes of vitamin B_{12} deficiency: hypersegmentation of neutrophils, marked anisocytosis, poikilocytosis with some large oval erythrocytes (megalocytes; thin arrow), and basophilic stippling (thick arrow). The serum vitamin B_{12} level was 8 pg per milliliter (6 pmol per liter; normal, >200 pg per milliliter [148 pmol per liter]), and a bone marrow biopsy showed marked megaloblastic changes consistent with the diagnosis of vitamin B_{12} deficiency. Although the mean corpuscular volume was very low for pure vitamin B_{12} deficiency of this severity and might have suggested an additional hematologic problem, most notably iron deficiency, no other abnormality was identified.

With parenteral vitamin B_{12} treatment, the patient's blood counts and mean corpuscular volume returned to normal and the megaloblastic bone marrow changes resolved.

Stephan Moll, M.D.

Duke University Medical Center
Durham, NC 27710

August 1, 1996

Correspondence

Megaloblastosis

December 26, 1996

To the Editor: The Image in Clinical Medicine of the peripheral-blood smear from a patient with vitamin B_{12} deficiency (Aug. 1 issue)[1] beautifully captures many of the features of megaloblastic anemia. The author mentions that the patient's mean corpuscular volume of 103 μm^3 was "very low for pure vitamin B_{12} deficiency of this severity and might have suggested an additional hematologic problem," but no additional abnormality was found. In fact, many patients with severe megaloblastic anemia have mean corpuscular volumes that are very elevated at first but later decline to the levels seen in this patient, while the red-cell–distribution width increases. Inspection of the peripheral-blood smear in such patients reveals the presence of schistocytes. The small size of the schistocytes lowers the mean corpuscular volume and raises the red-cell–distribution width. Schistocytes may be due to a further decline in the effectiveness of erythropoiesis in the bone marrow. The field shown in the image does not reveal schistocytes; however, they may be present in other fields.

Justine Meehan Carr, M.D.
Beth Israel Hospital
Boston, MA 02215

1. Moll S. Vitamin B_{12} deficiency. N Engl J Med 1996;335:323.

To the Editor: Moll describes a 72-year-old man with vitamin B_{12} deficiency and states that "a bone marrow biopsy showed marked megaloblastic changes consistent with the diagnosis of vitamin B_{12} deficiency." Your readers should not accept the idea that a bone marrow biopsy is the procedure of choice to confirm megaloblastosis. When Moll wrote that sentence, he was probably thinking of bone marrow aspiration. Evaluation of the cytoplasmic and nuclear morphology of hematopoietic precursors in aspirate smears allows precise assessment of megaloblastic changes. Bone marrow biopsy, which mainly provides histologic information, is not useful for this purpose.

José M. Raya, M.D.
Hospital Universitario de Canarias
38320 La Laguna, Spain

To the Editor: In the August 1 issue, which also included a review of the evaluation of dementia,[1] Dr. Moll tantalized us in the legend to the Image in Clinical Medicine by not divulging whether the patient's neuropsychiatric response matched his excellent hematologic response to replacement therapy.

Mark N. Lowenthal, M.B.
Soroka Medical Center and Ben Gurion University of the Negev
Beer Sheva 84101, Israel

1. Geldmacher DS, Whitehouse PJ. Evaluation of dementia. N Engl J Med 1996;335:330-6.

Correspondence Continued

Dr. Moll replies:

To the Editor: I am thankful to Dr. Carr for her comment on the contribution of schistocytes to the relatively low mean corpuscular volumes in some patients with severe vitamin B_{12} deficiency. In keeping with her observation, small, fragmented red cells were present on the blood film of our patient in areas not shown on the image. Her observation that the mean corpuscular volume in many patients is high early in the course of vitamin B_{12} deficiency and lower later in the course is interesting. An elevated mean corpuscular volume can decrease with worsening vitamin B_{12} deficiency if additional iron deficiency develops. If a patient with vitamin B_{12} deficiency is treated with folic acid only, the hematologic values often improve (the hemoglobin level increases and the mean corpuscular volume decreases), in spite of worsening vitamin B_{12} deficiency.[1] Progression from a high to a low mean corpuscular volume is otherwise not documented in the literature. Although Prentice and Evans[2] did note a steady increase in the mean corpuscular volume with worsening anemia, down to a red-cell count of 1.5×10^{12} per liter, and below this value a fall in the mean corpuscular volume, this decline was not statistically significant. Stabler et al.,[3] on the other hand, found a poor correlation between the degree of anemia and the mean corpuscular volume.

Raya correctly points out that bone marrow morphology is best evaluated by examination of bone marrow aspirates. To diagnose vitamin B_{12} deficiency, a bone marrow biopsy is not necessary. In fact, even bone marrow aspiration is, in many cases, unnecessary. The clinical presentation of a patient and the physical and laboratory findings may, however, require bone marrow examination to rule out leukemia or a myeloinfiltrative process.

The patient's short-term memory returned to normal after vitamin B_{12}–replacement therapy. A sensory examination to follow up on the loss of vibration sense was not reported by the patient's primary physician.

Stephan Moll, M.D.
Durham, NC 27705

1. Hall BE, Watkins CH. Experience with pteroylglutamic (synthetic folic) acid in the treatment of pernicious anemia. J Clin Lab Med 1947;32:622-34.
2. Prentice AG, Evans IL. Megaloblastic anaemia with normal mean cell volume. Lancet 1979; 1:606-7.
3. Stabler SP, Allen RH, Savage DG, Lindenbaum J. Clinical spectrum and diagnosis of cobalamin deficiency. Blood 1990;76:871-81.

Pseudothrombocytopenia

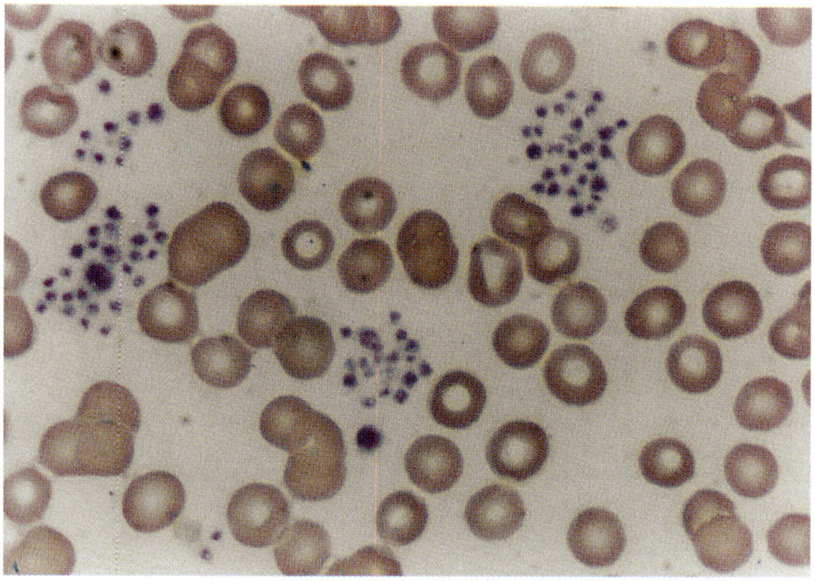

A

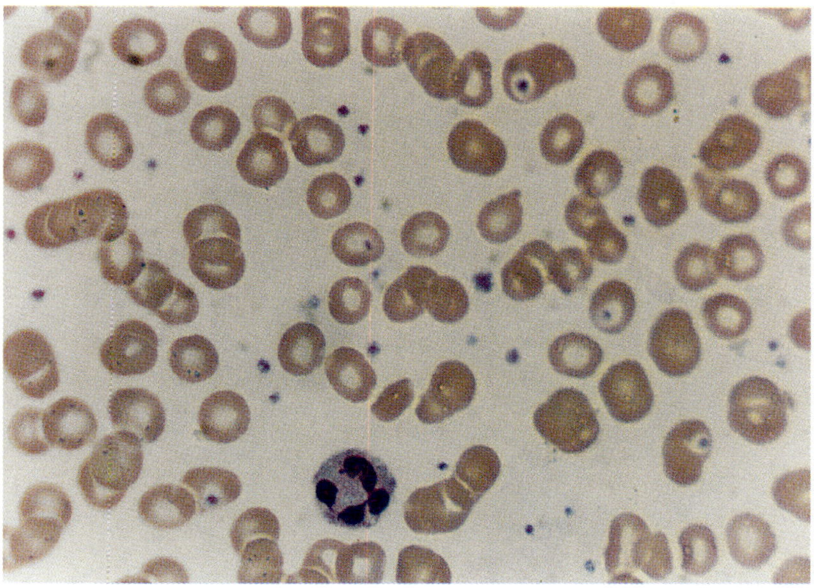

B

An electronic counting machine estimated the platelet count in a routine blood sample, anticoagulated with EDTA, at 44,000 per cubic millimeter. A peripheral-blood smear (Wright's stain, ×800) from the same blood sample (Panel A) shows three typical platelet clumps, each containing 20 to 30 platelets, which were misidentified by the machine as white cells. When a second blood sample from the same patient was anticoagulated with heparin, which prevented in vitro clumping and maldistribution of the platelets (Panel B; Wright's stain, ×800), the machine read the patient's true platelet count of 560,000 per cubic millimeter. This example is a salient reminder of the value of looking at blood smears.

Oded Shalev, M.D.
Anton Lotman, M.D.

Hadassah University Hospital
Mt. Scopus, Jerusalem, Israel

November 11, 1993

Some Features of Fanconi's Anemia

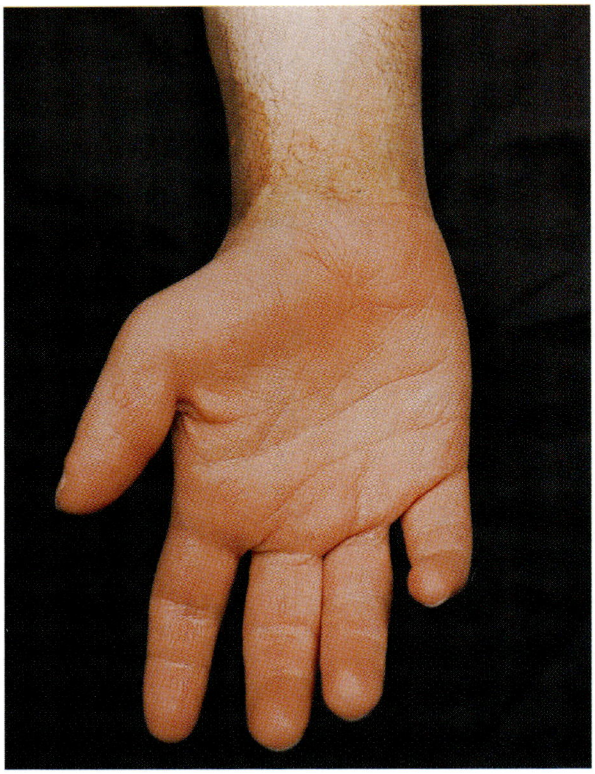

A

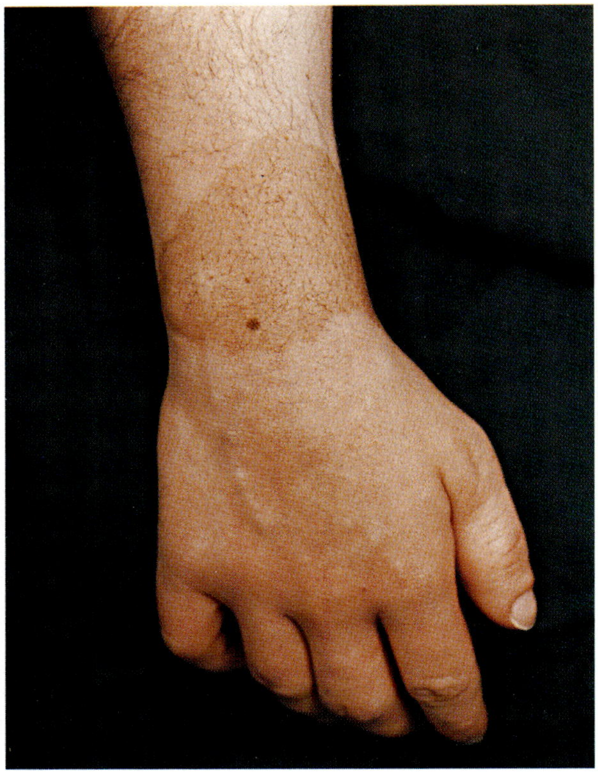

B

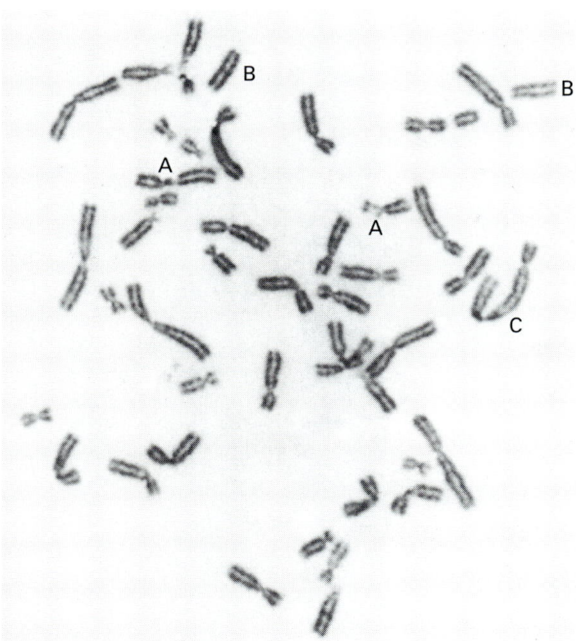

C

The physical and cytogenetic findings in some patients with Fanconi's anemia are shown. Panel A shows the characteristically short thumb; Panel B shows a café au lait spot; and Panel C shows chromosomal breaks as revealed by cytogenetic analysis (A indicates chromatid breaks, B chromatid fragments, and C a dicentric chromosome). Other common clinical manifestations include short stature, skin hyperpigmentation, pancytopenia, and renal anomalies.

Daniel A. Hagerman, M.D.
Gary P. Williams, M.D.

University of Wisconsin Medical School
Madison, WI 53792

October 14, 1993

Correspondence

Fanconi's Anemia

March 10, 1994

To the Editor: We have several comments on the Image in Clinical Medicine entitled "Some Features of Fanconi's Anemia" (Oct. 14 issue).[1] It is gratifying that efforts are being made to increase physicians' awareness of the clinical features of this disease; however, it is also important for readers to realize that there is extreme clinical heterogeneity among patients with Fanconi's anemia.

Recently, we analyzed clinical data from 370 patients with Fanconi's anemia who were enrolled in the International Fanconi Anemia Registry.[2] Of these, 220 (60 percent) represented probands with congenital malformations. In addition to the short stature, café au lait spots, and radial-ray and renal malformations described by Hagerman and Williams,[1] affected patients presented with cardiac, gastrointestinal, central nervous system, and various skeletal abnormalities. In addition, genital anomalies were common in male patients. Approximately 50 percent of the patients had radial-ray abnormalities. These ranged from bilateral absent thumbs and radii to a unilateral hypoplastic thumb or bifid thumb. Among the patients with congenital malformations, only 28 percent were given a diagnosis before the onset of hematologic manifestations.

In addition, we examined the clinical features of patients with Fanconi's anemia who did not have congenital malformations (a group constituting approximately one third of all patients enrolled in the International Fanconi Anemia Registry). Eighty-five percent of these patients had at least one of the following findings: skin-pigmentation abnormalities, microphthalmos, or height, weight, or head circumference in the lowest 5 percent for their age. Minor congenital anomalies were noted in approximately 20 percent of these patients.

We postulate that a lack of awareness of the full spectrum of abnormalities associated with Fanconi's anemia is responsible for the delayed diagnosis of this disorder among patients with congenital malformations. We believe that clinicians should realize that the clinical features of Fanconi's anemia are heterogeneous and the majority of patients do not have the "characteristic" features originally described by Fanconi.[3]

Philip F. Giampietro, M.D., Ph.D.
Jessica G. Davis, M.D.
Cornell University Medical College

Arleen D. Auerbach, Ph.D.
Rockefeller University
New York, NY 10021

1. Hagerman DA, Williams GP. Some features of Fanconi's anemia. N Engl J Med 1993; 329:1168.
2. Giampietro PF, Adler-Brecher B, Verlander PC, Pavlakis SG, Davis JG, Auerbach AD. The need for more accurate and timely diagnosis in Fanconi anemia: a report from the International Fanconi Anemia Registry. Pediatrics 1993;91:1116-20.
3. Fanconi G. Familial constitutional panmyelocytopathy, Fanconi's anemia (F.A.). I. Clinical aspects. Semin Hematol 1967;4:233-40.

Endoscopic Palliation of Malignant Dysphagia

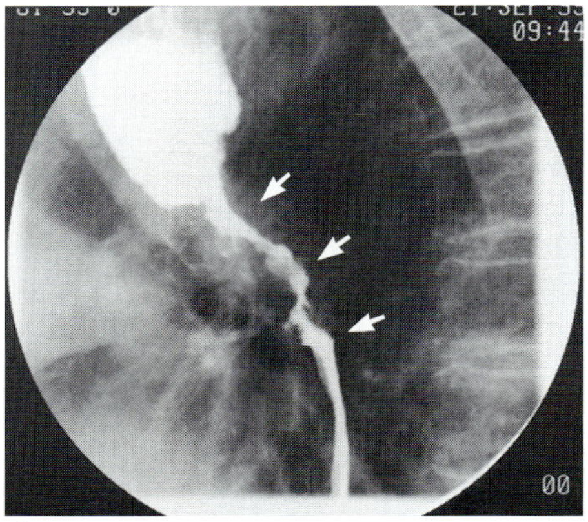

A

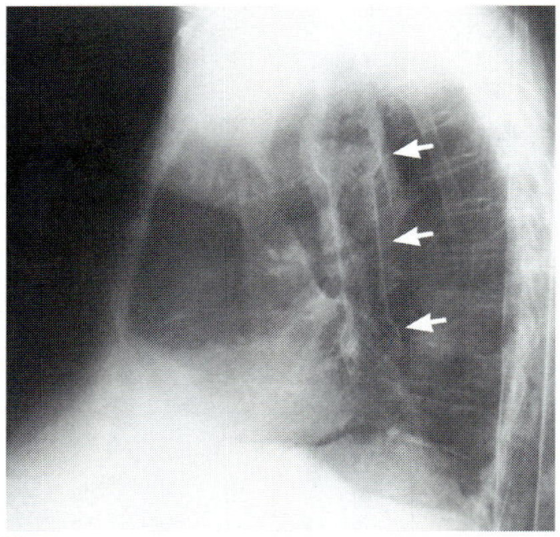

D

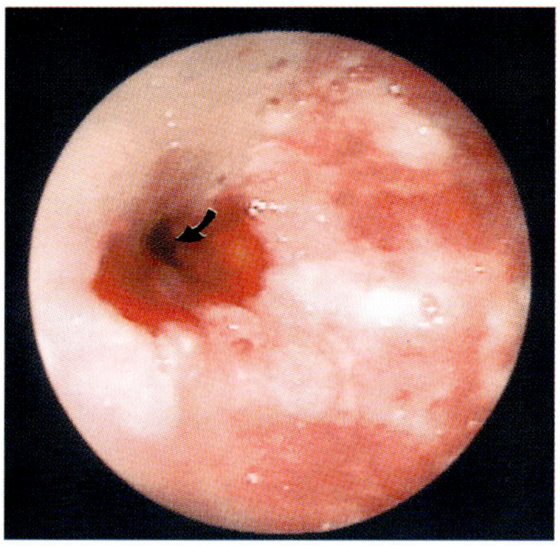

B

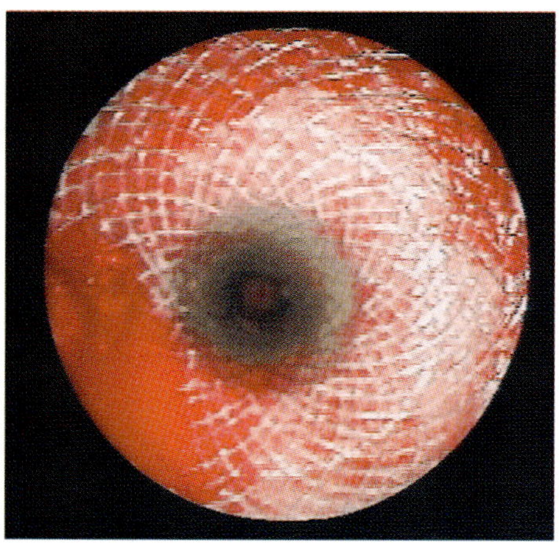

C

A 90-year-old woman presented with a three-month history of progressive dysphagia, postprandial vomiting, and weight loss. Barium contrast studies of the upper gastrointestinal tract showed an irregular narrowing in the midesophagus (Panel A, arrows). On the day upper gastrointestinal endoscopy was performed, the patient was unable to swallow her own saliva. Endoscopy showed a friable mass that almost totally obstructed the lumen of the midesophagus (Panel B, arrow). Biopsies disclosed invasive squamous-cell carcinoma. An expandable metallic esophageal endoprosthesis was endoscopically deployed (Panel C). A subsequent lateral chest x-ray film demonstrated a fully expanded endoprosthesis measuring 60 mm by 20 mm (Panel D, arrows). At follow-up nine months later, the patient was able to swallow liquids and pureed foods and was carrying on her usual daily activities.

Richard C.K. Wong, M.B., B.S.
Jacques Van Dam, M.D., Ph.D.

Brigham and Women's Hospital
Boston, MA 02115

August 15, 1996

Correspondence

Endoscopic Palliation of Malignant Dysphagia

January 23, 1997

To the Editor: In the Images in Clinical Medicine series (Aug. 15 issue),[1] Wong and Van Dam described a case in which an expandable metallic esophageal prosthesis spared their patient considerable discomfort and expense. Expandable metal stents, especially the latest "coated" ones that retard the ingrowth of tumors, are an important advance in the treatment of inoperable esophageal cancer. However, the placement of these stents is not without risk. My colleagues and I have encountered a high complication rate in our initial experience in 11 patients with the five types of expandable metallic stents currently available. Two patients had intractable substernal pain, and one had food impaction with aspiration. In one, the stent migrated, with subsequent uncontrollable gastric hemorrhage. In another, the stent eroded into the aorta, and the patient bled to death within 24 hours after placement of the stent. Six patients had no complications.

We believe that these stents should not be placed routinely after initial bougienage in patients with esophageal cancer but should be reserved for patients who have evidence of an esophageal perforation or tracheoesophageal fistula or those who require frequent bougienage and laser ablation.

Richard S. McCray, M.D.
St. Luke's–Roosevelt Hospital Center
New York, NY 10025

1. Wong RCK, Van Dam J. Endoscopic palliation of malignant dysphagia. N Engl J Med 1996;335:475.

The authors reply:

To the Editor: We thank Dr. McCray for his comments and agree that the use of expandable metallic endoprostheses (stents) for palliation of dysphagia in patients with malignant esophageal obstruction is not without risk. Dr. McCray's overall complication rate of 45 percent and procedure-related mortality rate of 18 percent are high and appear out of proportion to those reported in the original prospective, randomized trial by Knyrim et al.[1] In that study, palliation of malignant dysphagia using conventional plastic stents was compared with that achieved by the use of expandable metallic esophageal stents, and complications were significantly less frequent with the metallic stents than with the plastic stents (0 vs. 43 percent). However, more recent studies using metallic stents have revealed widely divergent complication and mortality rates. For example, Kozarek et al.[2] and Vermeijden et al.[3] reported stent-related mortality rates of 3 percent and 25 percent, respectively.

Kinsman et al.[4] identified the use of radiation, chemotherapy, or both before stent placement as a potential cause of increased morbidity and mortality. In their evaluation of 59 patients, Kinsman et al.[4] reported a stent-related mortality rate of 23 percent (5 of 22 patients) among those who had previously received radiotherapy, chemotherapy, or both, as compared with a rate of 0 percent (0 of 37) among those who had received no such prior therapy. Radiation and chemotherapy might induce tumor necrosis and vascular changes that could weaken the esophageal wall.[4,5]

Correspondence Continued

It is unclear whether the patients described by Dr. McCray had received radiation or chemotherapy before stent placement. If so, this could have resulted in higher-than-expected rates of complications and mortality. Also, the use of five different types of stents in 11 patients suggests a limited experience with any one stent design. We have limited the placement of these stents to patients who have not previously received radiation or chemotherapy. In addition, our post-stenting care entails advancing the patient's diet no further than to a soft solid diet (as tolerated), giving all patients acid-suppressive therapy, and instituting antireflux precautions. We believe that endoscopically deployed expandable metallic endoprostheses are an effective form of palliation for malignant dysphagia with an acceptable complication rate in experienced hands and when placed in selected patients.

Richard C.K. Wong, M.B., B.S
University Hospitals of Cleveland
Cleveland, OH 44106

Jacques Van Dam, M.D., Ph.D.
Brigham and Women's Hospital
Boston, MA 02115

1. Knyrim K, Wagner H-J, Bethge N, Keymling M, Vakil N. A controlled trial of an expansile metal stent for palliation of esophageal obstruction due to inoperable cancer. N Engl J Med 1993;329:1302-7.
2. Kozarek RA, Ball TJ, Brandabur JJ, et al. Expandable versus conventional esophageal prostheses: easier insertion may not preclude subsequent stent-related problems. Gastrointest Endosc 1996;43:204-8.
3. Vermeijden JR, Bartelsman JF, Fockens P, Meijer RC, Tytgat GN. Self-expanding metal stents for palliation of esophagocardial malignancies. Gastrointest Endosc 1995;41:58-63.
4. Kinsman KJ, DeGregorio BT, Katon RM, et al. Prior radiation and chemotherapy increase the risk of life-threatening complications after insertion of metallic stents for esophagogastric malignancy. Gastrointest Endosc 1996;43:196-203.
5. Bethge N, Sommer A, von Kleist D, Vakil N. A prospective trial of self-expanding metal stents in the palliation of malignant esophageal obstruction after failure of primary curative therapy. Gastrointest Endosc 1996;44:283-6.

Adenocarcinoma of the Esophagus

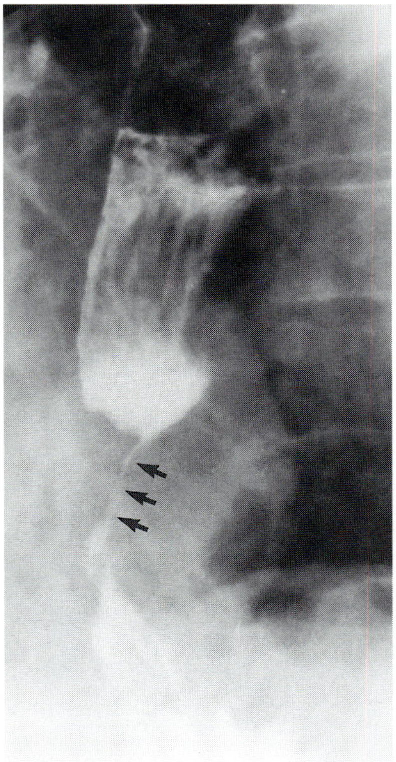

A

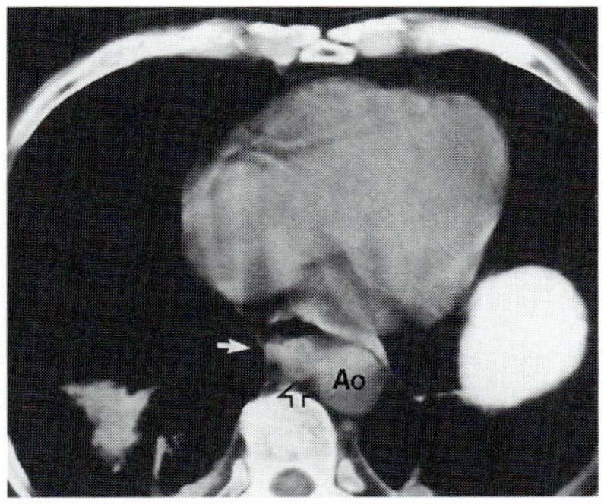

B

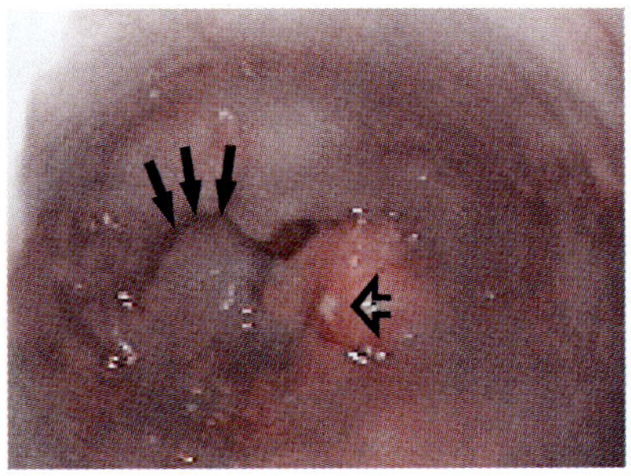

C

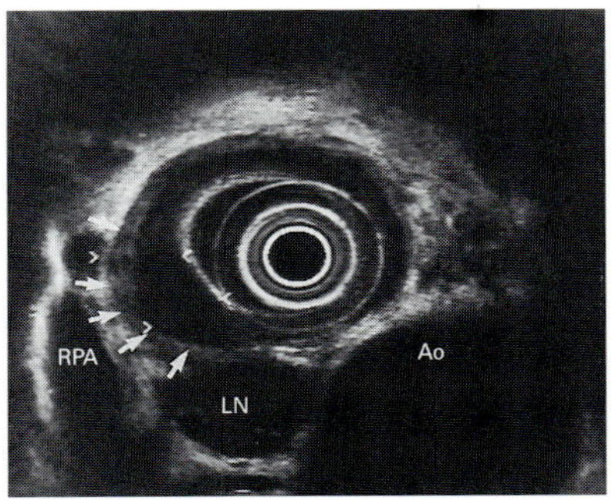

D

The esophagus of a 69-year-old man with progressive dysphagia was visualized by several methods. Barium esophagography (Panel A) demonstrated a long, irregular distal stricture (arrows) just proximal to the gastroesophageal junction. Computed tomographic scanning (Panel B) showed a thickened esophageal wall (large arrow) and an enlarged paraaortic node (small arrow); Ao denotes aorta. Endoscopy (Panel C) revealed narrowing of the distal esophagus (solid arrows); a biopsy of the nodule (open arrow) demonstrated adenocarcinoma. Endoscopic ultrasonography of the distal esophagus (Panel D), a new technique, showed several structures in cross-section, including the aorta, an irregular hypoechoic mass (arrows and V-shaped markers) that extended through the muscularis into the adventitia adjacent to the right pulmonary artery (RPA), and an enlarged adjacent lymph node (LN). The tumor was resected. Ordinarily, the diagnosis and management of esophageal cancer do not require all four of these procedures.

William R. Brugge, M.D.
Michael J. Lee, M.D.

Massachusetts General Hospital
Boston, MA 02114

September 1, 1994

Superior Vena Cava Syndrome

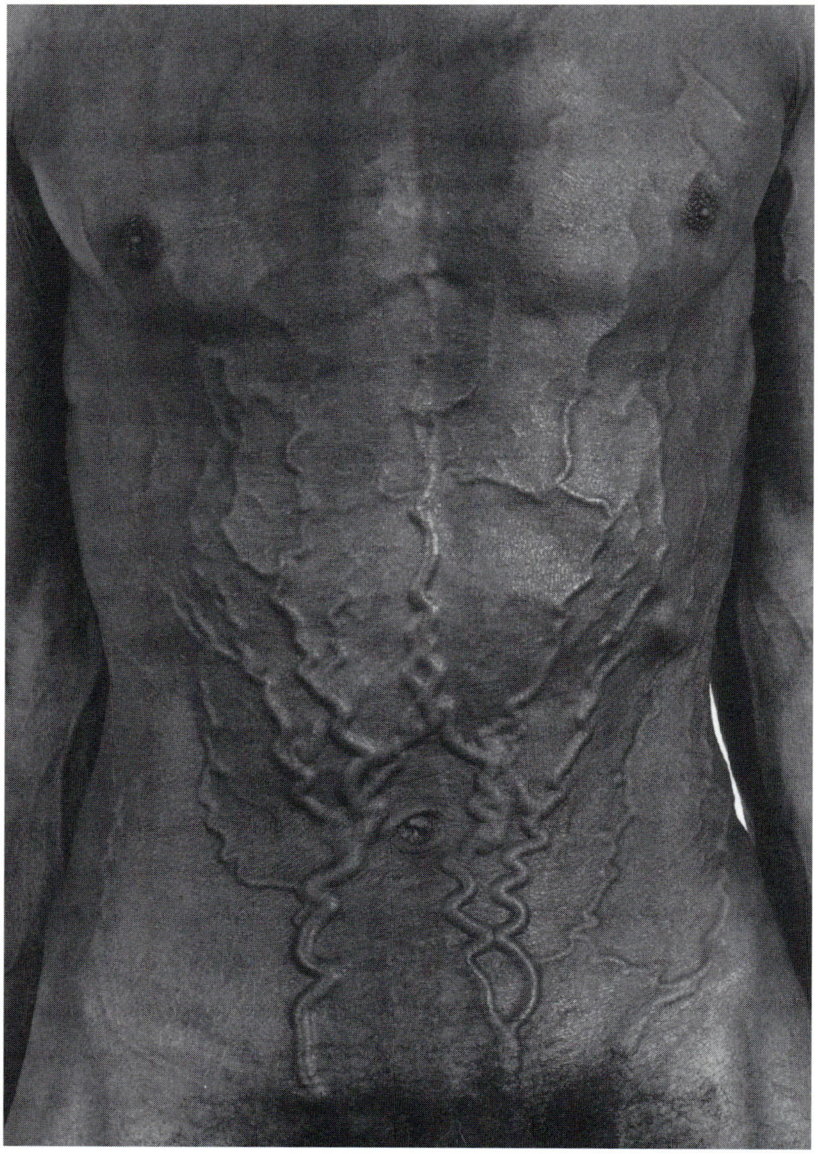

The photograph shows massive engorgement of collateral subcutaneous veins of the chest and abdomen in a 58-year-old man with partial obstruction of the superior vena cava caused by small-cell lung cancer. The patient also had distended neck veins but minimal facial edema. The venous dilatation improved transiently with radiation therapy. The patient died several weeks after the photograph was taken.

Ronald G. Kovacs, R.B.P.
Samuel M. Aguayo, M.D.

Atlanta Veterans Affairs Medical Center
Decatur, GA 30033

September 30, 1993

Correspondence

Vena Caval Obstruction by Tumor

February 24, 1994

To the Editor: In the September 30 issue the Image in Clinical Medicine[1] was alleged to be that of the superior vena cava syndrome. It showed the torso of a man with dilated superficial veins converging on the superficial inferior epigastric veins at the groin. The patient was also noted to have distended neck veins, but minimal facial edema. The veins of the patient's arms also appeared to be distended, and the ones of the upper part of the chest less so.

Although the patient probably had a partial obstruction of the superior vena cava, he must have had a serious obstruction of the inferior vena cava. If the superior vein was obstructed and the inferior one open, the veins of the most inferior portion of the abdominal wall should have been less distended rather than more so. Without belaboring the physics of the problem, the end of the vessel near the high-pressure source has a higher pressure, whereas the end near the lower-pressure sink has a lower pressure. The image and the accompanying legend indicate that the pressure in the inferior vena cava was greater than that in the superior.

Robert C. Luckey, M.D.
471 Williams, Suite 4
Richland, WA 99352

1. Kovacs RG, Aguayo SM. Superior vena cava syndrome. N Engl J Med 1993;329:1007.

To the Editor: The Image in Clinical Medicine in the September 30 issue shows massive engorgement of collateral subcutaneous veins of the chest and abdomen due to small-cell lung cancer. The patient was treated with radiotherapy, with transient improvement of venous dilatation, but he died some weeks later.

We suspect that radiotherapy was given in the belief that it is the treatment of choice in any patient with the superior vena cava syndrome due to a malignant tumor.[1,2] Yet there are data in the literature indicating that in certain instances a combination of chemotherapy and radiotherapy yields a higher response rate than radiotherapy alone.[3-5] On the basis of these data and our own experience, we suggest that chemotherapy should always be included in the treatment of superior vena cava syndrome due to malignant tumors, and in particular to small-cell lung cancer.

G.P. Stathopoulos, M.D.
E. Michailakis, M.D.
N.A. Malamos, M.D.
Hippokration Hospital
Athens 11528, Greece

1. Perez CA, Presant CA, Van Amburg AL III. Management of superior vena cava syndrome. Semin Oncol 1978;5:123-34.
2. Schraufnagel DE, Hill R, Leech JA, Pare JA. Superior vena caval obstruction: is it a medical emergency? Am J Med 1981;70:1169-74.

Correspondence Continued

3. Dombernowsky P, Hansen HH. Combination chemotherapy in the management of superior vena caval obstruction in small-cell anaplastic carcinoma of the lung. Acta Med Scand 1978;204:513-6.
4. Maddox AM, Valdivieso M, Lukeman J, et al. Superior vena cava obstruction in small cell bronchogenic carcinoma: clinical parameters and survival. Cancer 1983;52:2165-72.
5. Urban T, Lebeau B, Chastang C, Leclerc P, Botto MJ, Sauvaget J. Superior vena cava syndrome in small-cell lung cancer. Arch Intern Med 1993;153:384-7.

The authors reply:

To the Editor: Although we agree that the pressure in the inferior vena cava of this patient must have been increased, it is difficult to estimate whether the increase in pressure in the inferior vena cava was greater than that in the superior vena cava. Granted, when the superior vena cava is rapidly occluded, the predominant signs and symptoms are facial plethora and engorgement of the neck veins associated with dyspnea and headache. However, when the obstruction worsens gradually, an extensive collateral circulation may develop. The azygos venous system is still considered the most important alternative route of circulation, but there are other important collateral systems such as the internal thoracic veins, lateral thoracic veins, and the subcutaneous veins that were engorged in the patient. We also agree that most patients with the superior vena cava syndrome due to cancer should be considered for chemotherapy.

Samuel M. Aguayo, M.D.
Ronald G. Kovacs, R.B.P.
Atlanta Veterans Affairs Medical Center
Decatur, GA 30033

Nonpalpable Breast Carcinoma Detected by Screening Mammography

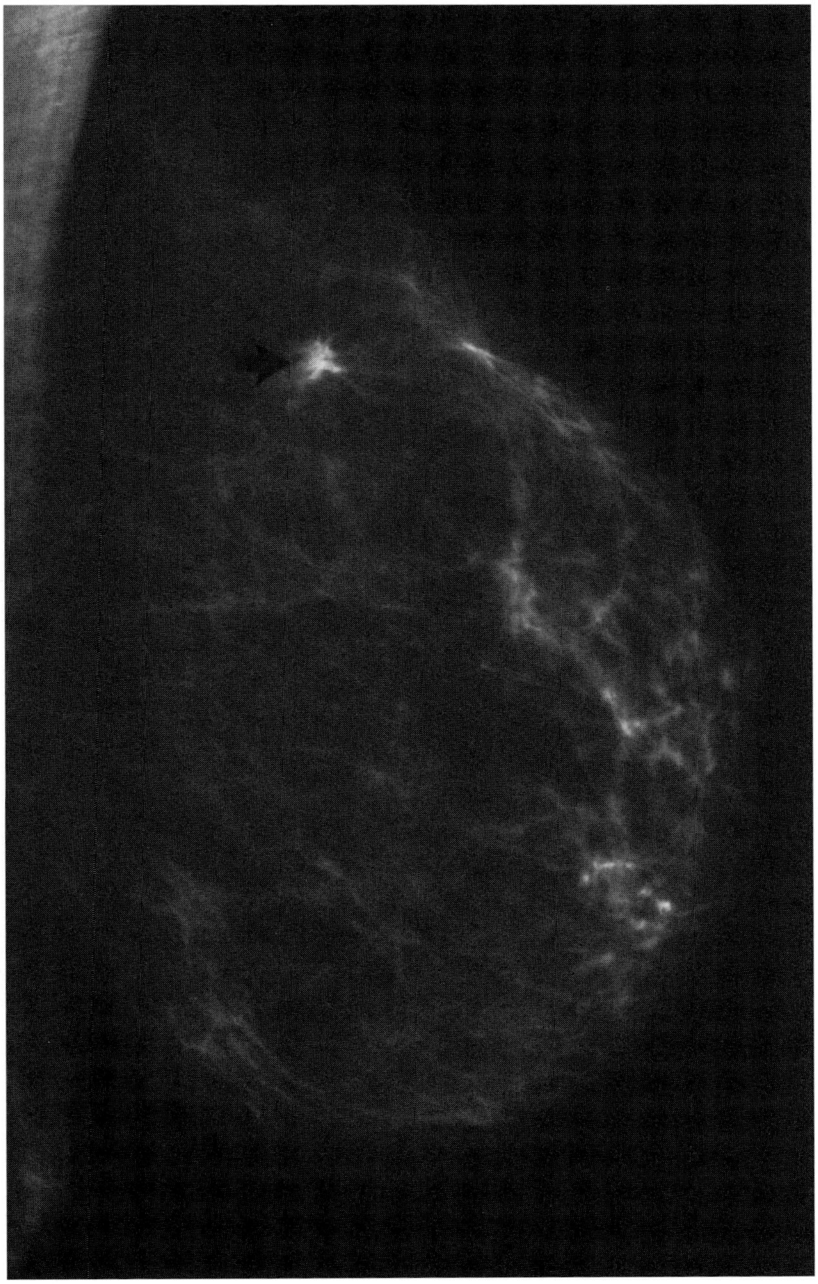

Breast cancer was identified on a routine screening mammogram (oblique view) in a 69-year-old woman. The mass, which measured 4 mm (arrow), was not palpable. Histologic examination revealed an infiltrating adenocarcinoma.

Marc J. Homer, M.D.

New England Medical Center
Hospital–Tufts University
Boston, MA 02111

June 3, 1993

A Metastasis Caught in the Act

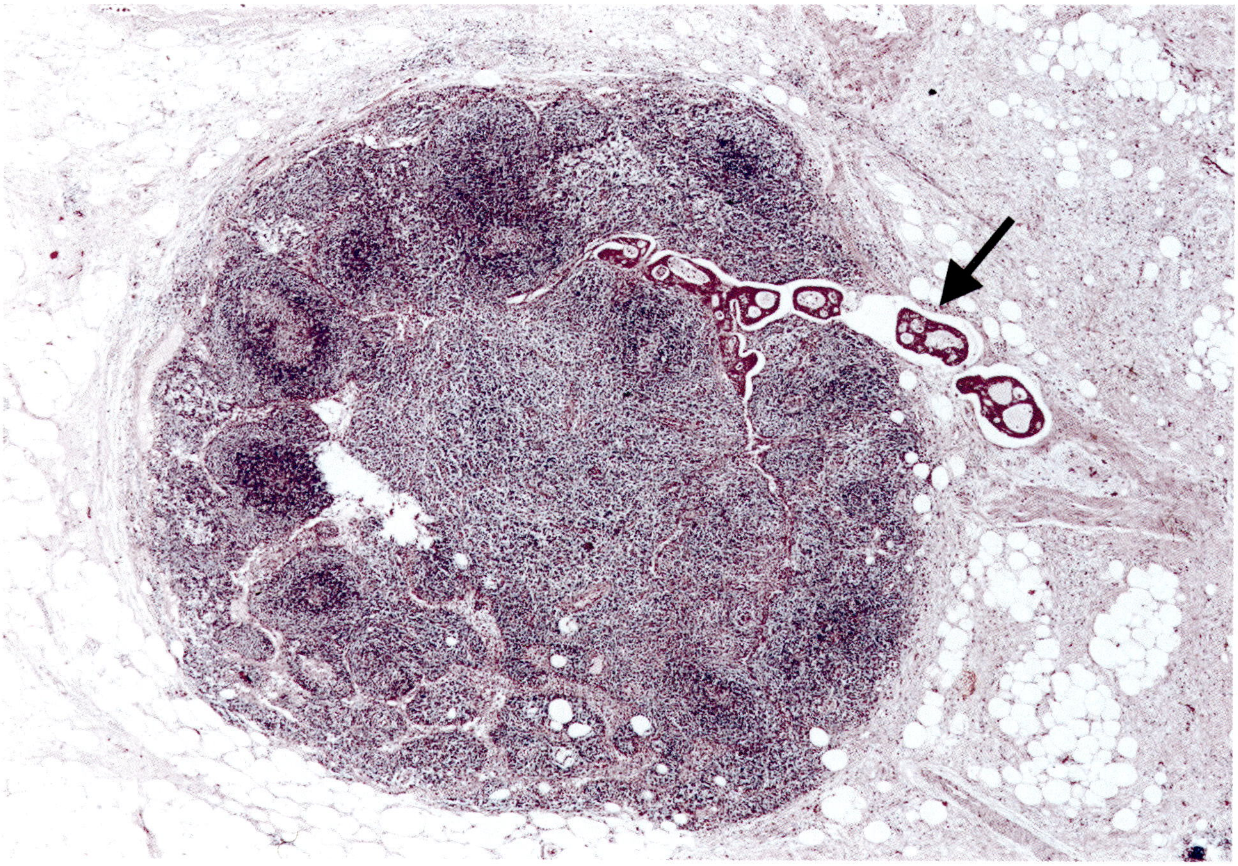

A 52-year-old man with no history of serious illness presented with abdominal pain, dark-colored urine, light-colored stools, and jaundice. Abdominal ultrasonography revealed dilatation of the intrahepatic and extrahepatic bile ducts. Surgical exploration and a pancreatoduodenectomy (Whipple's resection) were performed, revealing an infiltrating, poorly differentiated adenocarcinoma of the distal common bile duct. The carcinoma measured 2.0 cm in its greatest dimension. All margins of resection were negative for tumor. Fifteen lymph nodes were examined histologically for evidence of metastasis, and a single micrometastasis was identified (arrow). The carcinoma is present in sinusoids within the node and in a dilated lymphatic leading into the node (hematoxylin and eosin, ×62.5). The patient recovered uneventfully and was sent home on the 10th postoperative day. Two months after surgery, he began a course of radiation therapy and fluorouracil-based chemotherapy. At the most recent follow-up visit, he had no evidence of recurrence.

Daniel J. Brat, M.D., Ph.D.
Ralph H. Hruban, M.D.

Johns Hopkins Hospital
Baltimore, MD 21287

December 5, 1996

Bony Metastases

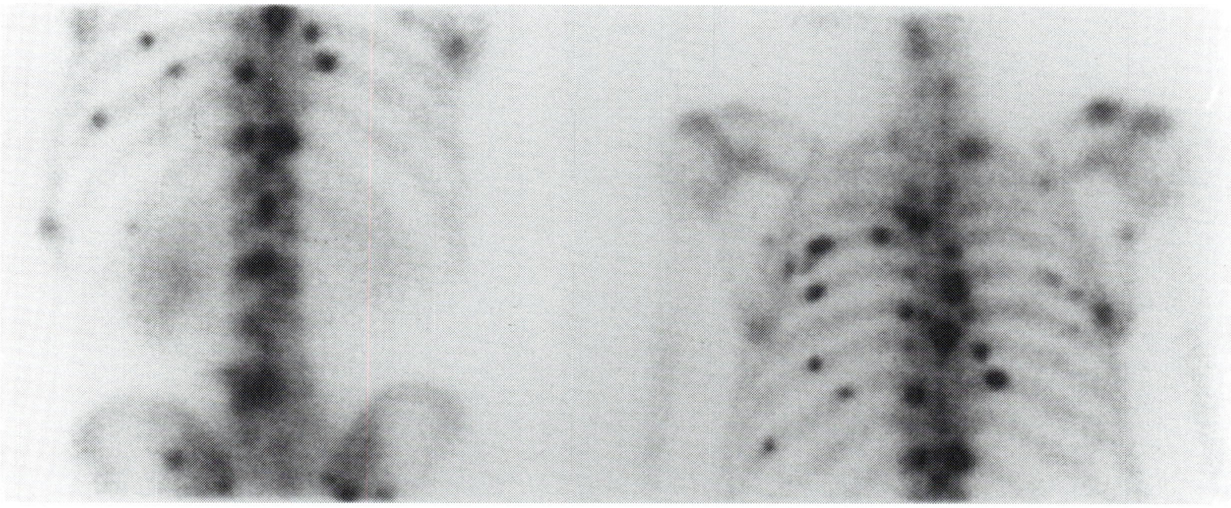

The results of whole-body bone scintigraphy in a 58-year-old man who reported backache are shown. Plain bone films were unremarkable. Scintigraphy revealed numerous foci of increased uptake of tracer ("hot spots"), a finding consistent with metastatic disease. Focally increased uptake reflects increased osteoblastic activity associated with the attempted repair of diseased bone. Subsequent studies revealed the tumor to be prostate cancer.

Mark Glazer, M.D.

University of Chicago
Chicago, IL 60637

Vidya V. Sagar, M.D.

Medical Center of Delaware
Newark, DE 19718

February 9, 1995

Sister Joseph's Node in Non-Hodgkin's Lymphoma

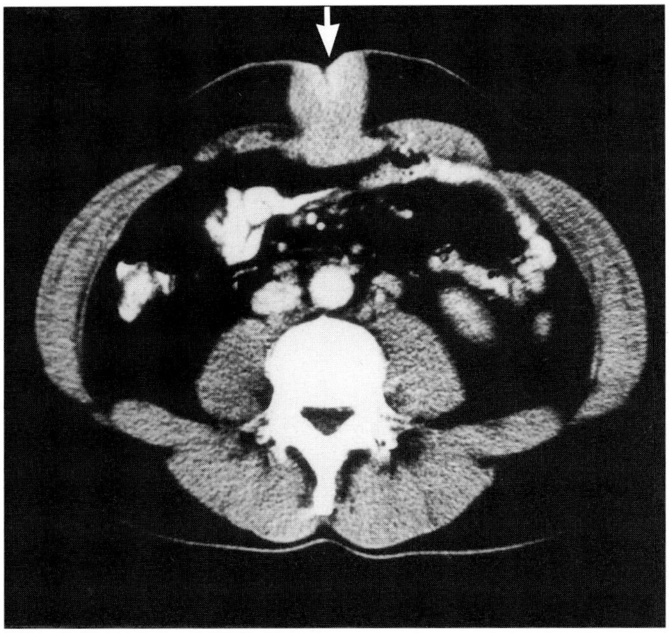

A

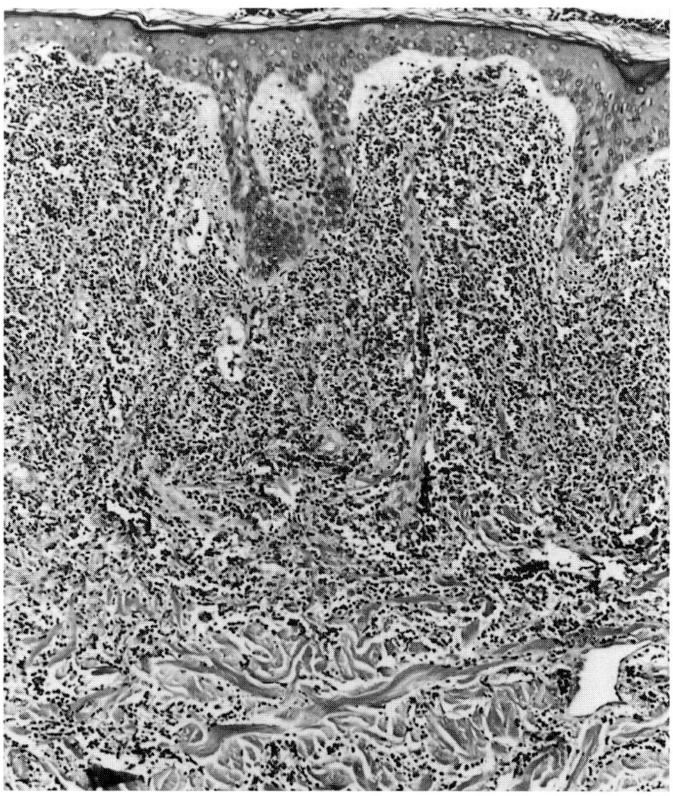

B

A 44-year-old man was found to have an umbilical tumor. Examination revealed the lesion to be firm and subcutaneous, approximately 5 cm in diameter, with erythema around the navel. The cervical and inguinal lymph nodes were enlarged. Computed tomography revealed an umbilical mass measuring 4.5 cm by 3.5 cm (Panel A, arrow) and multiple enlarged lymph nodes in the pelvis. A skin-biopsy specimen showed massive infiltration of the dermis by medium-sized, atypical lymphoid cells, which infiltrated between the bundles of collagen (Panel B; hematoxylin and eosin, ×200). Cells similar to those of the Sister Joseph's node were also seen in a biopsy specimen from an inguinal lymph node. The infiltrating cells were positive for B-cell markers. DNA extracted from the skin and the lymph node showed rearrangement of the immunoglobulin heavy-chain gene that was consistent with a B-cell lymphoma. The patient entered a complete remission after six courses of intensified therapy with cyclophosphamide, doxorubicin, vincristine, and prednisolone.

Keisuke Nagao, M.D.
Arata Kikuchi, M.D.

Keio University School of Medicine
Tokyo 160, Japan

November 21, 1996

Sister Joseph's Node in Carcinoma of the Cecum

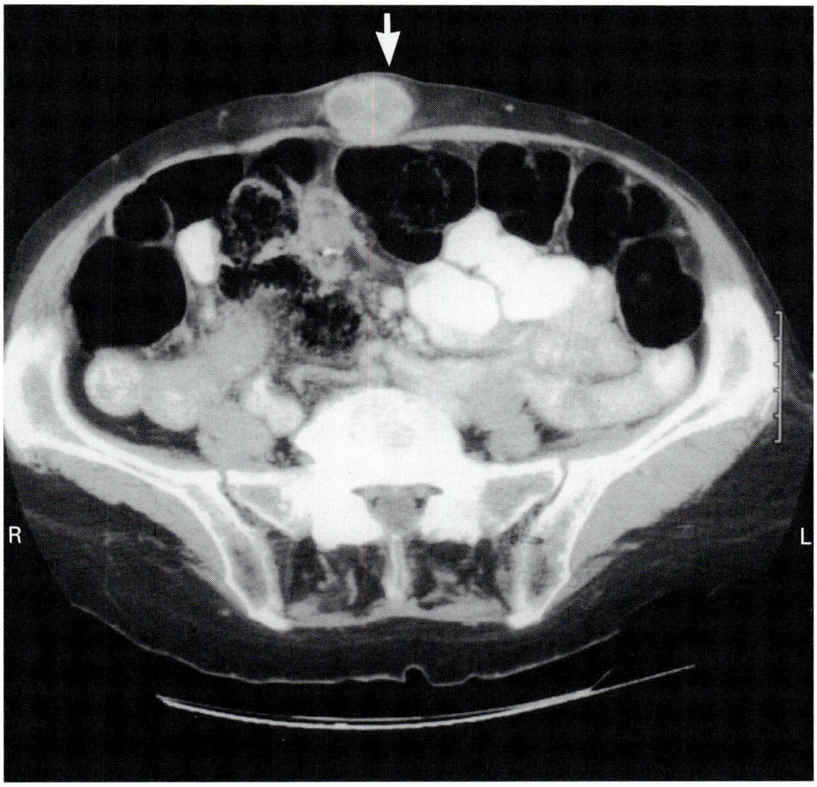

A 78-year-old woman who had undergone right hemicolectomy to treat carcinoma of the cecum with involvement of regional lymph nodes noticed a new periumbilical subcutaneous swelling two months after her surgery. Biopsy revealed an adenocarcinoma with the same histologic features as the original cecal tumor. The patient chose not to have any treatment. Two months later, the nodule had enlarged substantially, and abdominal and pelvic computed tomographic (CT) scans were obtained to assess the extent of metastatic disease before further treatment options were discussed.

The CT scan shows the periumbilical subcutaneous node (arrow), often referred to as Sister Joseph's node, for Sister Joseph, who in the early days of the Mayo Clinic noted periumbilical nodules in patients with intraabdominal cancer.

Other CT images obtained at the same time showed additional masses in the liver and pelvis (not visible here) that were compatible with metastatic disease. The patient decided against chemotherapy but received palliative radiation therapy to the abdominal wall in the region of the Sister Joseph's node, to prevent breakdown of the skin. There was no change in the node during this treatment. The patient died three weeks after the completion of the therapy.

Stephan Moll, M.D.

Duke University Medical Center
Durham, NC 27710

November 21, 1996

Double Uterus with Adenocarcinoma

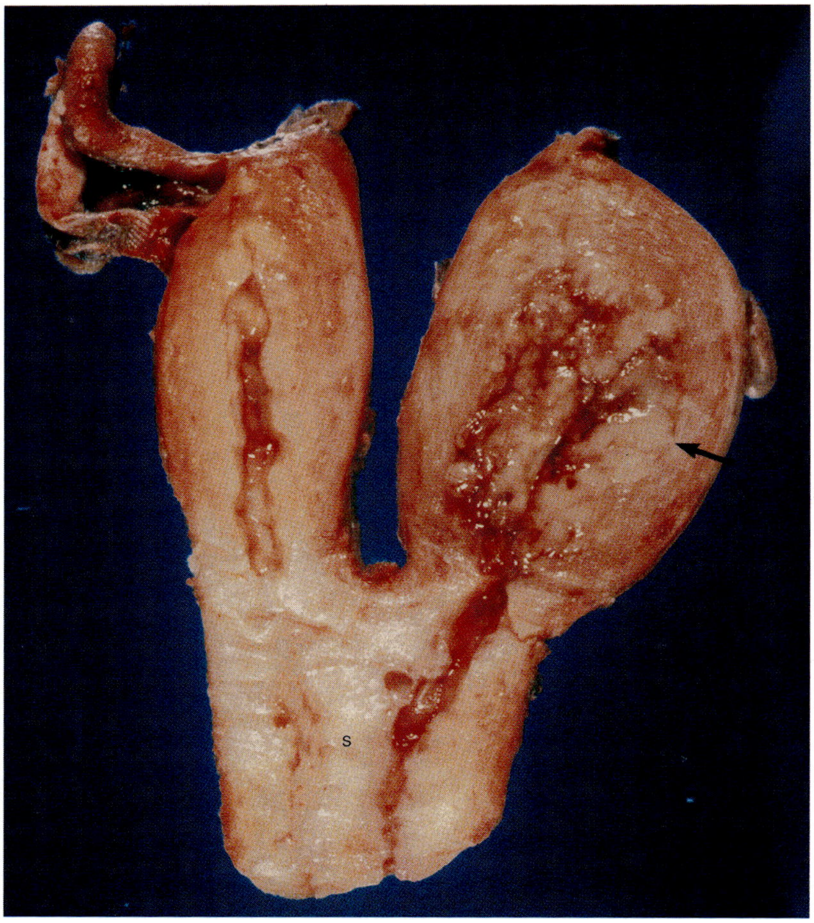

A posterior view of a double uterus from a 78-year-old woman with uterine bleeding is shown. On the right, an endometrial carcinoma (histologically classified as a grade II adenocarcinoma) has invaded the superficial third of the myometrium (arrow). The endometrium of the left fundus reveals cystic atrophy. The "s" indicates the septum between two endocervical canals.

Donald V. Pojman, M.D.
Jerome B. Taxy, M.D.

Lutheran General Hospital
Park Ridge, IL 60068

September 14, 1995

Neurofibromatosis Type 1

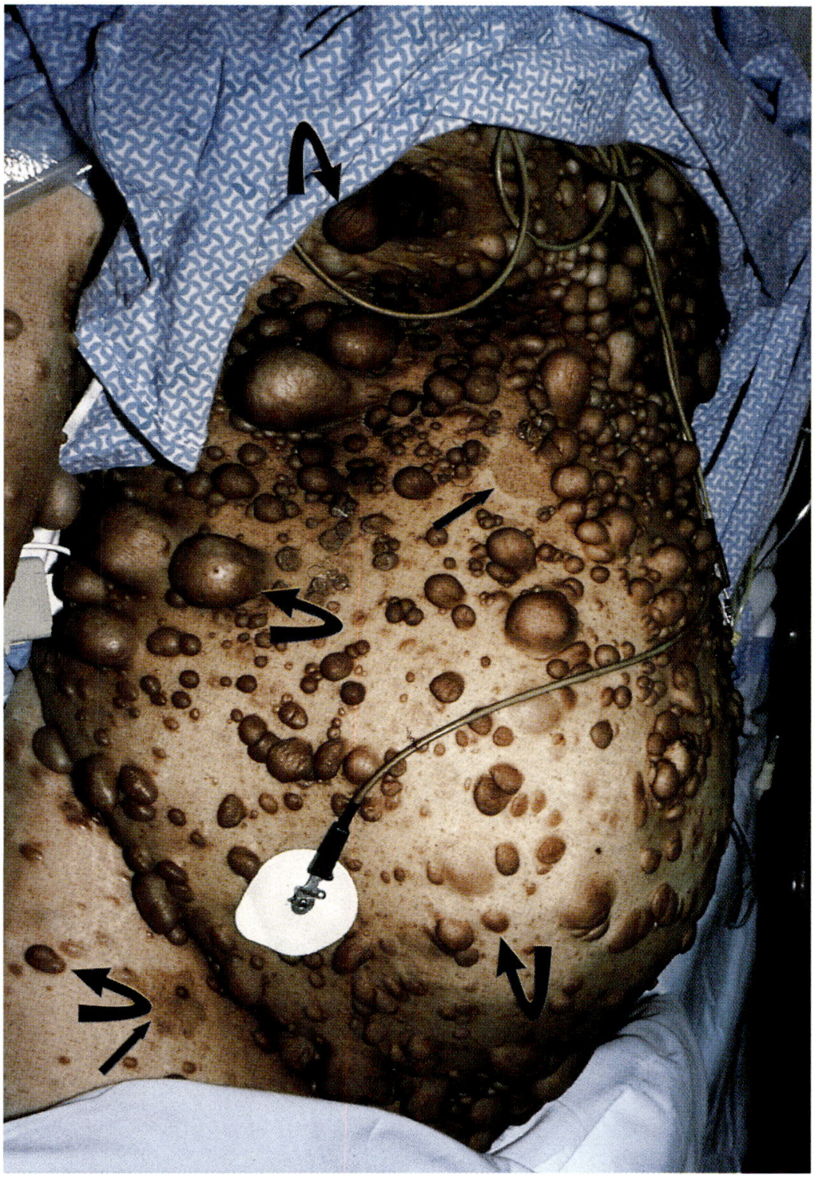

Severe neurofibromatosis type 1 is shown in a 45-year-old woman who was admitted for a severe exacerbation of asthma. Inguinal freckling (known as Crowe's sign), café au lait macules (straight arrows), and neurofibromas (curved arrows) are present. The café au lait macules were noted at birth; the neurofibromas began to appear during puberty.

Philip R. Cohen, M.D.

University of Texas Medical School
Houston, TX 77030

November 18, 1993

Retinopathy in Leukemia

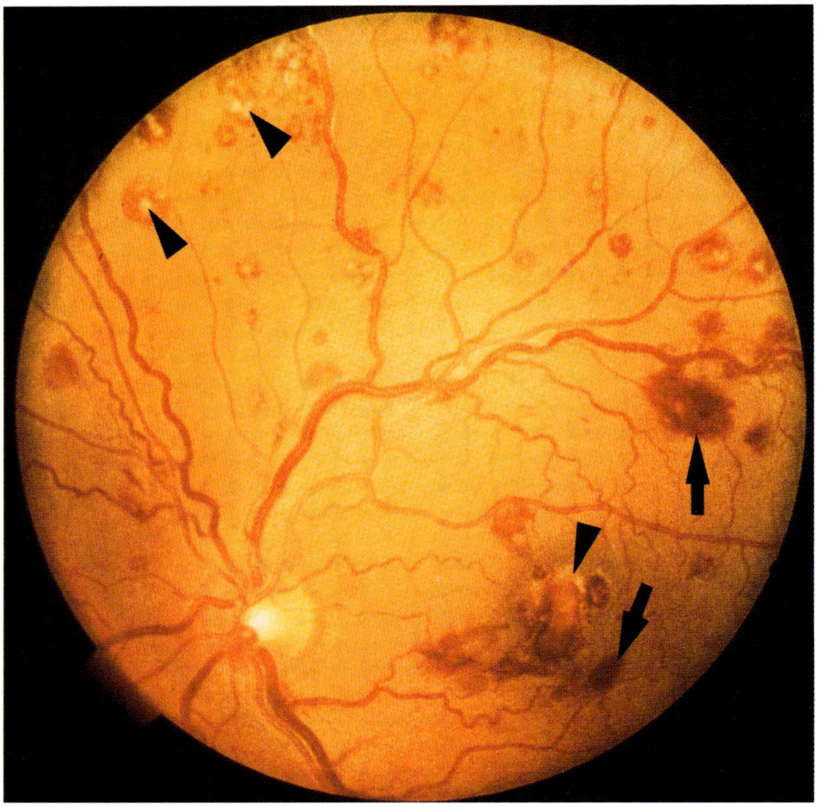

A 43-year-old man presented with blurred vision that had persisted for several days. Funduscopic examination of the retina revealed leukemic infiltrates (arrowheads) and hemorrhages (arrows). Bone marrow aspiration and biopsy confirmed the diagnosis of chronic myelogenous leukemia in blast crisis.

Mark A. Perazella, M.D.
John Magaldi, M.D.

Yale University School of Medicine
New Haven, CT 06510

October 6, 1994

Correspondence

Roth's Spots in Leukemic Retinopathy

February 2, 1995

To the Editor: Although the term "leukemic infiltrates" accurately describes the pertinent funduscopic findings in retinopathy in leukemia, which are strikingly pictured in the image by Perazella and Magaldi (Oct. 6 issue),[1] the legend fails to indicate that the distinctive hemorrhages with white centers are Roth's spots. Classically, Roth's spots have been linked with subacute bacterial endocarditis, but the association is not exclusive, since they occur in diverse conditions including leukemia and anemia.[2] Similarly, the pathologic basis of the pale white centers can be focal ischemia, inflammatory infiltrate, a colony of infectious organisms, fibrin and platelets, or an accumulation of neoplastic cells.[3]

Ironically, the white-centered hemorrhages recognized as Roth's spots by present-day clinicians may differ from the white retinal spots Moritz Roth described in 1872 and attributed to degeneration of the nerve-fiber layer.[4] Nevertheless, this dramatic photograph of leukemic retinopathy should underline the fact that the clinical usefulness of Roth's spots is not limited to the diagnosis of subacute bacterial endocarditis.

Frederick E. Lepore, M.D.
Robert Wood Johnson Medical School
New Brunswick, NJ 08903

1. Perazella MA, Magaldi J. Retinopathy in leukemia. N Engl J Med 1994;331:922.
2. Significance of fundus signs. In: Cogan DG. Ophthalmic manifestations of systemic vascular disease. Vol. 3 of Major problems in internal medicine. Philadelphia: W.B. Saunders, 1974:52.
3. Kaur B, Taylor D. Fundus hemorrhages in infancy. Surv Ophthalmol 1992;37:1-17.
4. Roth M. Ueber Netzhautaffectionen bei Wundfiebern. Dtsch Z Chim 1872;1:471-84.

Gingival Hypertrophy in Myelomonocytic Leukemia

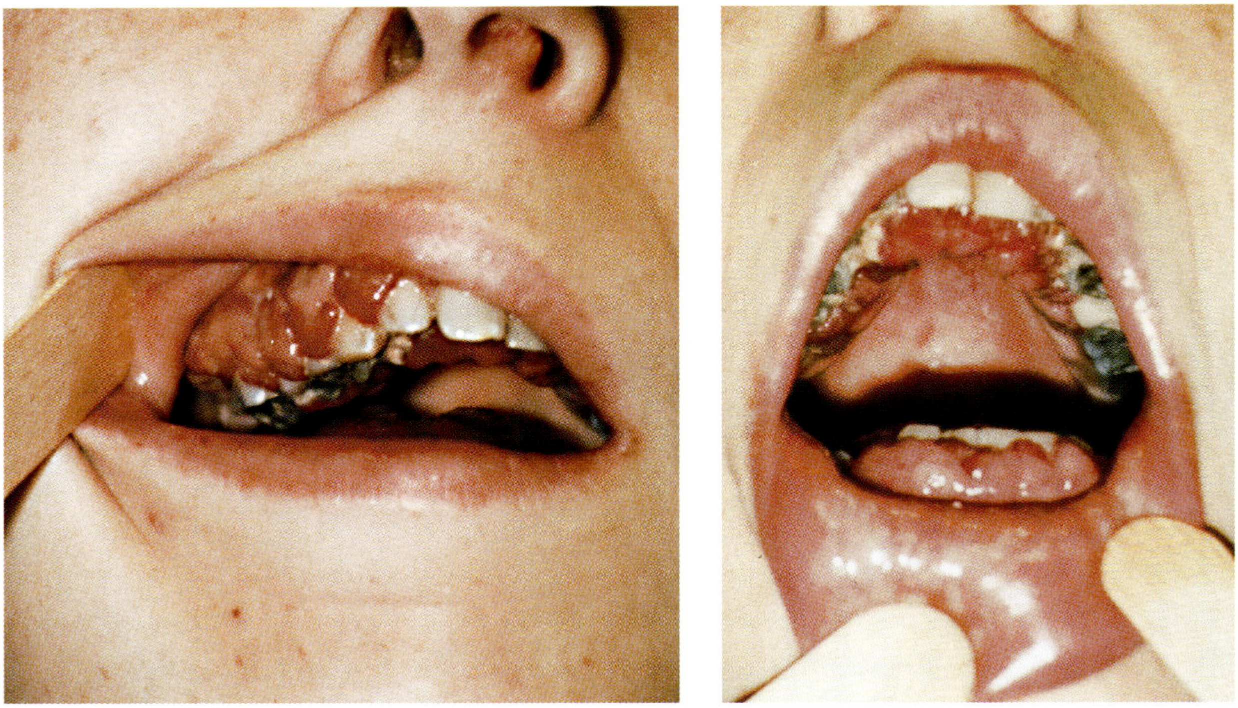

A 36-year-old woman with chronic myelomonocytic leukemia had marked gingival hypertrophy, thought to be due to infiltration of the gingiva by leukemic cells. The patient presented with a white-cell count of 28,800 per cubic millimeter, with 23 percent monocytes and 2 percent monoblasts, a hematocrit of 20 percent, and a platelet count of 156,000 per cubic millimeter. Treatment with etoposide, idarubicin, and cytarabine resulted in a clinical remission, with resolution of the gingival lesions.

Stan H.M. van Uum, M.D.

University Hospital
Nijmegen 6500 HB, the Netherlands

Jo-Jan Keuning, M.D., Ph.D.

Saint Joseph Hospital
Veldhoven 5500 MB, the Netherlands

March 24, 1994

Chemotherapy-Induced Acral Erythema

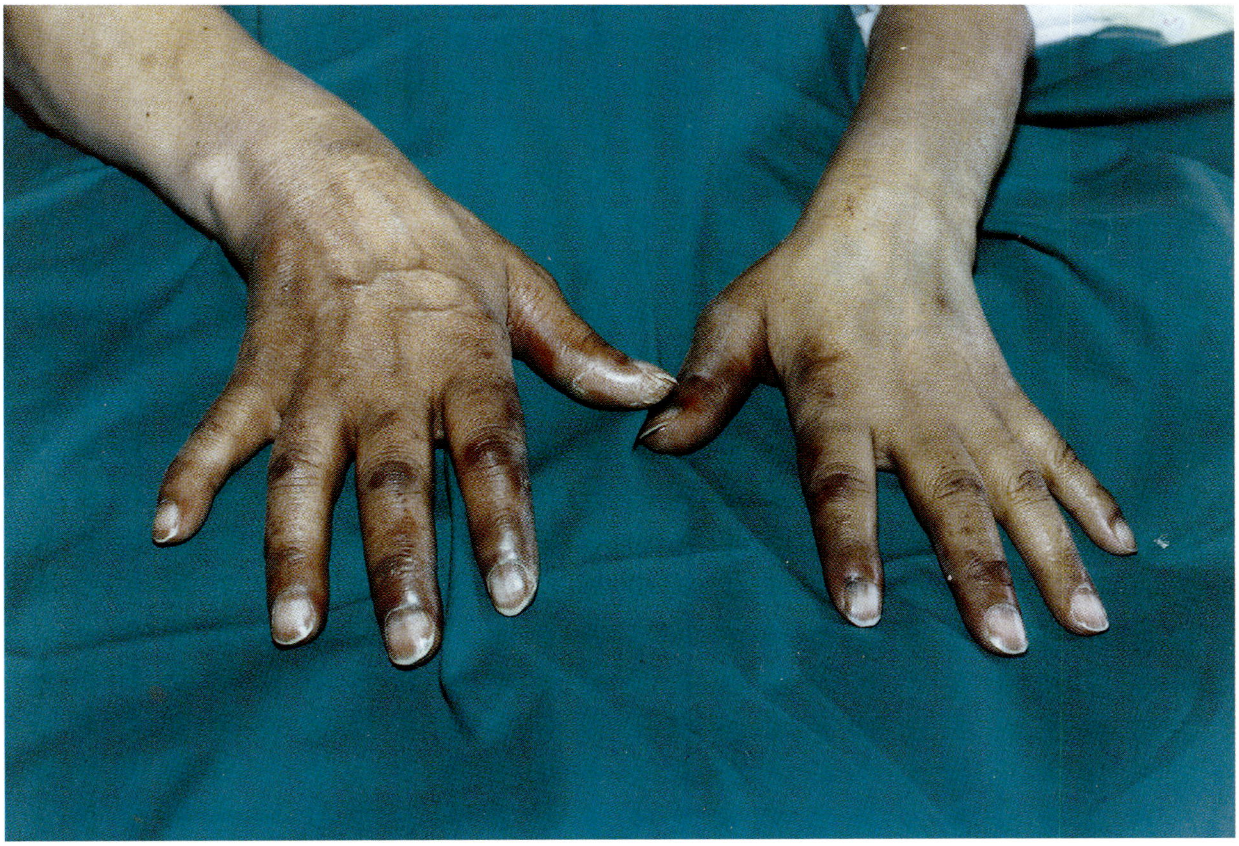

Acral cyanosis can be seen in a 61-year-old woman with non-Hodgkin's lymphoma. The lesions developed while the patient had severe neutropenia during a course of therapy consisting of methotrexate with leucovorin rescue, doxorubicin, cyclophosphamide, vincristine, prednisone, and bleomycin. The disorder is characterized by intense, painful erythema of the palms and soles, often culminating in the formation of vesicles or bullae. Chemotherapeutic agents are one of the known causes.

Mario Pirisi, M.D.
Giorgio Soardo, M.D.

Cattedra di Medicina Interna Università degli Studi
33100 Udine, Italy

May 5, 1994

Cyclic Fever in Hodgkin's Disease (Pel–Ebstein Fever)

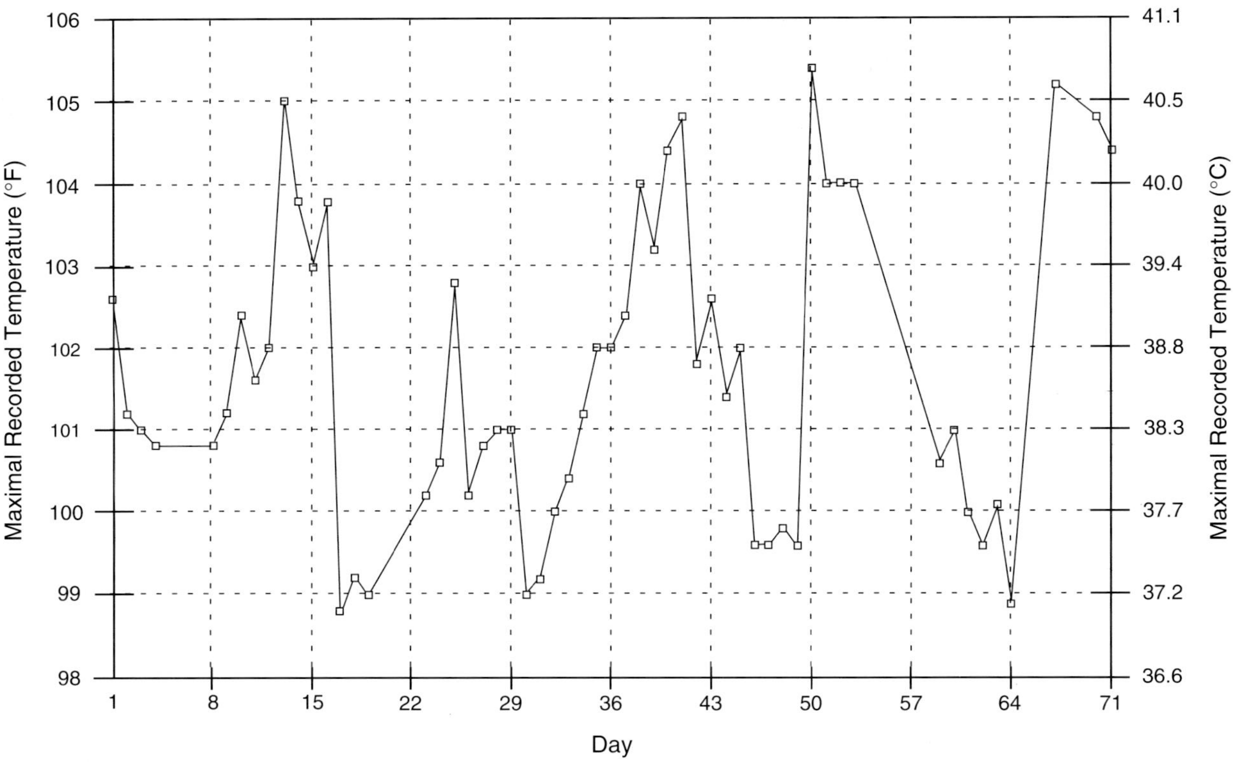

A 50-year-old man had fever, night sweats, and nonproductive cough for 10 weeks. He took antipyretic medications during the febrile periods. His wife recorded his temperatures, shown above, on 56 of the 71 days. Biopsy of a rapidly enlarging cervical lymph node revealed nodular sclerosing Hodgkin's lymphoma. The patient's fevers and other symptoms promptly disappeared after the first cycle of doxorubicin, bleomycin, vinblastine, and dacarbazine.

Gary R. Good, M.D.
Mark J. DiNubile, M.D.

Cooper Hospital–University Medical Center
Camden, NJ 08103

February 16, 1995

Correspondence

Pel–Ebstein Fever

July 6, 1995

To the Editor: The Images in Clinical Medicine in the February 16 issue[1] presents a temperature chart of cyclic fever in Hodgkin's disease, which the authors identify as Pel–Ebstein fever.

In his essay "Making Sense,"[2] Richard Asher refers specifically to Pel–Ebstein fever as a classic example of a condition that exists only because it has a name. As he points out, "Every student and every doctor knows that cases of Hodgkin's disease may show a fever that is high for one week and low for the next week and so on. Does this phenomenon really exist at all? If you collect the charts of 50 cases of Hodgkin's disease and compare them with the charts of 50 cases of disseminated malignant fever, do you really believe you could pick out even one or two cases because of the characteristic fever?" He then continues, "out of curiosity I looked up the original papers, and Dr. Burrows kindly translated them for me.[3,4] Both describe patients with chronic relapsing fever and splenomegaly but there is nothing in either paper to suggest any of them had Hodgkin's disease."

The *Journal* has indeed proved Asher's argument that "it does not matter whether or not Pel–Ebstein fever exists, my contention remains the same: the bestowal of a name upon a concept, whether real or imaginary, brings it into clinical existence."

Andrew J.W. Hilson, F.R.C.P.
Royal Free Hospital and School of Medicine, London NW3 2QG, United Kingdom

1. Good GR, DiNubile MJ. Cyclic fever in Hodgkin's disease (Pel–Ebstein fever). N Engl J Med 1995; 332:436.
2. Asher R. Richard Asher talking sense. London: Pitman Medical, 1972:21-2.
3. Pel PK. Zur Symptomatologie der Sog: Pseudo-Leukämie. Berl Klin Wochenschr 1885;22:3-7.
4. Ebstein W. Das chronische Rückfallsfieber, eine neue Infectionskrankheit. Berl Klin Wochenschr 1887; 24:565-8.

Dr. DiNubile replies:

To the Editor: Hilson questions the sensitivity and specificity of the cyclic pattern of fever known as Pel–Ebstein fever in Hodgkin's lymphoma. He contends that the disproportionate recognition of periodic fevers in patients with Hodgkin's disease occurs because this association has been specifically named "Pel–Ebstein fever" (even if the appellation is undeserved on the basis of the original reports). In his opinion, the association of cyclic fevers with Hodgkin's disease is no stronger than that of other causes of fever of unknown origin.

The predictive value of Pel–Ebstein fever obviously depends on the probability that a patient has lymphoma. In the setting of prolonged, unexplained fevers, in which the initial evaluation fails to disclose an infectious cause, my impression, shared by others,[1] is that a classic pattern of Pel–Ebstein fever is characteristic of (although not pathognomonic for) Hodgkin's disease. However, there are few published data to substantiate this impression.[2]

The indisputable power of naming[3] is even understood by young children,[4] who wait nervously for Sebastian to give the princess a new name in order to save Fantasia from "the Nothing" in *The Neverending Story.* Developmental psychologists, linguists, and theologians have taught us how inextricably bound a concept and its name are[5]; it is not always clear, as Hilson insightfully points out, which comes first — the name or the concept.

Mark J. DiNubile, M.D.
Cooper Hospital–Robert Wood Johnson Medical School, Camden, NJ 08103

1. Gelfand JA, Wolff SM. Fever of unknown origin. In: Mandell GL, Bennett JE, Dolin R, eds. Principles and practice of infectious diseases. 4th ed. Vol. 1. New York: Churchill Livingstone, 1995:544.
2. Colvett KL, Patel D, Smith JK. Multiple Beau's lines in a patient with fever of unknown origin. South Med J 1993;86:1424-6.
3. Isaiah. 43:1.
4. Akiyama MM, Wilcox SA. Naming as a function of linguistic form-class and object categories. J Child Lang 1993;20:419-35.
5. John. 1:1.

Periorbital Edema in Kaposi's Sarcoma

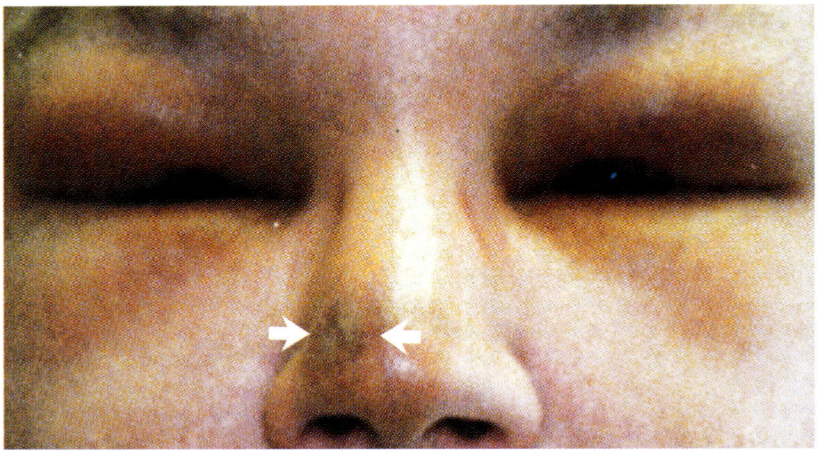

A

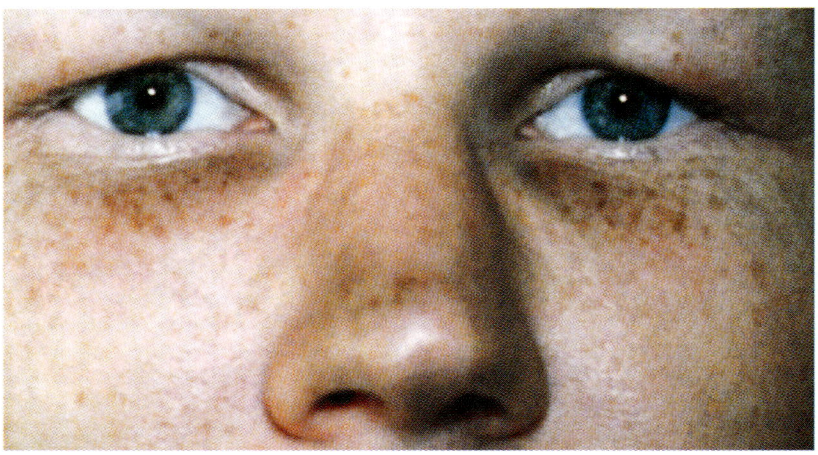

B

A 27-year-old man who was seropositive for the human immunodeficiency virus presented with severe periorbital and facial edema (Panel A) and generalized cutaneous Kaposi's sarcoma. Note the lesion (arrows) on the nose. Computed tomography (CT) of the head demonstrated thickening of the eyelids and the skin of the nose and face. The patient had neither superior vena cava syndrome nor nephrotic syndrome. Doxorubicin, vincristine, and bleomycin were administered intravenously every two weeks for four months. Facial and periorbital edema resolved rapidly (Panel B), as did the Kaposi's sarcoma. The CT findings also returned to normal. This type of edema, which occurs relatively frequently in patients with the acquired immunodeficiency syndrome and Kaposi's sarcoma, can be a source of major morbidity and can compromise vision. It is a clear-cut indication for systemic chemotherapy.

Bernard L. Zidar, M.D.

Medical College of Pennsylvania–
Hahnemann University,
Allegheny Campus
Pittsburgh, PA 15212

May 4, 1995

Correspondence

Periorbital Edema in Kaposi's Sarcoma

September 21, 1995

To the Editor: As Dr. Zidar notes in the legend accompanying the image of periorbital edema associated with AIDS-related Kaposi's sarcoma (May 4 issue),[1] edema is a common problem in patients with AIDS-associated Kaposi's sarcoma, especially those with advanced disease, with up to one fifth of patients having this problem.[2,3]

Edema is not, however, an absolute indication for systemic chemotherapy — especially a regimen as toxic as the combination of doxorubicin, bleomycin, and vincristine. We find that in the absence of other problems associated with Kaposi's sarcoma, periorbital edema responds well to local, wide-field, megavoltage irradiation. Systemic chemotherapy often condemns patients to a continuous regimen, and to its toxic effects, for the rest of their short lives. Irradiation offers a means of local treatment without the systemic side effects of chemotherapy. In our opinion, irradiation also offers a quicker means of relieving symptoms, especially in patients whose vision is threatened.

A fractionation regimen such as 20 Gy delivered in 10 fractions during a two-week period, with the use of internal eye shields, is easily tolerated, and marked symptomatic relief often occurs after only 2 or 3 fractions have been delivered. This approach also gives patients time to consider future options for therapy and, if the option of systemic therapy is chosen, allows time for base-line investigations to be properly completed.

A patient with other symptoms or signs of visceral or pulmonary Kaposi's sarcoma (i.e., abdominal pain or breathlessness) should, of course, receive the regimen of chemotherapy currently being used at the center where the patient is being treated. Radiotherapy still offers a quick means of relieving symptoms, especially if visual impairment is the main problem.

Mark Harrison, M.R.C.P., David Tomlinson, M.R.C.P., and Simon Stewart, M.D.
St. Mary's Hospital, London W2 1NY, United Kingdom

1. Zidar BL. Periorbital edema in Kaposi's sarcoma. N Engl J Med 1995;332:1204.
2. Bayley AC. Occurrence, clinical behaviour and management of Kaposi's sarcoma in Zambia. Cancer Surv 1991;10:53-71.
3. Harrison M, Tomlinson D, Stewart S. Liposomal-entrapped doxorubicin: an active agent in AIDS-related Kaposi's sarcoma. J Clin Oncol 1995;13:914-20.

Dr. Zidar replies:

To the Editor: The computed tomographic scans in our patient showed diffuse swelling not only of the periorbital area but also of the entire head and neck. Diffuse edema of the head, neck, and periorbital structures usually indicates serious involvement, with more aggressive and disseminated disease. We believe that this type of involvement is more amenable to systemic chemotherapy than to local irradiation, although we do not deny that in many cases of local edema, radiotherapy may be very effective. Unfortunately, there has not been a randomized trial comparing radiotherapy with chemotherapy in the treatment of edema related to Kaposi's sarcoma.

Radiotherapy, although effective, is not without its own inherent problems, including mucositis.[1,2] Krigel and Friedman-Kien have noted that complications are frequently encountered in the presence of moderate-to-severe edema and that long-standing tumor lesions and extensive confluent areas of Kaposi's sarcoma have been found to have reduced radiosensitivity.[3]

Bernard L. Zidar, M.D.
Medical College of Pennsylvania–Hahnemann University, Pittsburgh, PA 15212

1. Levine AM, Crawford J. AIDS-related malignancies: 1993. Amgen Journal Club presentation.
2. Northfelt DW, Kahn JO, Volberding PA. Treatment of AIDS-related Kaposi's sarcoma. Hematol Oncol Clin North Am 1991;5:297-310.
3. Krigel RL, Friedman-Kien AE. Kaposi's sarcoma in AIDS: diagnosis and treatment. In: DeVita VT, Hellman S, Rosenberg SA, eds. AIDS: etiology, diagnosis and prevention. 2nd ed. Philadelphia: J.B. Lippincott, 1988:255.

Mycosis Fungoides

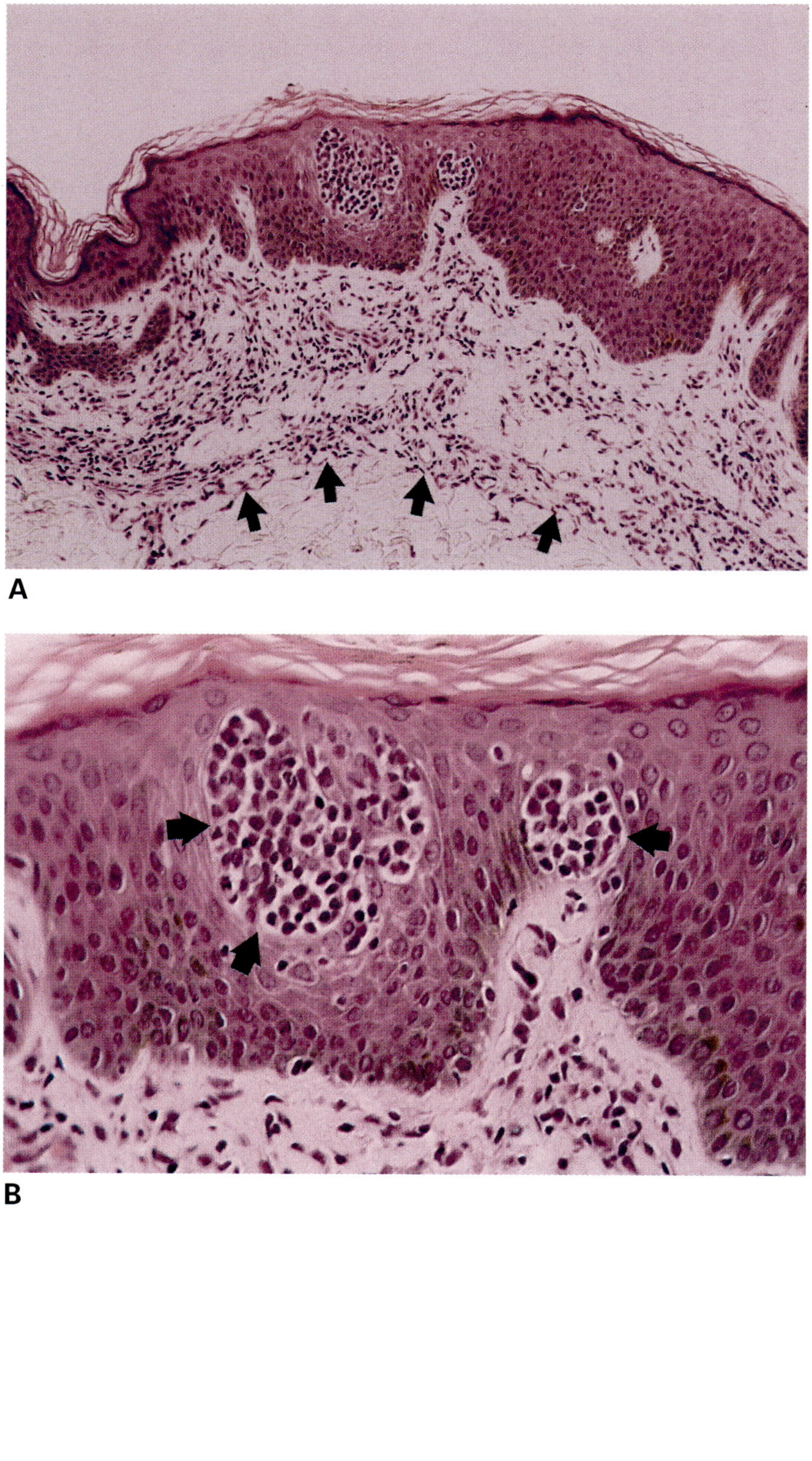

Mycosis fungoides is an epidermotropic variant of cutaneous T-cell lymphoma. The most notable histologic features in the plaque stage include a broad, band-like, cellular lymphoid infiltrate involving the densely fibrotic superficial dermis (arrows, Panel A). The lymphoid cells are small to medium in size and contain hyperconvoluted nuclei. The epidermis is involved when atypical lymphocytes form multiple nonspongiotic aggregates of Pautrier's microabscesses (arrows, Panel B). (Hematoxylin and eosin; Panel A, ×60; Panel B, ×240.)

Tai-Yuen Wong, M.D.
Martin C. Mihm, Jr., M.D.

Massachusetts General Hospital
Boston, MA 02114

December 30, 1993

Castleman's Disease

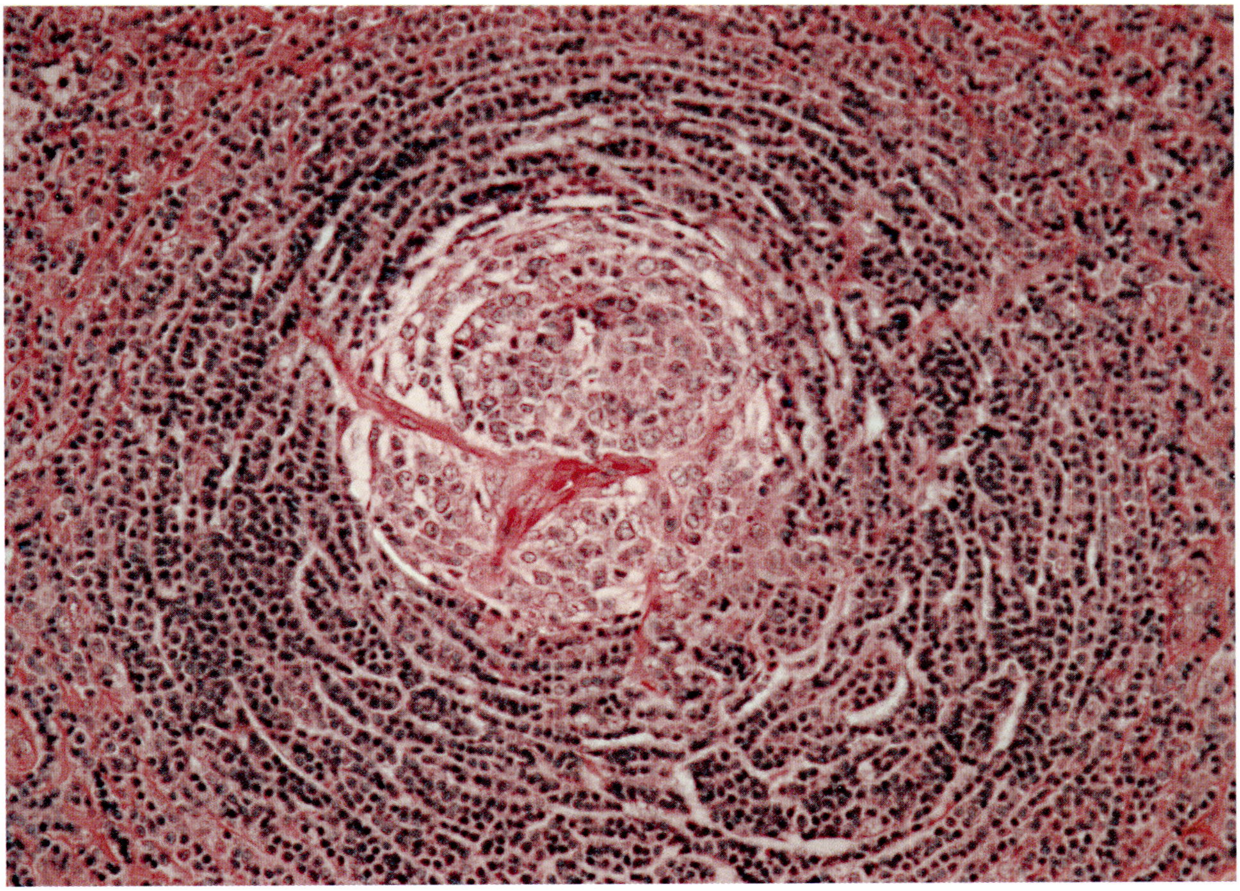

A 31-year-old woman who had had painless, right-sided cervical adenopathy for three months was given antibiotics, but the adenopathy persisted. She had no systemic symptoms and no other palpable lymph nodes, and the remainder of her physical examination was unremarkable. The results of all laboratory studies were normal. At surgery the node was 3 cm in diameter, tannish yellow, and rubbery. Histologic examination revealed numerous germinal centers pierced by capillaries emanating from a hypervascular pericortex and cuffed by small lymphocytes arranged in a concentric onion-skin pattern (hematoxylin and eosin, ×925). These morphologic features are characteristic of Castleman's disease.

Because of the benign nature of the condition, the patient received no further therapy. Ten years after the node appeared, the patient is well and has had no recurrence of lymphadenopathy.

Joshua Z. Sickel, M.D.

University of Rochester Medical Center
Rochester, NY 14642

September 21, 1995

Seasonal Hemolysis Due to Cold-Agglutinin Syndrome

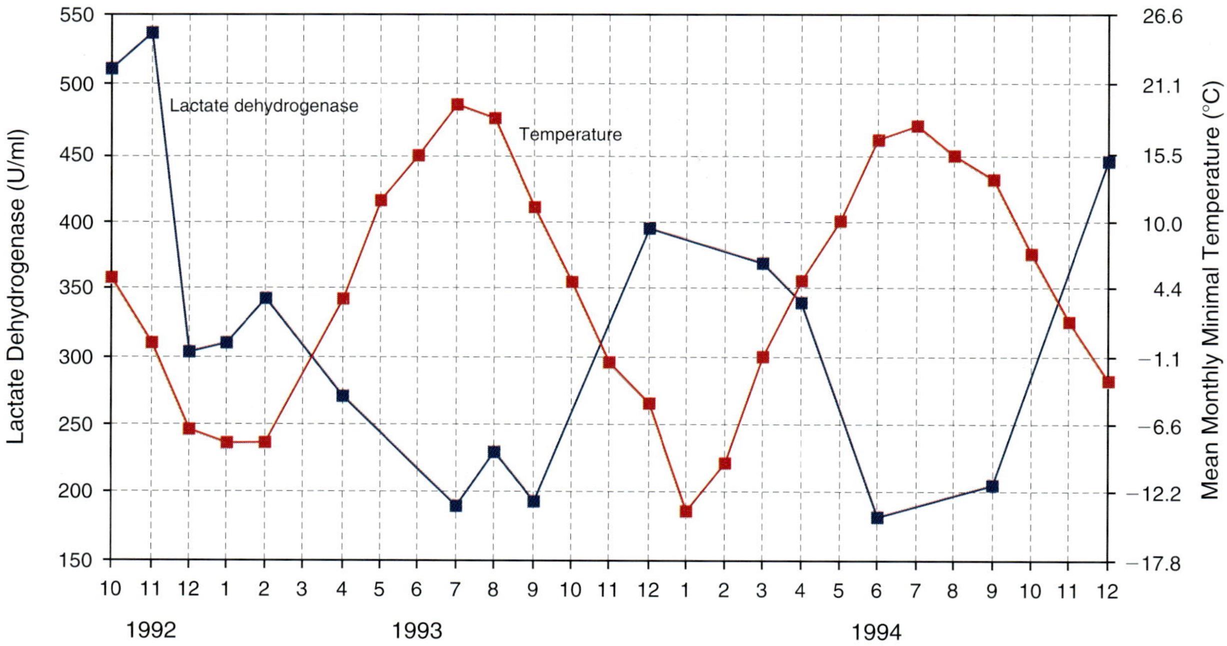

A 61-year-old roads inspector from Illinois presented in 1992 with hemolytic anemia and acrocyanosis and was found to have cold-agglutinin syndrome. He was treated with plasmapheresis, prednisone, and chlorambucil and then followed without therapy for two years. He continued to work, which involved spending the majority of time outdoors. The patient's cold-agglutinin titer exceeded 1:524,288, with a thermal maximum (the temperature at which agglutination occurs in vitro) of 37°C. The severity of the hemolysis, reflected by the lactate dehydrogenase concentration, was related to the ambient temperature, as illustrated. He is currently well and asymptomatic.

Laurie J. Lyckholm, M.D.
Michael B. Edmond, M.D., M.P.H.

University of Iowa
Iowa City, IA 52242

February 15, 1996

Multiple Myeloma

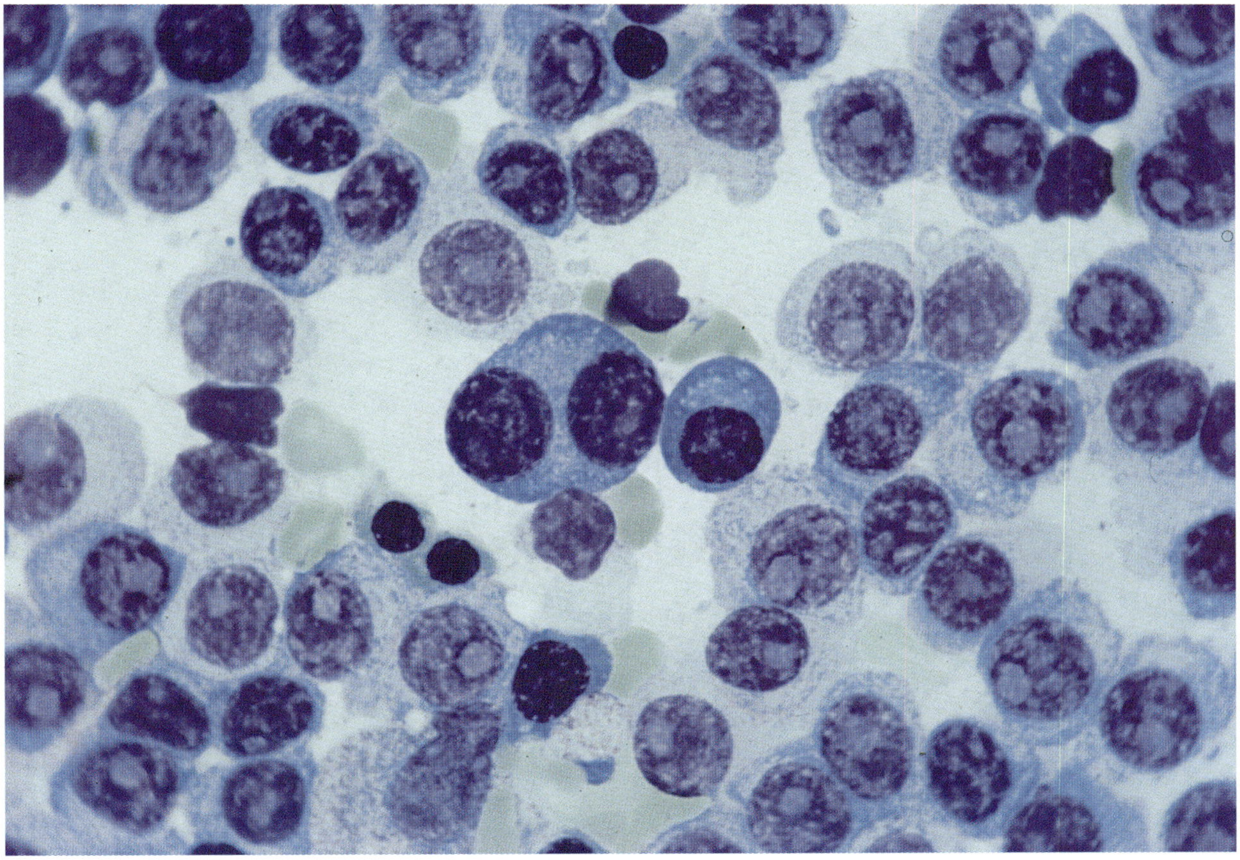

Dysplastic plasma cells are visible in the bone marrow of a patient with multiple myeloma. Many of the nuclei contain nucleoli. A binucleated plasma cell can be seen in the center of the field (Wright–Giemsa stain).

Robert S. Schwartz, M.D.

Deputy Editor

February 17, 1994

Gastroenterology

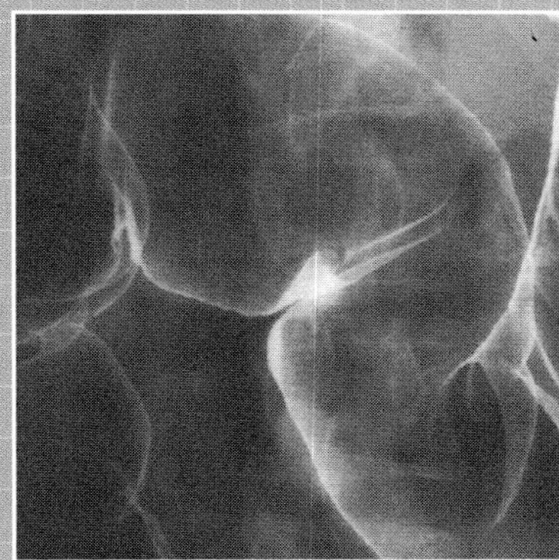

Giant Esophageal Ulcers

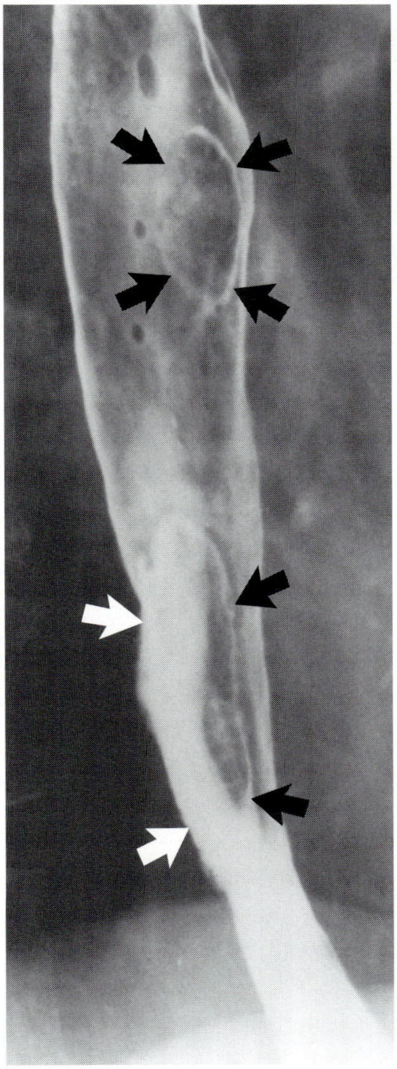

A

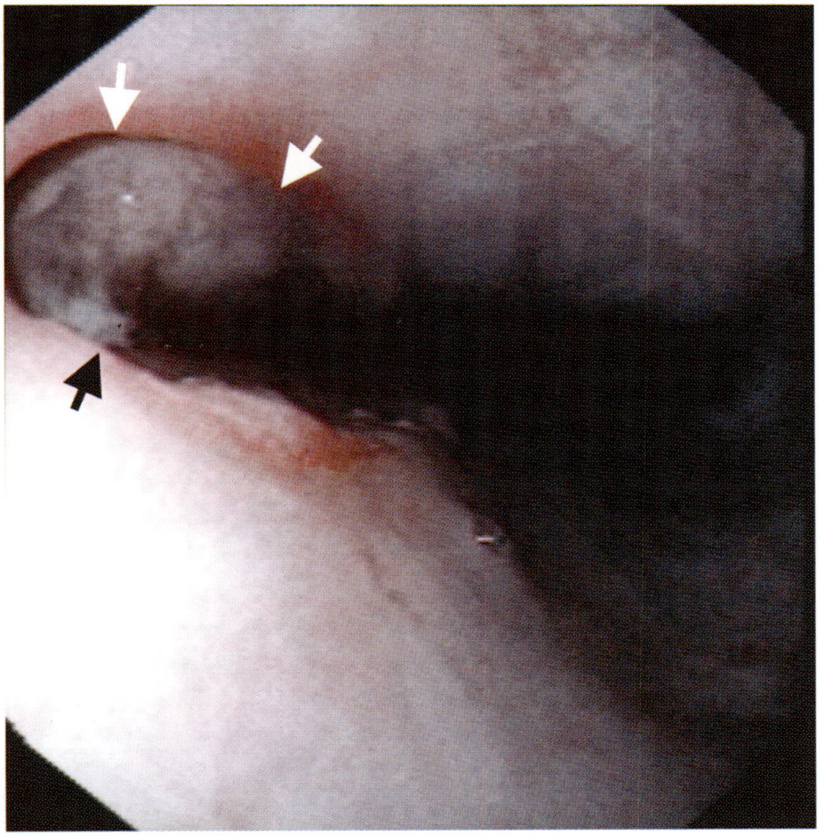

B

Acute, severe odynophagia developed in a 52-year-old man known to be positive for the human immunodeficiency virus (HIV). A double-contrast esophagogram (Panel A) shows two giant, ovoid ulcers (arrows) measuring 3 cm and 6 cm in length in the middle and distal thirds of the esophagus, respectively. An endoscopic photograph of the mid-portion of the esophagus (Panel B) shows the proximal ulcer to be a deep lesion with well-demarcated margins (arrows). The distal ulcer had a similar appearance, and the mucosa between the lesions was grossly normal, without exudates or plaques. Endoscopic brushings, biopsy specimens, and cultures obtained from the ulcer margins and ulcer beds were negative for cytomegalovirus, so the patient was assumed to have HIV esophagitis. His symptoms resolved in less than two weeks with 40 mg of prednisone daily.

Raymond A. Rubin, M.D.

Thomas Jefferson
University Hospital
Philadelphia, PA 19107

Marc S. Levine, M.D.

Hospital of the University
of Pennsylvania
Philadelphia, PA 19104

April 18, 1996

Helicobacter pylori in a Gastric Pit

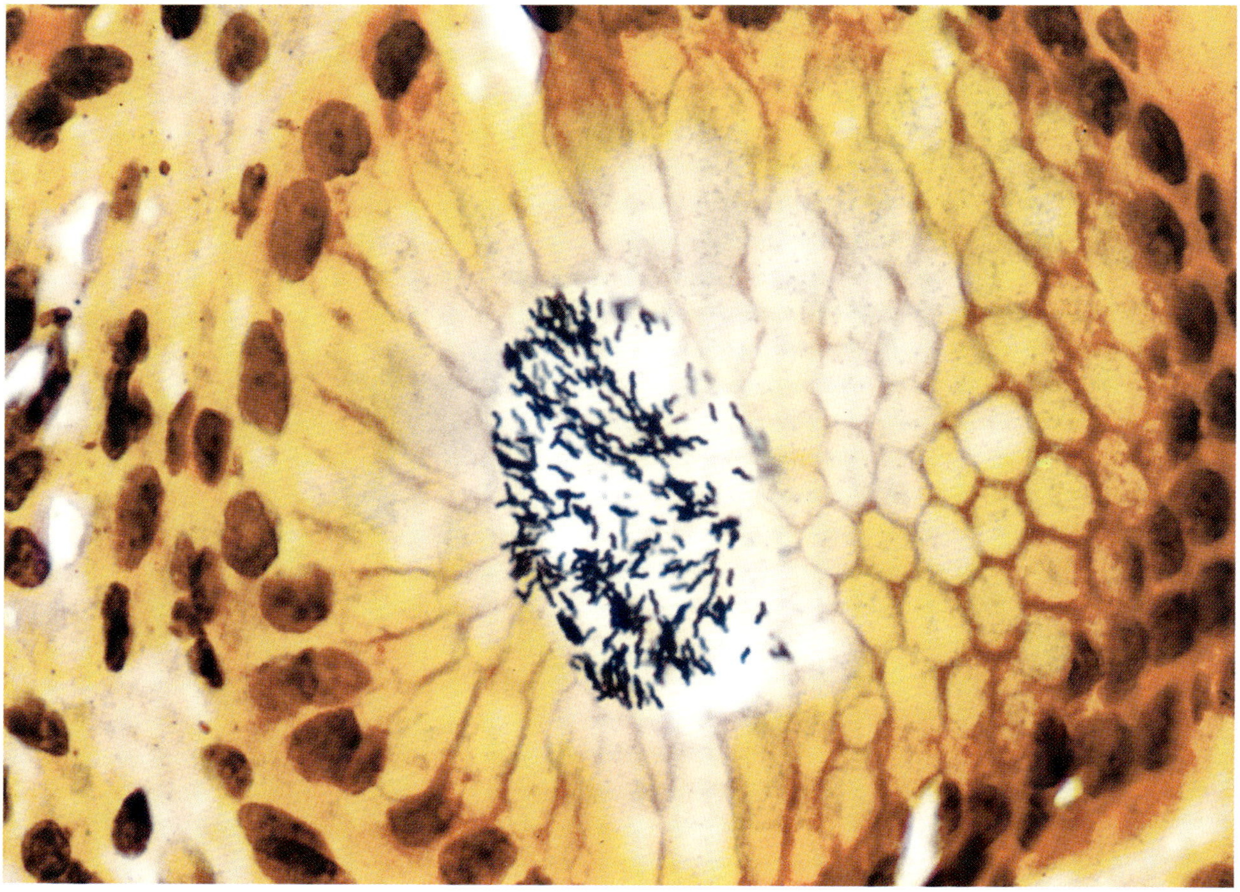

A 35-year-old man presented with epigastric pain of several months' duration. An esophagogastroduodenoscopy revealed an active duodenal ulcer. Biopsy of the gastric antrum showed chronic active gastritis with innumerable *Helicobacter pylori* organisms on the gastric mucosa. This photomicrograph of a section of an antral-biopsy specimen (×1000) stained with the Genta stain (a triple stain consisting of a modified Steiner, hematoxylin and eosin, and Alcian blue; pH 2.5) shows a gastric pit virtually filled with *H. pylori*. Culture confirmed that the infecting organism was *H. pylori*. The patient was treated for two weeks with omeprazole, clarithromycin, and metronidazole. Endoscopy eight weeks later showed healing of the duodenal ulcer. The cure of *H. pylori* infection was confirmed by the absence of *H. pylori* in any of three gastric-biopsy specimens obtained at this time and by a negative urea breath test.

Robert M. Genta, M.D.
David Y. Graham, M.D.

Veterans Affairs Medical Center
Houston, TX 77030

July 25, 1996

Correspondence

Treatment of Helicobacter pylori *Infection*

December 12, 1996

To the Editor: I enjoyed seeing the excellent photomicrograph of *Helicobacter pylori* provided by Genta and Graham in Images in Clinical Medicine (July 25 issue).[1] They describe a 35-year-old man with a duodenal ulcer who received triple therapy with omeprazole, clarithromycin, and metronidazole for two weeks. Why did the patient undergo endoscopy eight weeks later, as well as a urea breath test? Documentation of the eradication of *H. pylori* is not currently warranted in clinical practice.[2] The best evidence of a cure is the absence of recurrent symptoms of an ulcer. I suspect that the patient was enrolled in a therapeutic study. If this was the case, it should have been mentioned.

Klaus E. Mönkemüller, M.D.
University of Alabama at Birmingham
Birmingham, AL 35294

1. Genta RM, Graham DY. *Helicobacter pylori* in a gastric pit. N Engl J Med 1996;335:250.
2. Walsh JH, Peterson WL. The treatment of *Helicobacter pylori* infection in the management of peptic ulcer disease. N Engl J Med 1995;333:984-91.

The authors reply:

To the Editor: The gastric-biopsy specimen was from a patient who participated in a study designed to compare the reliability of the urea breath test with that of the histologic examination for the detection of *H. pylori* infection. We did not mention this in the description of our photomicrograph because we view the Images in Clinical Medicine section as a vehicle for illustrating particularly attractive visual aspects of medicine rather than as a forum for the dissemination of diagnostic or therapeutic opinions.

We take exception to Dr. Mönkemüller's statement, "The best evidence of a cure [of *H. pylori* infection] is the absence of recurrent symptoms of an ulcer." Although this strategy may be the cheapest one, it may not be the best. Patients with ulcers in whom a combined regimen consisting of an antibiotic and a proton-pump inhibitor has failed to eradicate *H. pylori* may still have prolonged relief of symptoms, and the ulcer may then recur with a classic presentation or, in some patients, with a catastrophic event, such as an upper gastrointestinal hemorrhage. The possibility of such consequences should be a factor in the equation used to assess the cost effectiveness of a procedure or a test.

We do not believe that post-treatment upper endoscopic examinations or urea breath tests are needed in all patients, but using a reliable and relatively inexpensive noninvasive test such as the urea breath test may be better than letting treatment failures announce themselves catastrophically.

Robert M. Genta, M.D.
David Y. Graham, M.D.
Veterans Affairs Medical Center
Houston, TX 77030

Porcelain Gallbladder

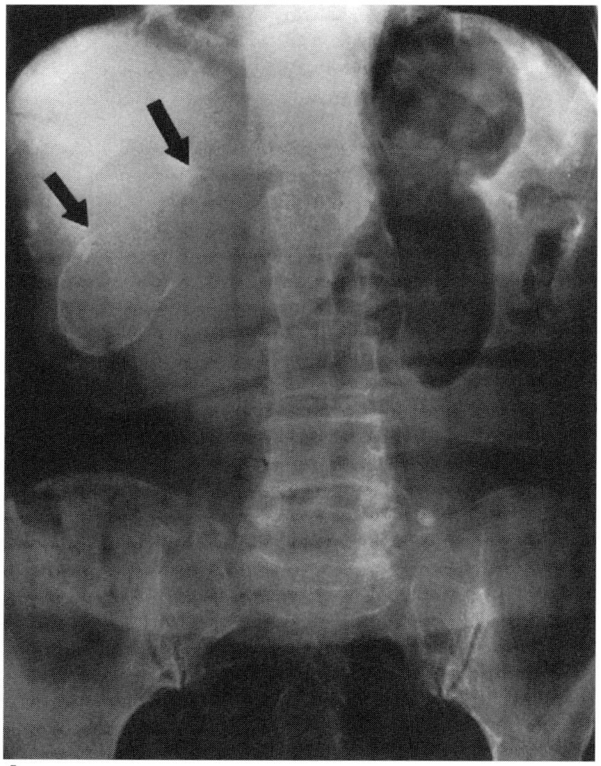
A

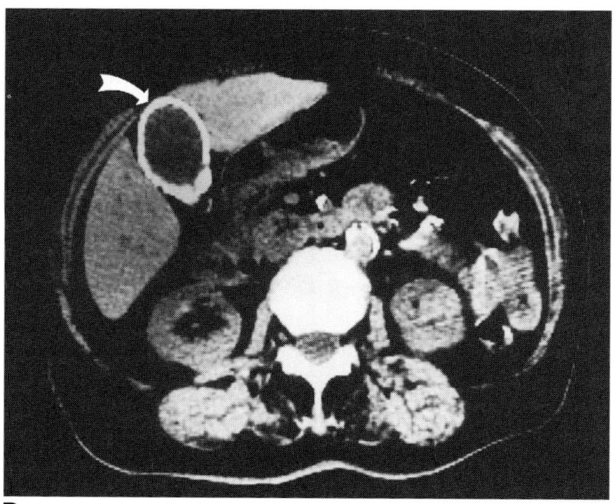
B

The entire wall of the gallbladder is calcified in an 86-year-old woman with anemia probably caused by a slowly bleeding hiatal hernia. The patient had no abdominal symptoms. The border of the gallbladder is evident on a plain film of the abdomen (Panel A, arrows). The calcified rim can be seen on a computed tomographic scan without contrast enhancement (Panel B, arrow). Gallstones are not present.

Tze Shien Lo, M.D.
Masanobu Okada, M.D.

Nagoya Tokushukai Hospital
Aichi 487, Japan

February 10, 1994

Correspondence

Porcelain Gallbladder

June 30, 1994

To the Editor: In the clinical image of porcelain gallbladder (Feb. 10 issue),[1] Lo and Okada state, "The entire wall of the gallbladder is calcified. . . ." This statement is not entirely correct. The calcifications in porcelain gallbladder are seen often in the wall of the corpus and less frequently in the fundus. Typically, the ostium of the gallbladder is spared; therefore, porcelain gallbladder presents radiographically as a U-shaped calcification with a cephalad open end, as shown in the plain film of the abdomen in Panel A (lower arrow). Therefore, the upper arrow in Panel A does not indicate part of a calcified gallbladder wall but, in my opinion, either calcified rib cartilage or, less likely, a small gallstone in the fundus.

Only the single, large, calcified gallstone (*Tonnenstein*) — the main other entity in the differential diagnosis of porcelain gallbladder — presents as a closed ring of calcification.

This particular condition was named porcelain gallbladder because of the blue discoloration and brittle consistency of the gallbladder wall.[2,3]

Martin C. Freund, M.D.
Mannheim Hospital
D-68135 Mannheim, Germany

1. Lo TS, Okada M. Porcelain gallbladder. N Engl J Med 1994;330:402.
2. Osler W. The principles and practice of medicine. 10th ed. St. Louis: C.V. Mosby, 1925: 1214-5.
3. Berk RN, Burhenne HJ. Radiology of the gallbladder. In: Margulis AR, Burhenne HJ, eds. Alimentary tract radiology. 4th ed. Vol. 2. St. Louis: C.V. Mosby, 1989:1214-5.

The authors reply:

To the Editor: Dr. Freund points out that the upper arrow in Panel A of our image does not point to the calcified gallbladder wall but, in his opinion, either to calcified rib cartilage or to a small gallstone in the fundus. However, judging from the shape and the position of the area in Panel A, the likelihood of its being calcified rib cartilage is very low.

We sliced the gallbladder in 5-mm sections from the neck to the fundus, using computed tomographic scanning, but no gallstone was found inside the gallbladder. Therefore, what looks like a round gallstone in the neck of the gallbladder (the upper arrow in Panel A) is actually part of the neck of the calcified bladder shown in a cross-sectional view.

We think that this case of porcelain gallbladder is rare in the sense that it does not contain any gallstones. It is known that gallstones are present in nearly all instances of porcelain gallbladder.[1]

Tze Shien Lo, M.D.
Masanobu Okada, M.D.
Nagoya Tokushukai Hospital
Aichi 487, Japan

1. Berk RN, Maglinte DDT. Conventional radiology of the biliary tract. In: Berk JE, ed. Bockus gastroenterology, 4th ed. Vol. 6. Philadelphia: W.B. Saunders, 1985:3520-1.

Cholelithiasis and Choledocholithiasis

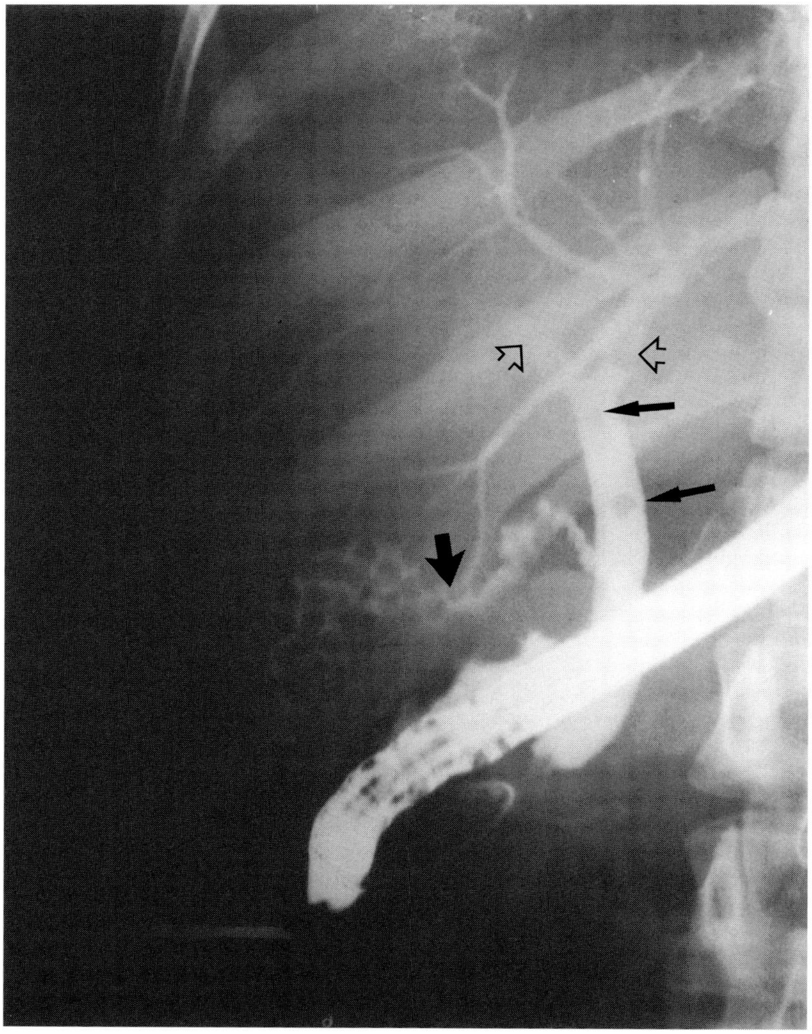

An endoscopic retrograde cholangiogram from a 20-year-old woman with pain in the right upper quadrant and jaundice reveals stones in the left and right hepatic ducts (open arrows) and the common bile duct (small arrows) and multiple stones in the gallbladder (large arrow). The common bile duct is dilated, but the intrahepatic ducts are normal. A sphincterotomy was performed, the stones were extracted, and the patient had an uneventful laparoscopic cholecystectomy the following day.

Alexandra L. Gibas, M.D.
Craig Philpot, M.D.

Case Western Reserve University
Cleveland, OH 44106

February 11, 1993

Impacted Stone in the Ampulla of Vater

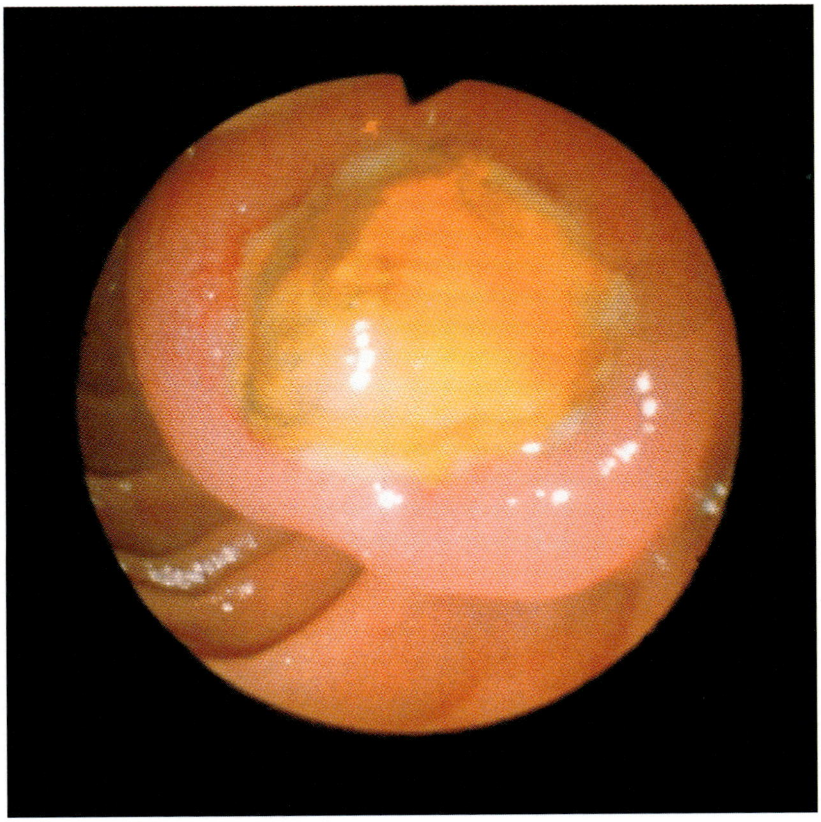

An impacted common-duct stone is visible in the ampulla of Vater in a patient with suppurative cholangitis. White or tan pus can be seen draining around the margin of the calculus.

P. Gregory Foutch, D.O., M.S.

Desert Samaritan Medical Center
Mesa, AZ 85202

January 28, 1993

Gallstone Ileus

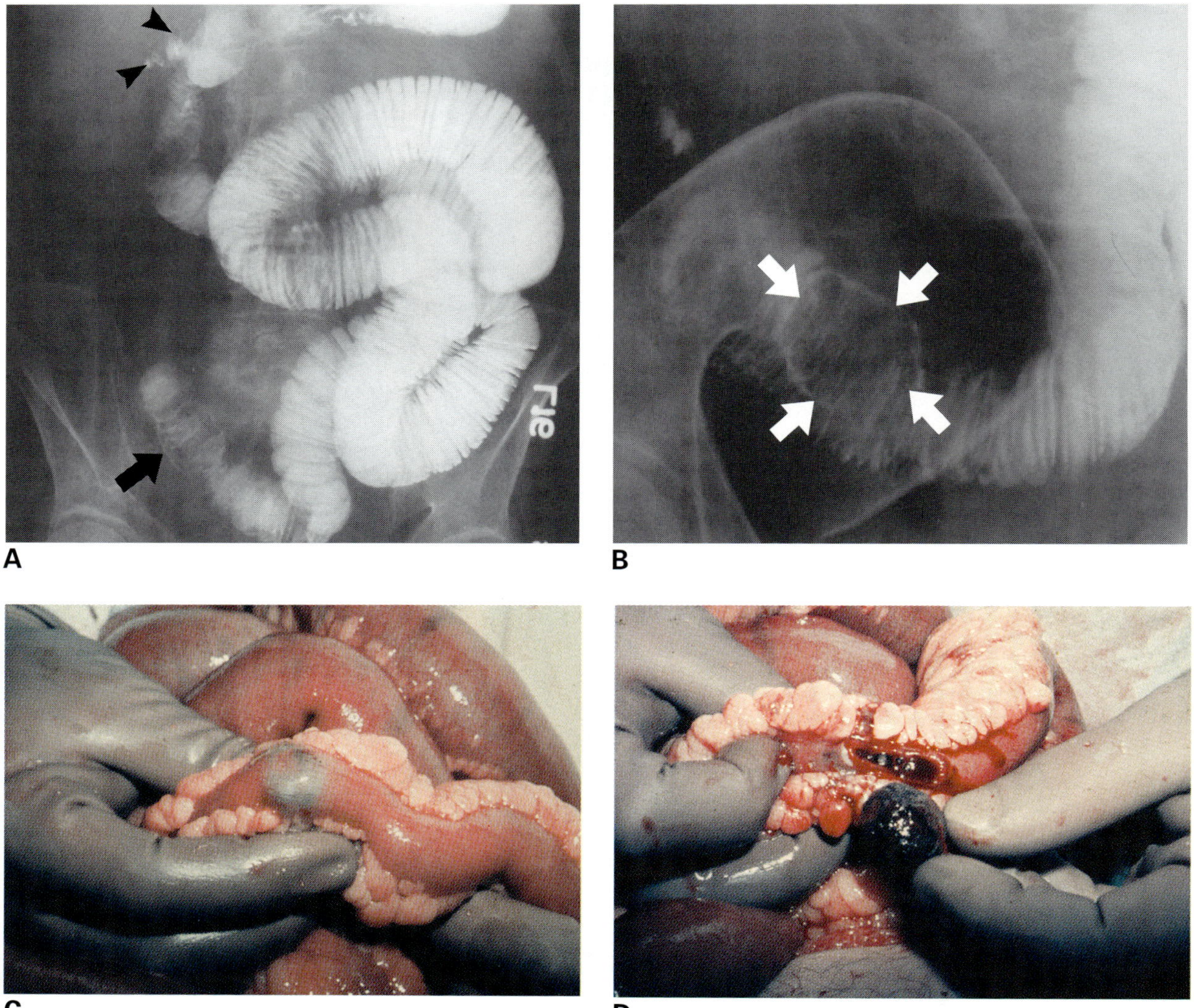

Seven days before admission, nausea and crampy abdominal pain developed in a 65-year-old woman with a history of cholecystitis and cholelithiasis. Two days before admission, the pain became more intense, and she vomited, had no bowel move-ments, and passed no gas. A posteroanterior radiograph obtained during a barium examination of the small bowel shows an irregular collection of barium in the right upper quadrant (Panel A, arrowheads), representing partial filling of the cystic duct. Both jejunum and ileum are markedly dilated, with dilution of the barium in a pattern consistent with small-bowel obstruction. There is abrupt termination of the barium column at the site of an oval intraluminal filling defect (Panel A, arrow). A view of the end of the barium column shows luminal obstruction by a smooth intraluminal mass (Panel B, arrows) with faint calcification of the peripheral rim. Exploratory laparotomy revealed a foreign body in the terminal ileum that was 4 cm by 4 cm and felt hard (Panel C). A gallstone was extracted through a transverse incision (Panel D). The entire length of the intestine was examined in search of other gallstones, but none were found. The patient recovered uneventfully.

Ernesto P. Molmenti, M.D.

Washington University
School of Medicine
St. Louis, MO 63110

September 26, 1996

Correspondence

Gallstone Ileus

March 20, 1997

To the Editor: Gallstone ileus results in considerable morbidity and mortality. Ileus is due to obstruction of the bowel by a large biliary stone that wedges in the terminal ileum or any other intestinal location (e.g., the colon). Prior formation of a cholecystoenteric fistula is common and has usually resulted from gallstone perforation of the duodenum or the colon. The occurrence of subsequent pneumobilia provides a strong clue to the diagnosis of gallstone ileus, but it is not found in all patients. Nonetheless, barium examination should be avoided in cases of acute abdominal illness.

First, barium administration in a patient such as the one described in Images in Clinical Medicine (Sept. 26 issue)[1] is inappropriate. The patient had prolonged complete ileus, since she had had two days without bowel movements or passage of gas. In such circumstances, barium administration may aggravate symptoms of ileus as a result of barium-induced impaction, particularly in a paralytic bowel or in the presence of a prestenotic colon segment.

Second, this approach should not be used if there is a possibility of impaired intestinal viability or gastrointestinal perforation, because extravasation of barium into the peritoneal cavity can precipitate a severe and potentially fatal inflammatory response.[2]

Finally, in a patient with a two-day history of complete ileus, treatment should not be delayed any further by time-consuming imaging studies. But, on the basis of the history, clinical findings, and sonograms and plain abdominal radiographs showing possible pneumobilia or an ectopic gallstone, the patient should undergo emergency surgery (open laparotomy or laparoscopy[3]) shortly after admission, regardless of whether a definitive diagnosis has been established preoperatively.

Andreas M. Kaiser, M.D.
University Hospital
CH-8091 Zurich, Switzerland

1. Molmenti EP. Gallstone ileus. N Engl J Med 1996;335:942.
2. Yamamura M, Nishi M, Furubayashi H, Hioki K, Yamamoto M. Barium peritonitis: report of a case and review of the literature. Dis Colon Rectum 1985;28:347-52.
3. Montgomery A. Laparoscope-guided enterolithotomy for gallstone ileus. Surg Laparosc Endosc 1993;3:310-4.

Dr. Molmenti replies:

To the Editor: Dr. Kaiser bases his arguments on an isolated case report[1] of barium peritonitis after a double-contrast colonic enema treated with irrigation and urokinase solution. He fails to justify avoiding the performance of a diagnostic upper gastrointestinal study in our patient, who presented without peritoneal signs, pneumobilia, or a history of surgery. Furthermore, initial films on admission showed a small amount of air in the colon and mostly fluid in the small bowel.

A search of the literature reveals multiple references to the use of contrast studies (such as the one we used) in the diagnosis of gallstone ileus.[2-4]

Correspondence Continued

Dr. Kaiser also suggests that in a patient such as ours emergency surgery would have been appropriate. As stated in a textbook of modern surgical practice,[5] "a patient in whom fluid and electrolyte imbalance develops after several days of illness may profit from 18 to 24 hours of preoperative preparation." Indeed, the chief threat to the life of a patient such as ours may lie in the performance of "emergency surgery" without further preoperative preparation rather than in an imaging study. Our patient underwent surgery 18 hours after admission.

Ernesto P. Molmenti, M.D.
University of Pittsburgh
Pittsburgh, PA 15213

1. Yamamura M, Nishi M, Furubayashi H, Hioki K, Yamamoto M. Barium peritonitis: report of a case and review of the literature. Dis Colon Rectum 1985;28:347-52.
2. Reisner RM, Cohen JR. Gallstone ileus: a review of 1001 reported cases. Am Surg 1994;60:441-6.
3. Morrissey KP, McSherry CK. In: Blumgart LH, ed. Surgery of the liver and alimentary tract. 2nd ed. New York: Churchill Livingstone, 1994.
4. Clavien PA, Richon J, Burgan S, Rohner A. Gallstone ileus. Br J Surg 1990;77:737-42.
5. Jones RS. Intestinal obstruction. In: Sabiston DC, ed. Textbook of surgery: the biological basis of modern surgical practice. 15th ed. Philadelphia: W.B. Saunders, 1997:919.

Vasculitis and Cryoglobulinemia Related to Hepatitis C

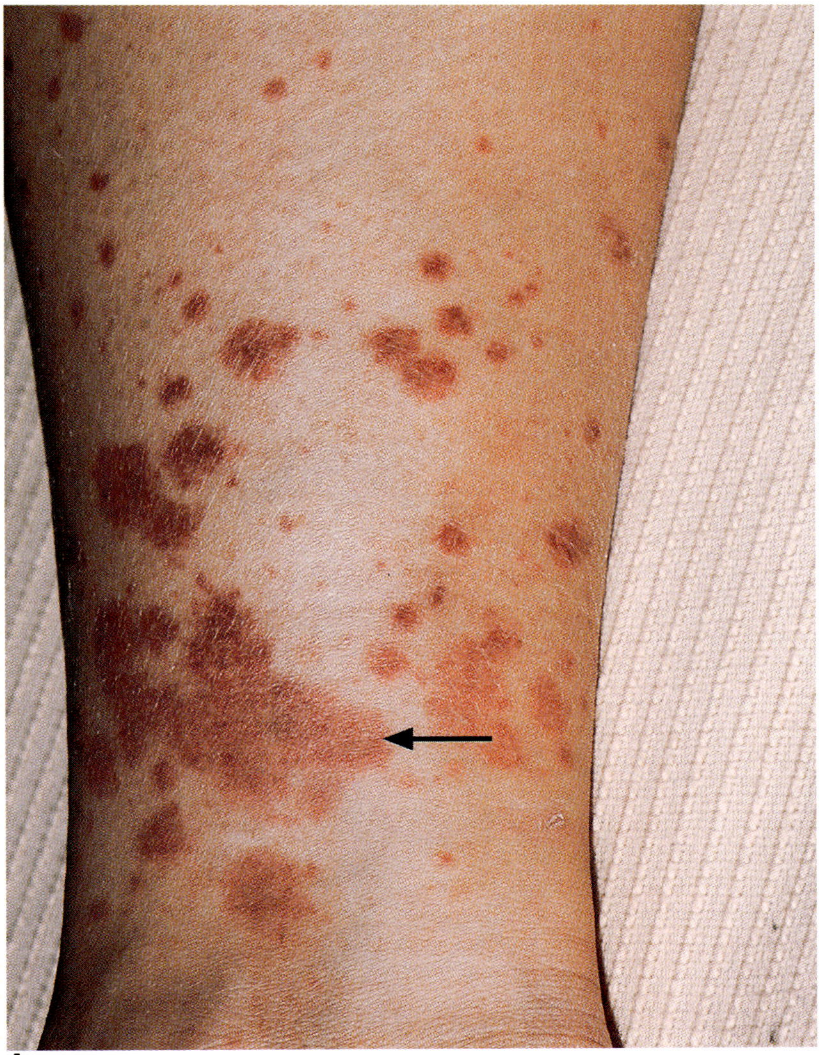

A

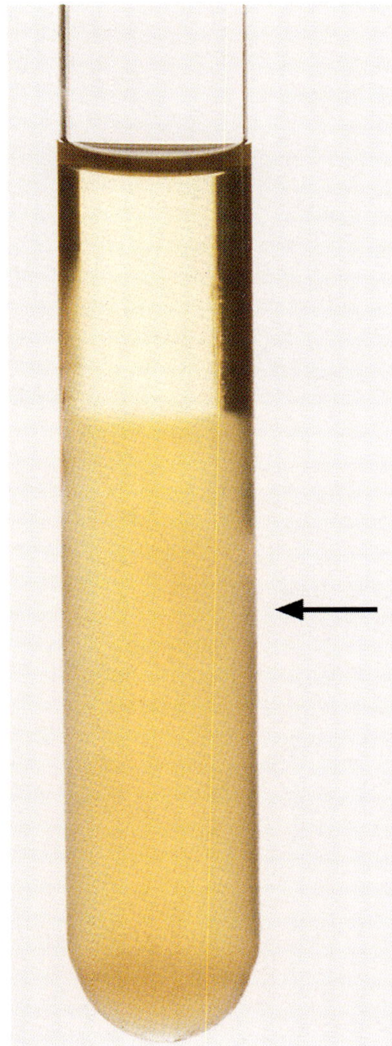

B

A 51-year-old woman with chronic hepatitis C virus (HCV) infection and type II cryoglobulinemia reported fatigue, pain in her ankles, and recurrent crops of superficial vasculitic lesions on her legs. She had no evidence of renal involvement. Antibodies to HCV and HCV RNA were detectable in serum, and serum aminotransferase concentrations were elevated.

Panel A shows the medial aspect of the patient's lower leg; the arrow indicates an area of palpable purpura approximately 2 cm by 3 cm. Panel B shows the patient's uncentrifuged serum after 48 hours at 4°C; the arrow indicates cryoprecipitate. After centrifugation, the cryocrit was 6 percent. Subsequent evaluation showed that the cryoglobulins were composed of polyclonal IgG and IgM kappa chains. The patient was treated with interferon alfa (3 million units three times weekly) for six months. Mild fatigue persisted after treatment began, but joint pains subsided within a few weeks and the skin lesions disappeared within three months. Serum aminotransferase concentrations never returned to normal. When interferon alfa was discontinued, the joint pains and skin lesions recurred.

A. Obaid Shakil, M.D.

Adrian M. Di Bisceglie, M.D.
National Institutes of Health
Bethesda, MD 20892

December 15, 1994

Primary Biliary Cirrhosis

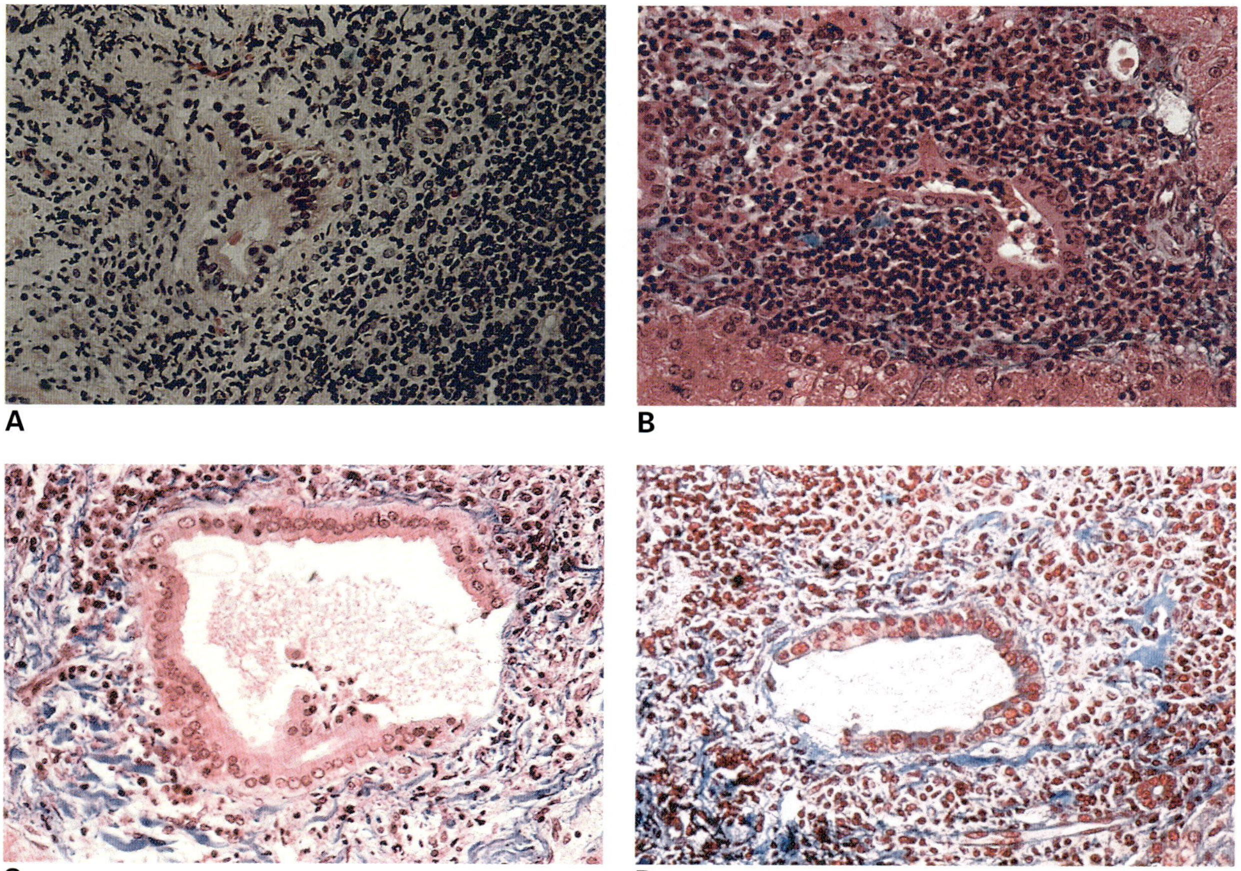

A B C D

Stage I lesions in primary biliary cirrhosis are seen in these slides, with typical destruction of small bile ducts by lymphocytes. In Panels A and B, a small bile duct is surrounded and infiltrated by lymphocytes. In Panels C and D, there is eccentric destruction of bile-duct cells. As the disease progresses, more bile ducts are destroyed, and in the late stages of the disease there is a characteristic paucity of bile ducts.

Marshall M. Kaplan, M.D.

New England Medical Center
Boston, MA 02111

April 29, 1993

Bleeding Esophageal Varices

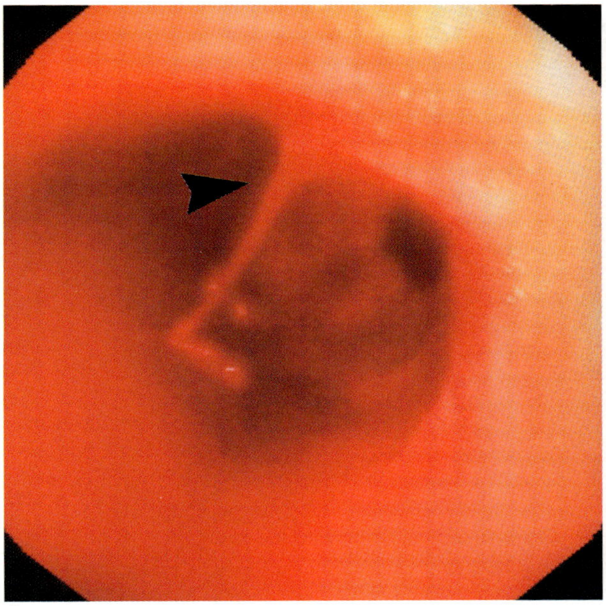

A

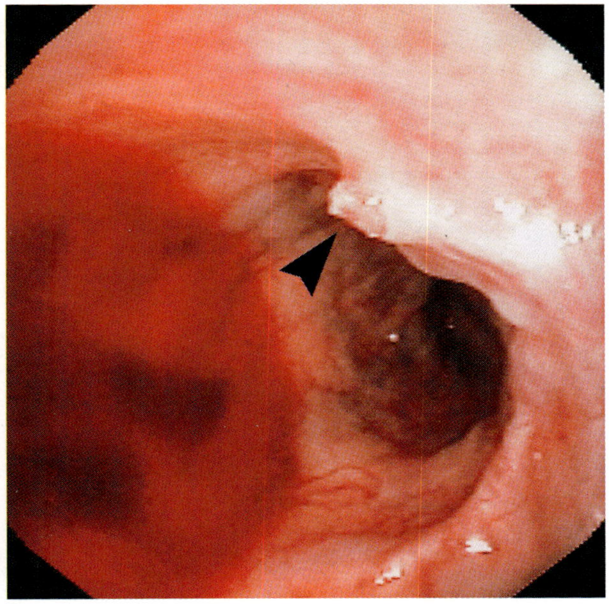

B

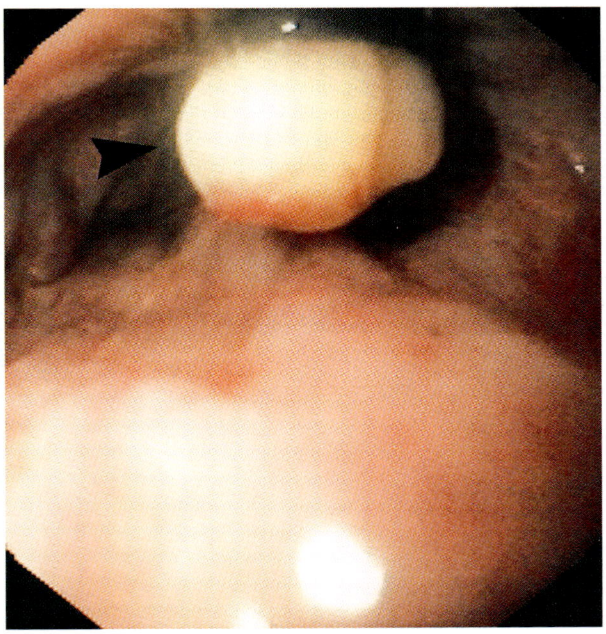

C

In an endoscopic photograph of the esophagus of a 56-year-old alcoholic man with massive hematemesis, blood can be seen spurting from a ruptured varix (arrow, Panel A). After injection sclerotherapy of the variceal trunk and immediate hemostasis, the source of bleeding was revealed as a white nipple, which represents what was thought to be a fibrin–platelet plug (arrow, Panel B). Endoscopic variceal ligation was performed for recurrent bleeding from the same source three weeks after the initial episode. The white object in Panel C (arrow) is the remnant of a banded varix.

Victor Navarro, M.D.
Adrian Reuben, M.B., B.S.

Yale University School of Medicine
New Haven, CT 06510

October 27, 1994

Transjugular Intrahepatic Portosystemic Shunt

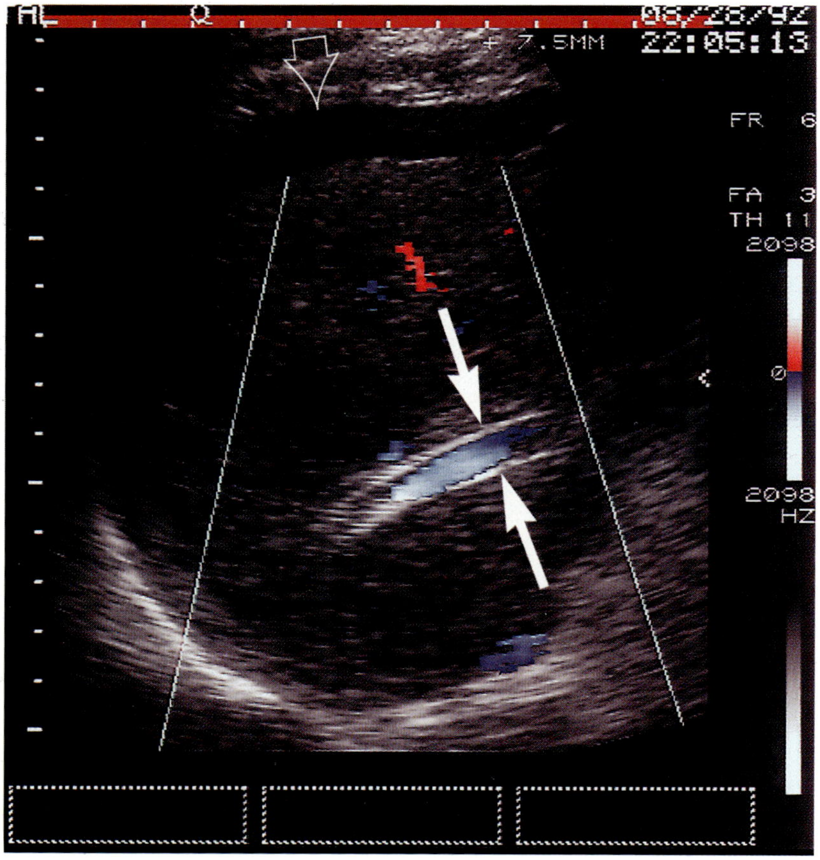

This hepatic Doppler sonogram in a 55-year-old man with alcoholic cirrhosis and portal hypertension shows the successful placement of a transjugular intrahepatic portosystemic shunt. The procedure was performed because of refractory and debilitating ascites. The shunt shows characteristic echogenicity (solid arrows), along with an intense (blue) signal from the shunted blood. Ascites (open arrow) is present anterior to the liver. After the placement of the shunt, the patient's esophageal varices regressed and the ascites improved without further therapy, until the shunt became thrombosed eight months later. The patient is currently awaiting liver transplantation.

Michael A. Sadler, M.D.
Robert S. Shapiro, M.D.

Mount Sinai School of Medicine
New York, NY 10029-6574

January 20, 1994

Infarct Cavities in a Hepatic Allograft

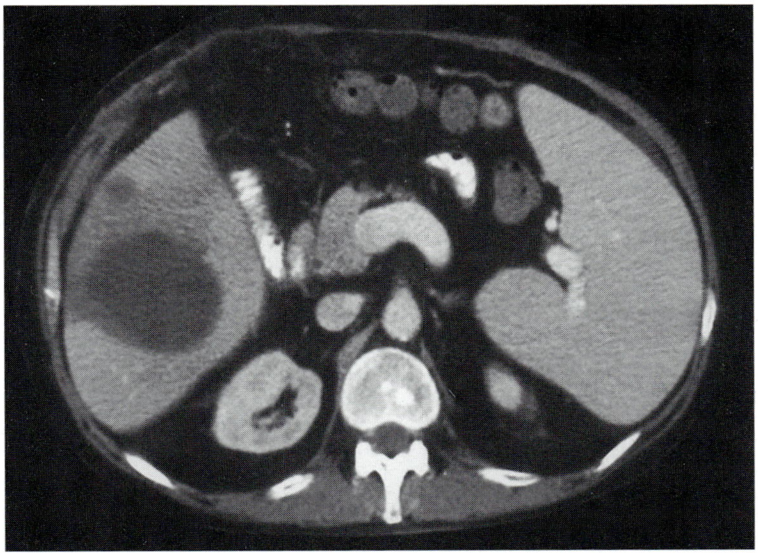

A

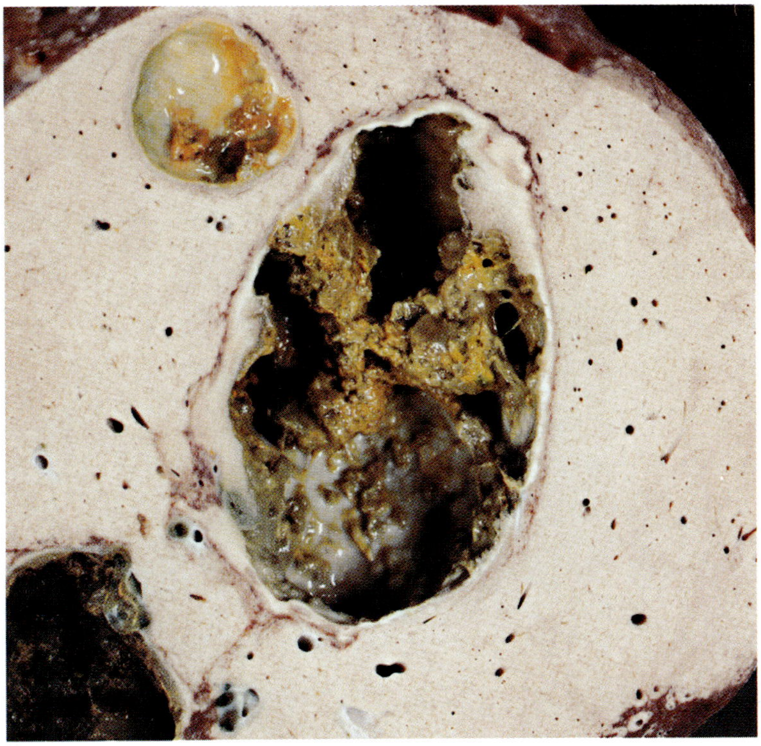

B

A 49-year-old man underwent liver transplantation in 1989 for alcoholic cirrhosis. In 1994, ischemic cholangitis developed with strictures and signs of ascending cholangitis, leading to a second transplantation. Three weeks later, blood cultures were positive for *Clostridium clostridiiforme.* Angiography and ultrasonography revealed hepatic-artery thrombosis. A computed tomographic scan (Panel A) of the second allograft showed intrahepatic cavities. A culture from a cavity contained *Enterococcus faecalis* and coagulase-negative staphylococci. Because of these complications, the second allograft had to be removed. The specimen contained large, multiloculated ischemic infarcts with extensive central cavitation (Panel B). The patient is doing well nine months after receiving his third allograft.

Jurgen Ludwig, M.D.
Gregory J. Gores, M.D.

Mayo Clinic
Rochester, MN 55905

October 26, 1995

Polyp of the Appendix

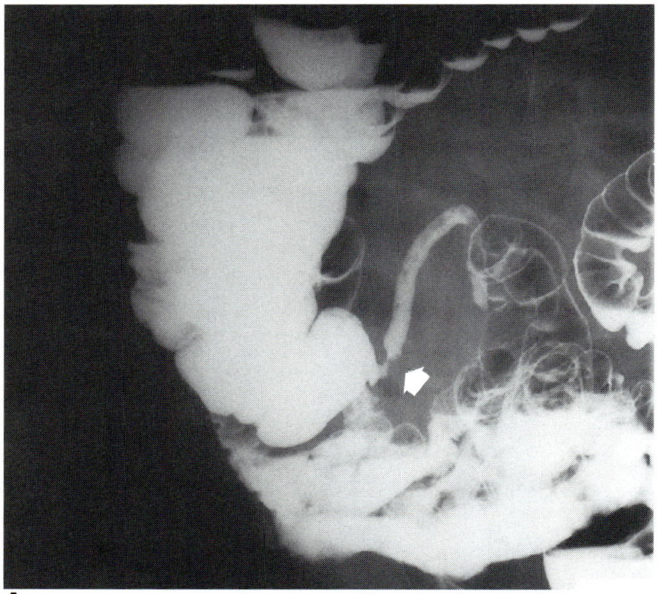

A

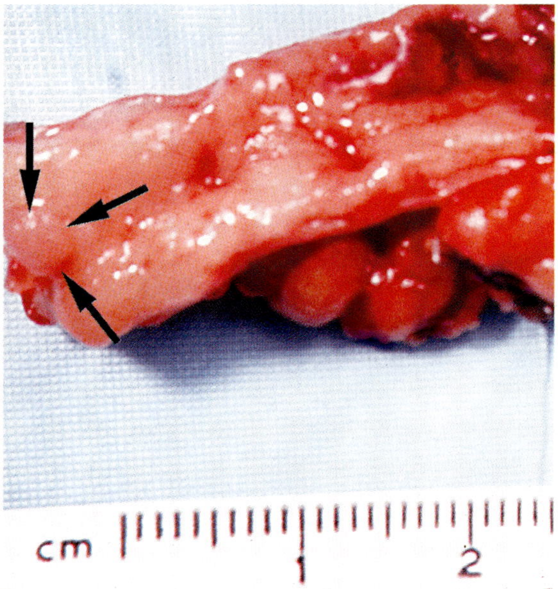

B

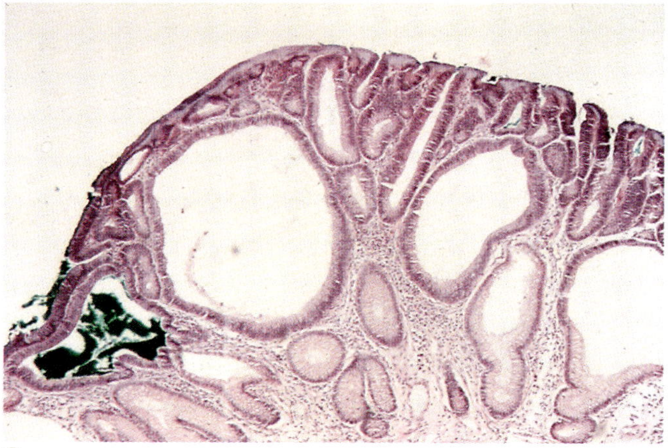

C

An asymptomatic filling defect of the appendix was discovered during a barium enema (arrow, Panel A) in a 72-year-old woman during an evaluation for persistently guaiac-positive stools. After laparoscopic appendectomy, a 5-mm sessile polypoid lesion was found at the base of the appendix (arrows, Panel B). (The specimen was opened longitudinally.) Histologic analysis (Panel C) showed the lesion to be an adenomatous polyp (hematoxylin and eosin, ×10). Extensive studies of the gastrointestinal tract failed to disclose the source of bleeding, but it was thought to be due either to the use of nonsteroidal antiinflammatory agents or to diverticulitis of the left colon. The appendiceal polyp was probably not the cause of bleeding.

Robert P. Sticca, M.D.
Michael L. Palmer, M.D.

Roswell Park Cancer Institute
Buffalo, NY 14263

December 2, 1993

Correspondence

Polyp of the Appendix

April 21, 1994

To the Editor: The case of a polyp of the appendix described by Sticca and Palmer in the Images in Clinical Medicine section (Dec. 2 issue)[1] reflects what is terribly wrong with American medicine today. First of all, most would agree that persistently guaiac-positive stools should be evaluated colonoscopically, not radiographically, since such an examination would detect angiodysplasias and allow therapeutic maneuvers such as polypectomy. Furthermore, the authors state that the tiny appendiceal polyp was probably not the cause of bleeding. Why, therefore, was the patient subjected to a laparoscopic appendectomy? Finally, diverticulitis is generally not an asymptomatic condition and is not generally associated with guaiac-positive stools but rather with occasional torrential hemorrhage.

Thus, although the radiograph obtained after a barium enema and the views of the pathological specimen certainly demonstrate an interesting curiosity, the clinical vignette that accompanies them suggests that an inappropriate diagnostic test resulted in an inappropriate therapeutic intervention.

Steven Brozinsky, M.D.
752 Medical Center Court
Chula Vista, CA 91911

1. Sticca RP, Palmer ML. Polyp of the appendix. N Engl J Med 1993;329:1709.

The authors reply:

To the Editor: The patient we described had persistent guaiac-positive stools over a two-year period, and she was evaluated endoscopically through both the upper and lower gastrointestinal tracts on her initial presentation. The cause of the occult blood loss was not found, and after a prolonged period a barium enema was ordered. The mass in the appendix was an incidental finding, and colonoscopy was performed to attempt to visualize the mass, obtain a biopsy specimen, and possibly remove the lesion. When the lesion could not be removed through the endoscope, appendectomy was performed, because we were concerned that the polyp might be malignant or premalignant. We recognized, of course, that the incidence of adenocarcinoma of the appendix and adenomatous polyps of the appendix is low, approximately 0.1 percent in most series.[1,2]

We believe that any lesion with a malignant potential in an otherwise healthy patient should be removed whether it is an incidental finding or a cause of clinical symptoms.

Robert P. Sticca, M.D.
Greenville Hospital System
Greenville, SC 29605

Michael L. Palmer, M.D.
Foxhall Surgical Associates
Washington, DC 20016

1. Collins DC. 71,000 Human appendix specimens: a final report, summarizing forty years' study. Am J Proctol 1963;14:365-81.
2. Wolff M, Ahmed N. Epithelial neoplasms of the vermiform appendix (exclusive of carcinoid). II. Cystadenomas, papillary adenomas, and adenomatous polyps of the appendix. Cancer 1976;37:2511-22.

Giant Colonic Diverticulum

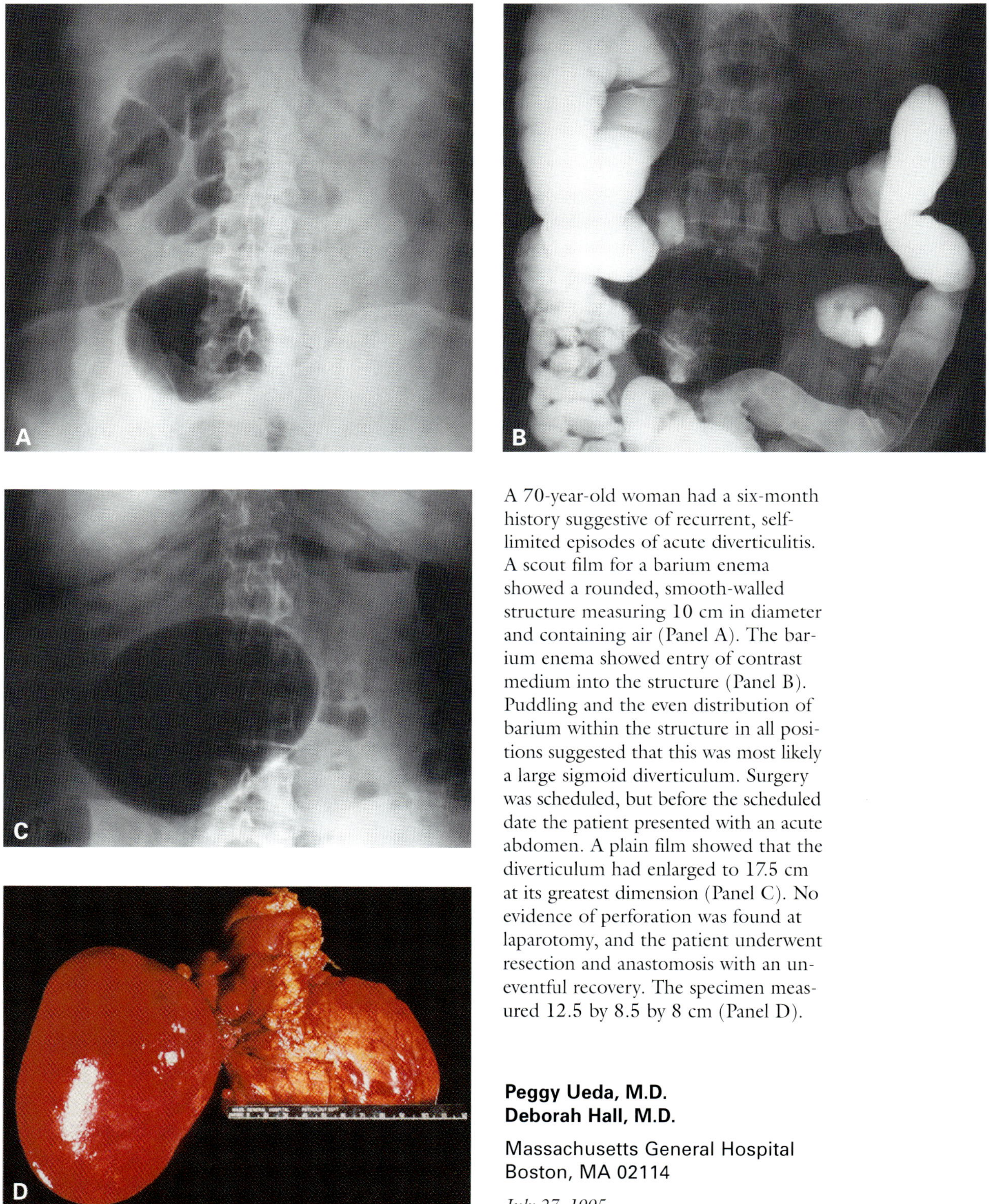

A 70-year-old woman had a six-month history suggestive of recurrent, self-limited episodes of acute diverticulitis. A scout film for a barium enema showed a rounded, smooth-walled structure measuring 10 cm in diameter and containing air (Panel A). The barium enema showed entry of contrast medium into the structure (Panel B). Puddling and the even distribution of barium within the structure in all positions suggested that this was most likely a large sigmoid diverticulum. Surgery was scheduled, but before the scheduled date the patient presented with an acute abdomen. A plain film showed that the diverticulum had enlarged to 17.5 cm at its greatest dimension (Panel C). No evidence of perforation was found at laparotomy, and the patient underwent resection and anastomosis with an uneventful recovery. The specimen measured 12.5 by 8.5 by 8 cm (Panel D).

Peggy Ueda, M.D.
Deborah Hall, M.D.

Massachusetts General Hospital
Boston, MA 02114

July 27, 1995

Correspondence

Giant Colonic Diverticulum

December 14, 1995

To the Editor: The legend to the Image in Clinical Medicine by Ueda and Hall showing a giant colonic diverticulum (July 27 issue)[1] suggests that the patient's recurrent episodes of pain were causally related to the giant diverticulum of the sigmoid colon. Although that may be true, a noninflamed diverticulum that has not undergone torsion, even if it has enlarged, is unlikely to cause such acute episodes of pain.

The term "acute abdomen" used to describe the circumstances that led to an emergency operation is an unfortunate one, giving no clue to the cause of the pain. The barium enema shows an extremely redundant ascending colon and hepatic flexure, and a cecum and ileum high in the right abdomen, an anatomical precursor of so-called cecal volvulus. Did the surgeon assess this area at operation (although spontaneous detorsion may have occurred), and has the patient had further attacks of pain?

William Silen, M.D.
Robert G. Sheiman, M.D.
Beth Israel Hospital
Boston, MA 02215

1. Ueda P, Hall D. Giant colonic diverticulum. N Engl J Med 1995;333:228.

Dr. Ueda replies:

To the Editor: These questions present the opportunity to fill out this patient's history, which was quite interesting.

The patient told a curious story of a feeling of warmth in the pelvic area, with chills in the extremities, that had occurred four times over the previous year. The onset of these symptoms always followed a normal void, and the symptoms lasted two days and were accompanied by a temperature reaching 38.3°C. She also said that for six months she had felt as if she had a lump in her lower abdomen that seemed to move from side to side and was particularly noticeable with recumbency. She had long-standing constipation. The abdominal examination on this first visit did raise a question of a mass in the right lower quadrant, with tympany to percussion over this area. A pelvic examination was normal. Pelvic ultrasonography showed a hypoechoic uterine mass, probably representing a fibroid in the right adnexa.

Before further evaluation was undertaken, the patient presented at the end of a typical episode. She described a temperature of 38.9°C two days earlier, possibly with a rigor, and dysuria, crampy right-lower-quadrant and suprapubic pain, and one episode of vomiting. Her symptoms were relieved by acetaminophen. At the visit she was afebrile and had no other signs of systemic infection. Her examination was notable only for moderate tenderness in the right lower quadrant, with flatness to percussion and mild right costovertebral tenderness. An examination of urinary sediment was unremarkable (and a culture subsequently negative), and a complete blood count was normal.

Correspondence Continued

At this point I asked whether the patient's symptoms could be explained simply by recurrent episodes of self-limited diverticulitis. A barium enema was performed in the hope of clarifying the situation, as well as to rule out more serious bowel disease. The finding of the giant diverticulum was frankly a surprise, but in retrospect it may indeed explain her symptoms. Specifically, the Valsalva maneuver involved in voiding may have forced additional colonic gas into an already enlarged diverticulum, with resulting acute distention and transient bacteremia.

At surgery, in addition to the giant diverticulum, moderate sigmoid diverticulosis was found. It is entirely possible that any of these diverticula may have accounted for previous symptomatic episodes. None were inflamed at laparotomy, and the colon was otherwise normal. The rectosigmoid was resected, along with the right fallopian tube and ovary, because the giant diverticulum adhered to these structures. Since her surgery, which occurred almost three years ago, the patient has had no further symptoms.

Peggy Ueda, M.D.
Massachusetts General Hospital
Boston, MA 02114

Multiple Jejunoileal Diverticula

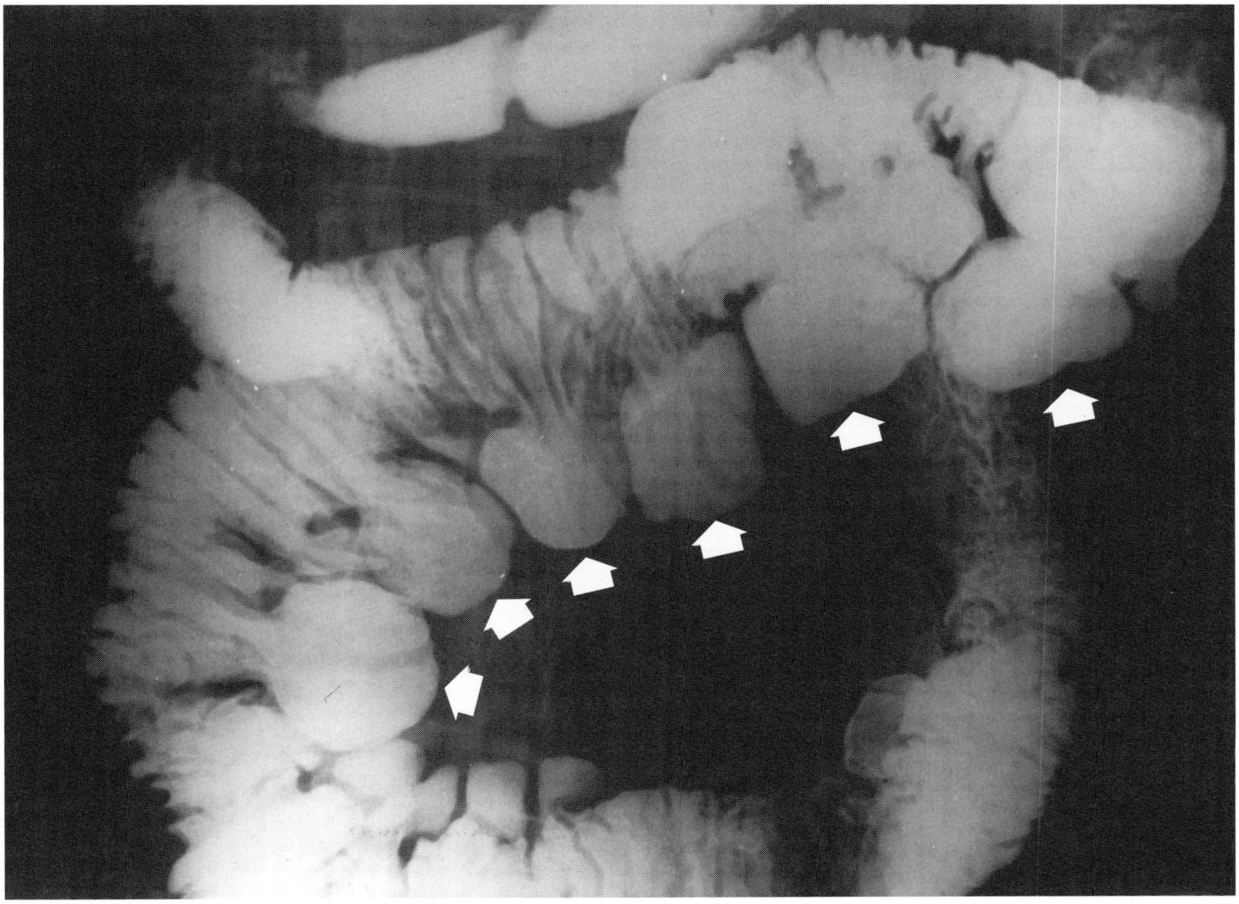

An 82-year-old man with a one-year history of diarrhea, steatorrhea (20 g of fat per day), and massive weight loss (20 kg) was suspected of having pancreatic carcinoma. The results of gastroduodenoscopy and an abdominal computed tomographic scan were normal. Multiple jejunoileal diverticula, without duodenal diverticula, were detected on x-ray films of the small bowel (arrows); their presence doubled the size of the bowel wall. The patient responded dramatically to oral antibiotics, which are an effective treatment for the bacterial overgrowth syndrome associated with small-intestine diverticula.

Claude Matuchansky, M.D.
Yves Lenormand, M.D.

St. Lazare Hospital
Paris, France

January 6, 1994

Diverticulitis

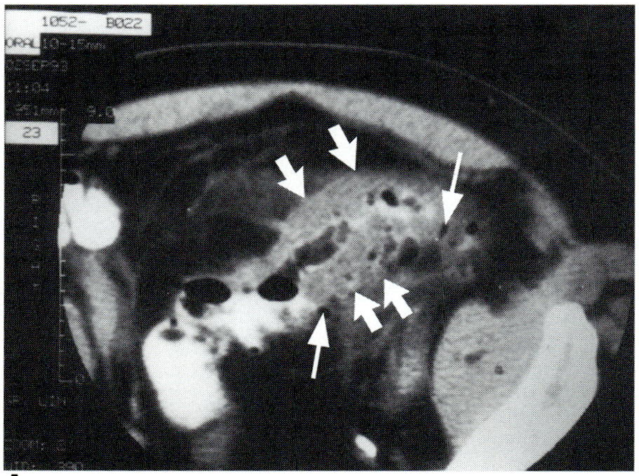

A

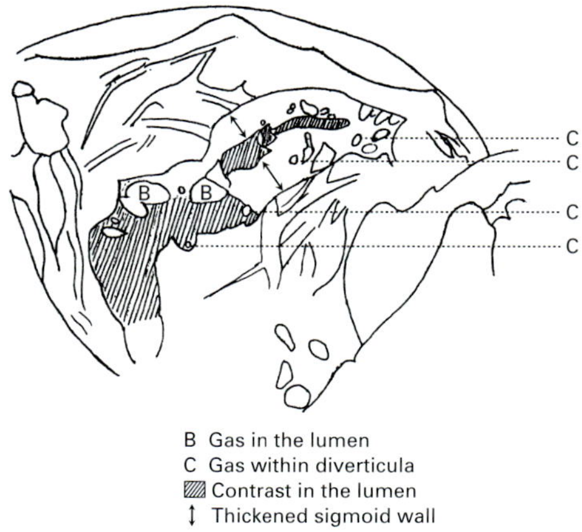

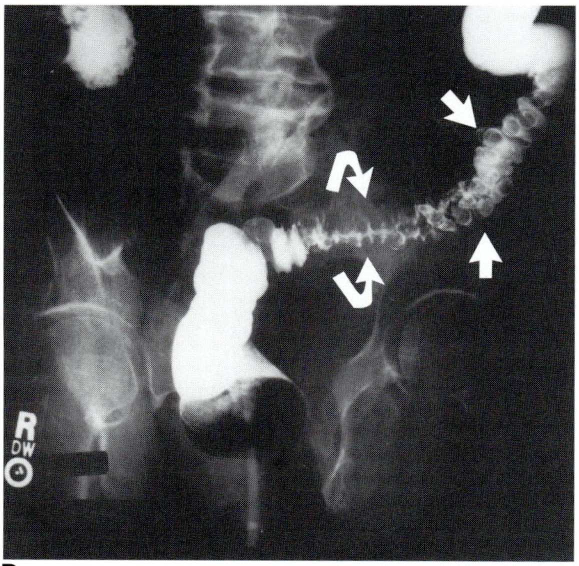

B

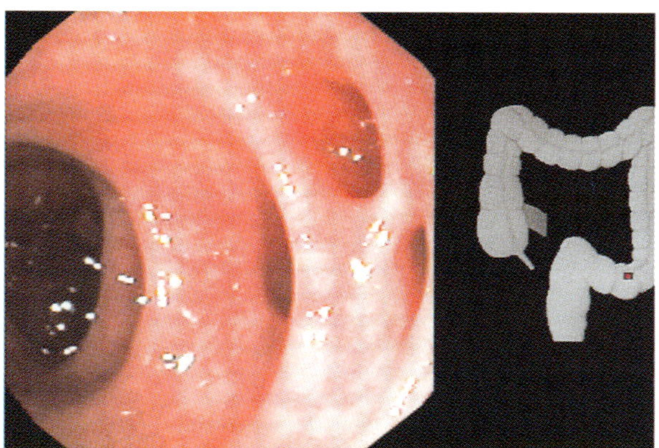

C

A 70-year-old, previously healthy man had had sudden, colicky lower abdominal pain and increased urinary frequency for four days. He had marked suprapubic tenderness but no other abnormal physical findings. There was mild leukocytosis and a slight leftward shift; the results of urinalysis were unremarkable. A computed tomographic (CT) scan of the pelvis obtained on the first hospital day (Panel A and adjacent sketch) shows thickening of the sigmoid colon (thick arrows). The dark areas represent gas in the lumen, and the white areas represent contrast material. The small dark areas (thin arrows) represent gas in diverticula. A low-pressure barium enema (Panel B) performed on the same day revealed moderate narrowing of the distal sigmoid colon due to mucosal thickening and spasm (curved arrows), corresponding to the CT findings, and multiple diverticula in the proximal sigmoid colon (arrows). Within 48 hours of the initiation of therapy with metronidazole and clindamycin, the patient's pain, tenderness, and urinary frequency decreased. Three weeks later, when he was symptom-free, flexible sigmoidoscopy, carried out because of his concern about cancer, revealed wide-mouth diverticula with normal mucosa (Panel C). The patient remained well during 15 months of follow-up.

Rakesh Nanda, M.D.
Jafar Amini, M.D.

Dwight D. Eisenhower Medical Center
Leavenworth, KS 66048

August 24, 1995

Correspondence

Diverticulitis

December 28, 1995

To the Editor: We disagree with some aspects of the studies and therapy of the 70-year-old man with diverticulitis reported by Drs. Nanda and Amini (Aug. 24 issue).[1] We question the need for a barium enema, especially one performed on the same day as the computed tomography (CT). CT is the single best test for the diagnosis of diverticular inflammation. In one study,[2] it revealed inflammation of pericolic fat 98 percent of the time. CT also reveals unsuspected extraluminal disease, such as an abscess, without the risk of barium peritonitis, which may result from a barium enema.

We also question treatment with both metronidazole and clindamycin. This therapy is redundant — one drug or the other should be used, but not both. We use metronidazole because it is much cheaper and involves less risk of pseudomembranous colitis. In addition, we almost always give a drug that protects against gram-negative organisms.[3]

Jonathan David, M.D.
Lisa A. Ozick, M.D.
College of Physicians and Surgeons of Columbia University
New York, NY 10037

1. Nanda R, Amini J. Diverticulitis. N Engl J Med 1995;333:498.
2. Hulnick DH, Megibow AJ, Balthazar EJ, Naidich DP, Bosniak MA. Computed tomography in the evaluation of diverticulitis. Radiology 1984;152:491-5.
3. Ozick LA, Salazar CO, Donelson SS. Pathogenesis, diagnosis, and treatment of diverticular disease of the colon. Gastroenterologist 1994;2:299-310.

To the Editor: The images obtained in a patient with diverticulitis are illustrative and elegant. It is important to point out, however, that the routine use of CT in patients with uncomplicated diverticulitis adds cost without clinical benefit. In the case described, plain abdominal radiography, empirical antibiotic therapy, and observation would have sufficed, with CT reserved for patients with clinical deterioration or a poor response to treatment. Sigmoidoscopy and barium enema are warranted to rule out cancer and confirm the diagnosis of diverticulitis. The proliferation of readily obtainable, noninvasive tests has contributed greatly to the increasing cost of medical care, often with no proof that patients' outcomes are improved.

William Harford, M.D.
Walter L. Peterson, M.D.
University of Texas Southwestern Medical Center
Dallas, TX 75235

To the Editor: Nanda and Amini report using a low-pressure barium enema in a patient with clinical evidence of acute diverticulitis. In such situations, the use of barium is contraindicated. If a perforation is present or if one is created by the instillation of barium, barium peritonitis may result. If there is concern about the diagnosis of acute diverticulitis, a water-soluble material (e.g., Gastrografin,

Correspondence Continued

Squibb) should be used. Wexner and Dailey[1] reported that the early use of an enema containing such material is the most cost-effective means of establishing the diagnosis.

Virendra A. Parikh, M.D.
Parkview Memorial Hospital
Fort Wayne, IN 46805

1. Wexner SD, Dailey TH. The initial management of left lower quadrant peritonitis. Dis Colon Rectum 1986;29:635-8.

The authors reply:

To the Editor: These letters raise important issues in the management of diverticulitis. We agree that CT should be the first test performed if diverticulitis is suspected. If a barium enema is considered, it should be performed by an experienced radiologist under controlled conditions, with a low volume of contrast material at low pressure, and provided there is no contraindication, such as peritonitis or suspected perforation. The radiologist should be asked to limit the study to the colonic segment in question. If there is evidence of severe disease, perforation, or systemic symptoms, treatment with antibiotics should include those that affect gram-negative organisms.

The role of CT as compared with barium enema remains controversial in the diagnosis of diverticulitis.[1,2] Some authors suggest that CT yields a high rate of false negative results and should be reserved for patients whose conditions do not respond to medical treatment or in whom the diagnosis is uncertain.[3] Barium enemas are safe and underused.[1,4] In a study of 102 patients with acute diverticulitis who had barium enemas, there were no complications.[4] Thus, earlier studies do not substantiate the traditionally perceived concern about complications of such enemas.[1,4]

Regarding the type of contrast material used, we believe that contrast enemas can be performed safely with either barium or water-soluble contrast material.[4] Such studies are not indicated if there is any suspicion of a perforation or leak in the colon. In treating our patient, we thought that barium enema would complement the findings of CT, because the diagnosis was in doubt. We believe that the selection of the test really depends on experience, expertise, and availability.

We agree that the second antibiotic (clindamycin) did not particularly add to the spectrum of treatment. On the basis of the CT scan, at the time of drug administration we felt more comfortable providing additional protection against anaerobic microbes. Clindamycin covers some additional gram-positive organisms. In hindsight, we agree that this clinical decision was an empirical one.

Jafar Amini, M.D.
Rakesh Nanda, M.D.
Dwight D. Eisenhower Veterans Affairs Medical Center
Leavenworth, KS 66048

1. Naitove A, Smith RE. Diverticular disease of the colon. In: Sleisenger MH, Fordtran JS, eds. Gastrointestinal diseases: pathophysiology, diagnosis, management. 5th ed. Vol. 2. Philadelphia: W.B. Saunders, 1993:1347-63.
2. Case 16: diverticulitis: In: Stephen DH, ed. Gastrointestinal disease (fourth series) test and syllabus. Reston, Va.: American College of Radiology, 1990:252-64.
3. Schoetz DJ Jr. Uncomplicated diverticulitis: indications for surgery and surgical management. Surg Clin North Am 1993;73:965-74.
4. Johnson CD, Baker ME, Rice RP, Silverman P, Thompson WM. Diagnosis of acute colonic diverticulitis: comparison of barium enema and CT. AJR Am J Roentgenol 1987;148:541-6.

Hepatic Venous Obstruction by a Membranous Web

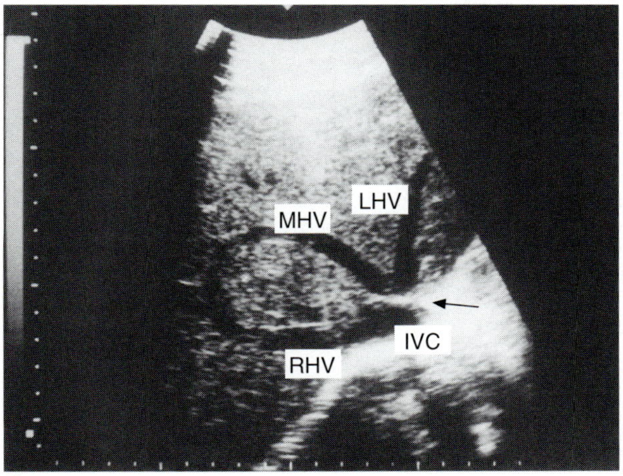

A

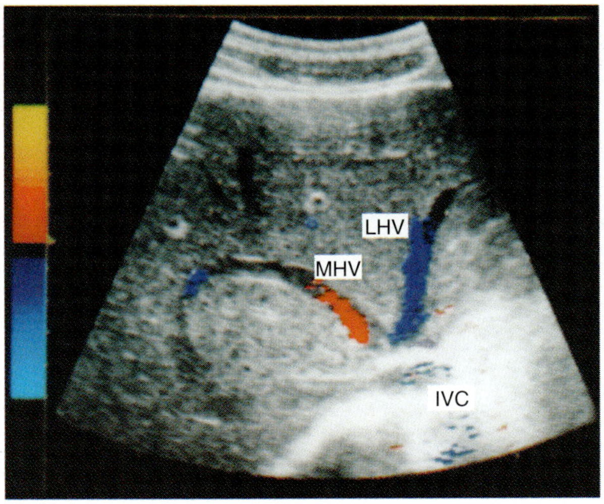

B

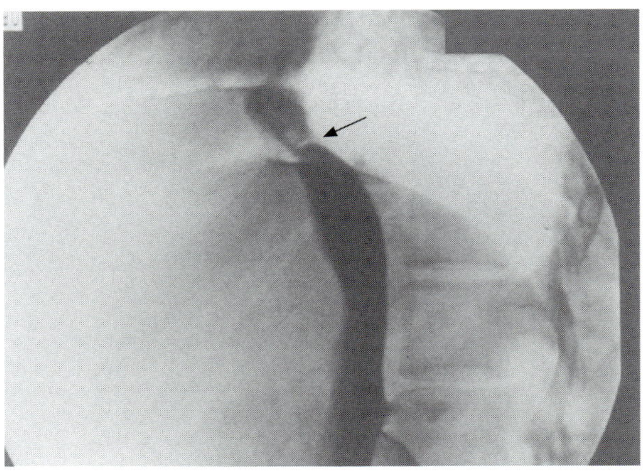

C

Abdominal ultrasonography in a 25-year-old man who reported pain in the right upper quadrant on exertion (Panel A) revealed communicating vessels between the right (RHV) and middle (MHV) hepatic veins and a membranous septum (arrow) at the confluence of the middle and left (LHV) hepatic veins and the inferior vena cava (IVC). Color Doppler imaging confirmed the presence of reversed blood flow in the middle hepatic vein (red segment in Panel B), suggesting the Budd–Chiari syndrome. The diagnosis was confirmed by inferior venacavography (Panel C), which revealed a membranous septum (arrow), about 1 mm thick, above the level of the liver. The patient was treated with percutaneous transluminal angioplasty. Abdominal pain completely disappeared after the procedure, as did the pressure gradient between the thoracic and abdominal inferior vena cava. He remains free of the symptoms 10 months later.

Kenji Kakizaki, M.D.
Hidemi Yamauchi, M.D.

Sendai National Hospital
Sendai 983, Japan

May 9, 1996

Colocolic Fistula

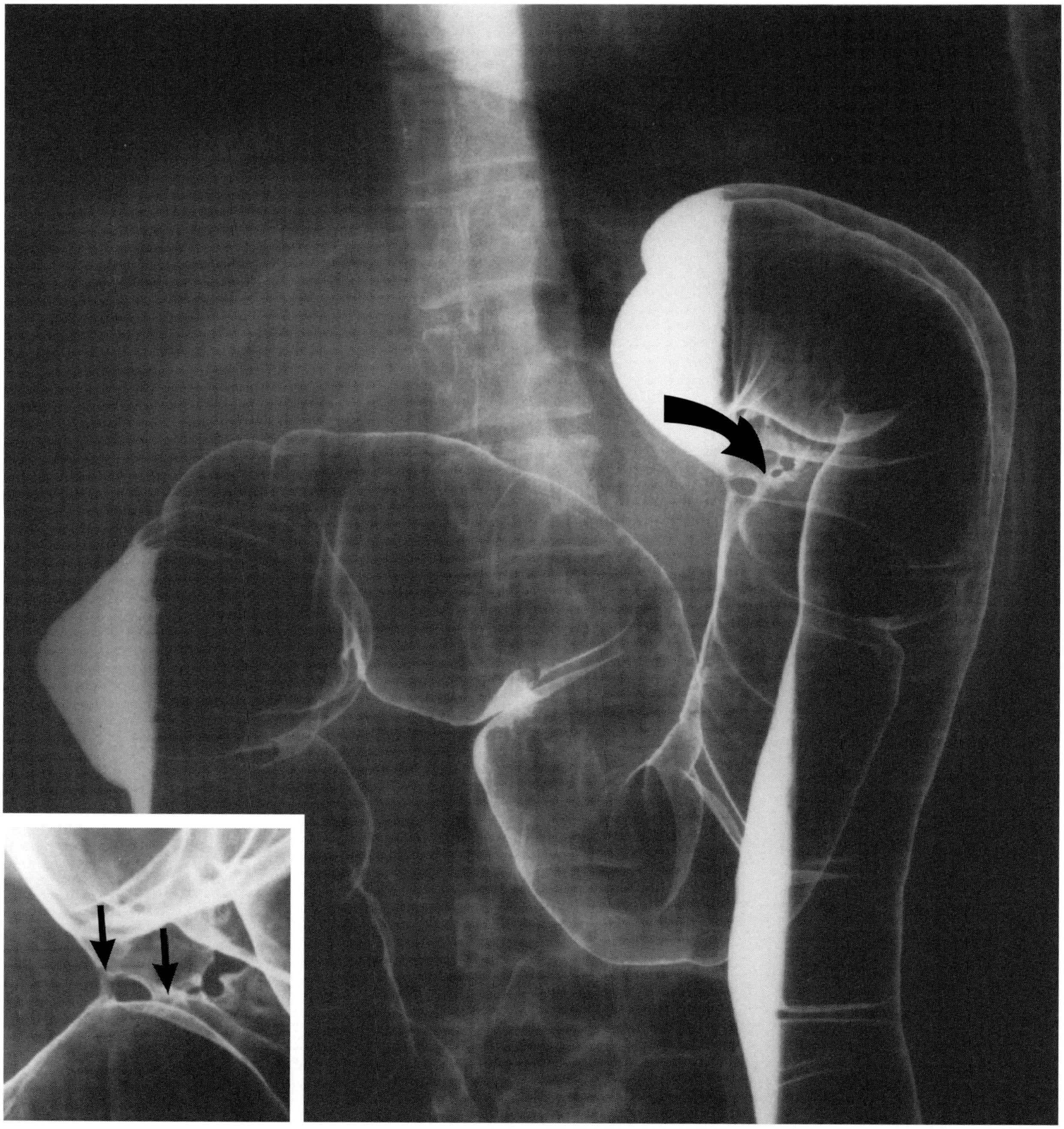

A double-contrast barium enema in an asymptomatic 31-year-old woman with a history of Crohn's colitis shows a colocolic fistula in the transverse colon (curved arrow). The inset shows the fistula at a higher magnification. The remainder of the colon is normal.

David B. Bach, M.D., F.R.C.P.C.
University Hospital
London, ON N6A 5A5, Canada

June 17, 1993

Correspondence

Colocolic Fistula

December 30, 1993

To the Editor: The Image in Clinical Medicine "Colocolic Fistula" (June 17 issue)[1] is a splendid radiographic demonstration of a typical complication of Crohn's disease. For a clinician, however, this nice image also raises an important question: Why would a doctor ask for a study using a double-contrast barium enema in an asymptomatic 31-year-old woman with a history of Crohn's colitis? In view of the potential hazards of radiation and recent discussions about the cost of health care[2] and health care reform,[3] it would seem appropriate to view such an imaging study critically from the perspective of its clinical relevance and, more important, the medical indication for its performance.

Hubert E. Blum, M.D.
Eike Walter, M.D.
University Hospital
CH-8091 Zurich, Switzerland

1. Bach DB. Colocolic fistula. N Engl J Med 1993;328:1758.
2. Relman AS. The health care industry: where is it taking us? N Engl J Med 1991;325:854-9.
3. Angell M. How much will health care reform cost? N Engl J Med 1993;328:1778-9.

Dr. Bach replies:

To the Editor: The barium enema was performed to explain the observation on colonoscopy of two channels at the splenic flexure of the colon. The colonoscopist thought that this might represent a sinus or fistula and that an associated inflammatory process might explain the patient's abdominal pain. Because a colocolic fistula would not have accounted for the patient's symptoms, the term "asymptomatic" was used in the caption.

The concern of Dr. Blum and Dr. Walter about radiation hazards is misplaced. The risks to the patient from a barium-enema study are substantially less than those from colonoscopy.[1] The most serious complication, perforation, has a risk of approximately 1 in 5000,[1,2] as compared with 2 in 1000 for colonoscopy.[3]

David B. Bach, M.D., F.R.C.P.C.
University Hospital
London, ON N6A 5A5, Canada

1. Williams SM, Harned RK. Recognition and prevention of barium enema complications. Curr Probl Diagn Radiol 1991;20:123-51.
2. Han SY, Tishler JM. Perforation of the colon above the peritoneal reflection during the barium-enema examination. Radiology 1982;144:253-5.
3. Ransohoff DF, Lang CA. Screening for colorectal cancer. N Engl J Med 1991;325:37-41.

Nephrology

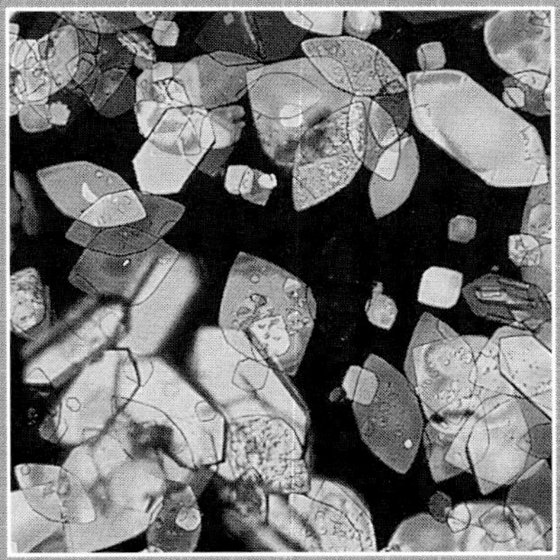

Polycystic Liver and Kidney Disease

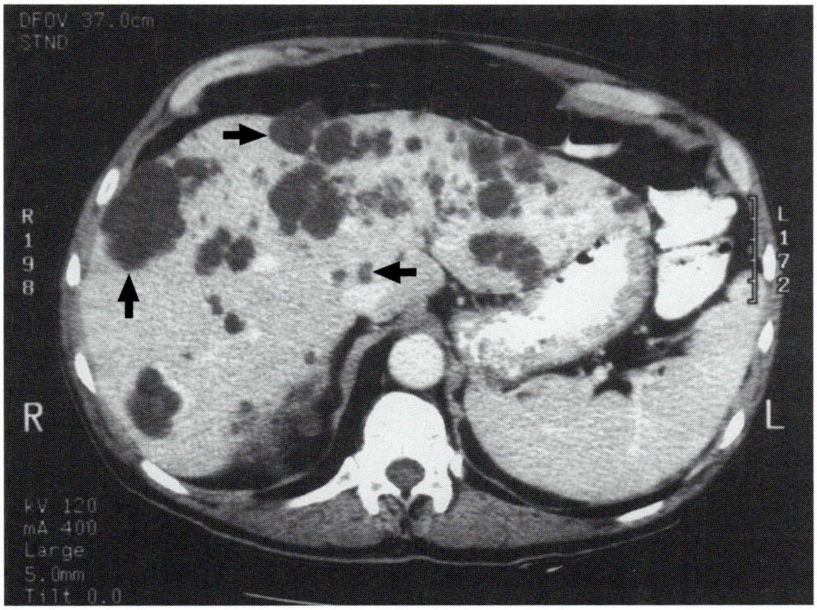

A

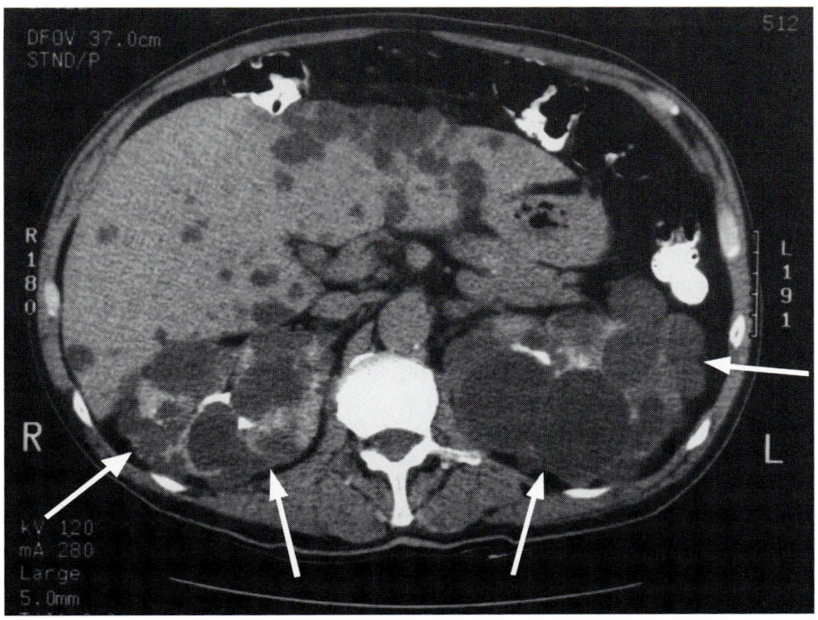

B

An asymptomatic 63-year-old man was found on routine physical examination to have palpable hepatic nodules and ballotable kidneys. Contrast-enhanced abdominal computed tomography showed many hepatic masses of various sizes (arrows, Panel A), whose measured density was consistent with that of water. Both kidneys (arrows, Panel B) also contained numerous cystic masses similar to those in the liver. The patient had microscopic hematuria and a serum creatinine concentration of 1.9 mg per deciliter (168 μmol per liter). The results of other laboratory studies, including liver-function tests, were normal. The patient had no family history of liver or kidney disease, received no treatment, and remains well.

Herbert L. Fred, M.D.
Iqbal Siddique, M.D.

University of Texas
Health Science Center
Houston, TX 77030

July 6, 1995

Uric Acid Crystals

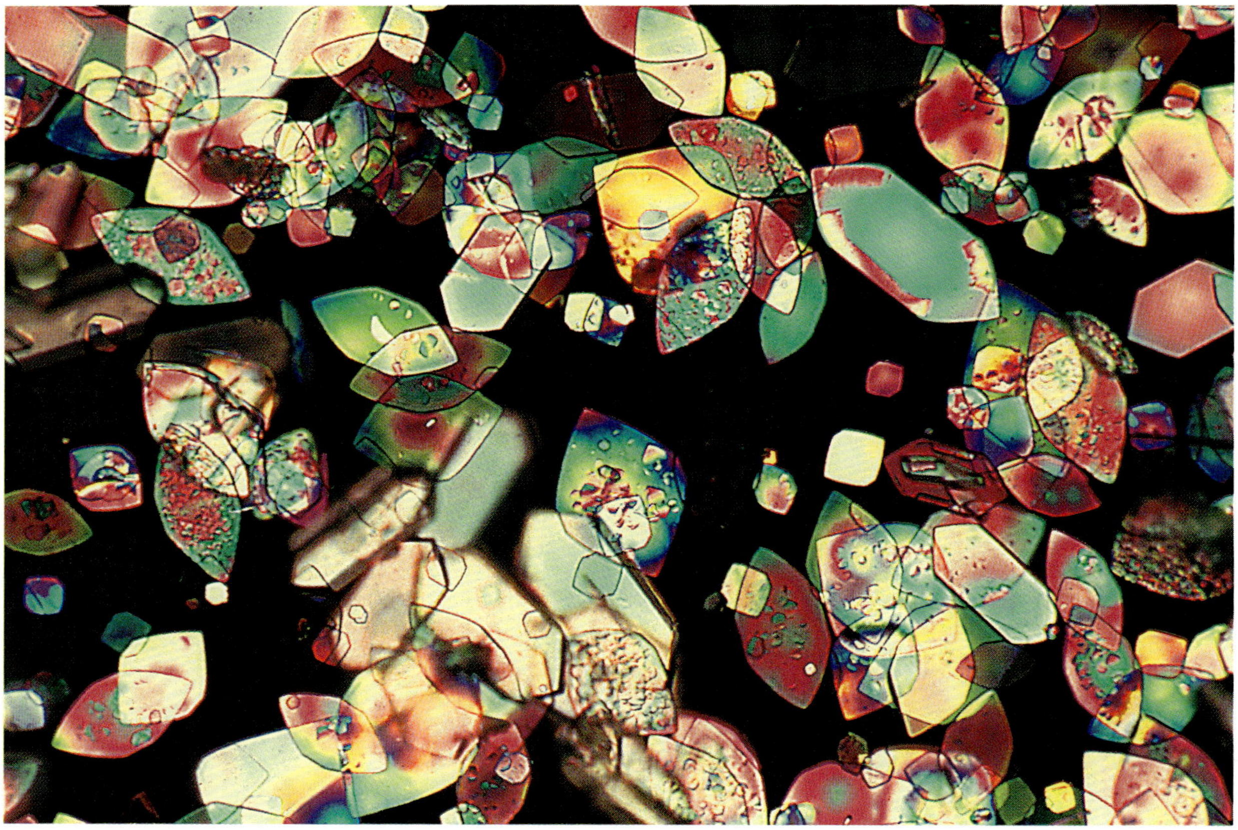

Typical uric acid crystals from fresh, centrifuged urinary sediment are shown through polarized light (×400).

F. Bruder Stapleton, M.D.

State University of New York at Buffalo
Buffalo, NY 14222

Michael A. Linshaw, M.D.

Tufts University School of Medicine
Boston, MA 02111

March 17, 1994

Uric Acid Stones in Crohn's Disease

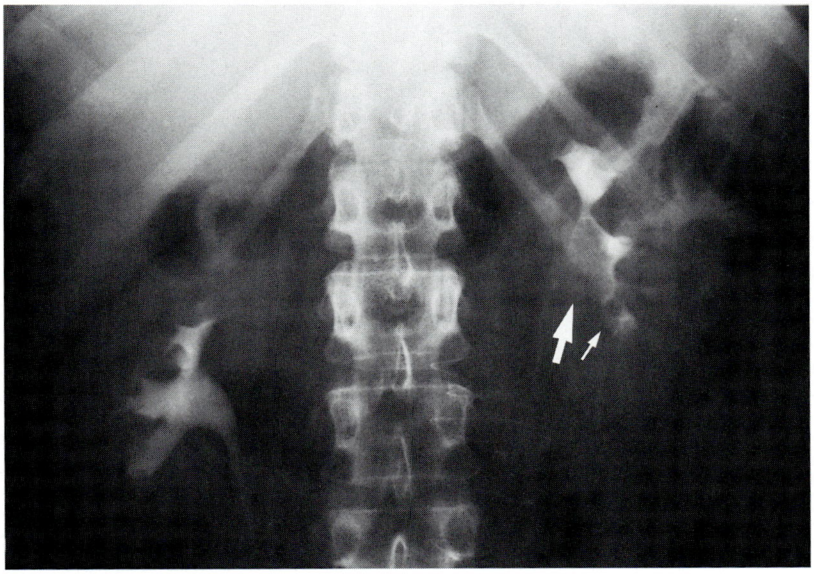

An intravenous urogram was obtained in a 37-year-old woman with persistent watery diarrhea. She had had Crohn's disease for 11 years, and most of her colon and part of her ileum had been removed 4 years earlier. A large radiolucent defect occupies most of the left renal pelvis (large arrow), and a smaller defect obstructs the lower pole calix of the left kidney (small arrow). The right kidney appears to be normal. Three years after this study was performed, similar stones developed in the right kidney. These were found to contain uric acid.

Carlos D. Flombaum, M.D.

Memorial Sloan-Kettering Cancer Center
New York, NY 10021

Extraintestinal Manifestations of Crohn's Disease

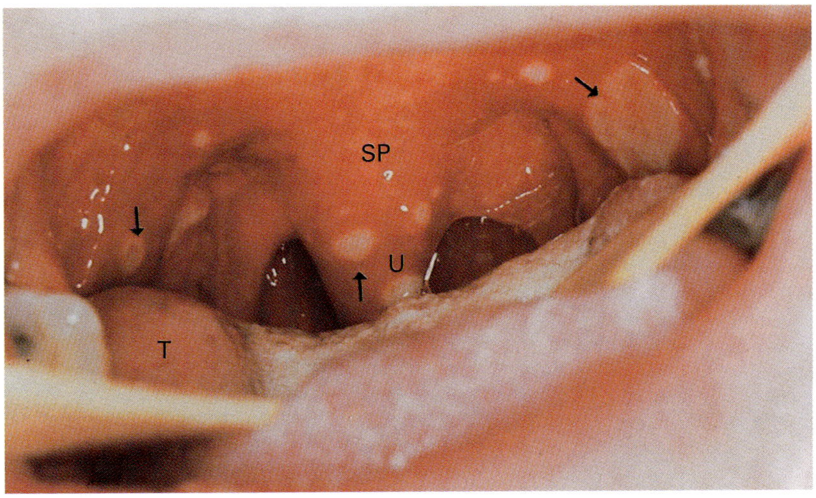

A

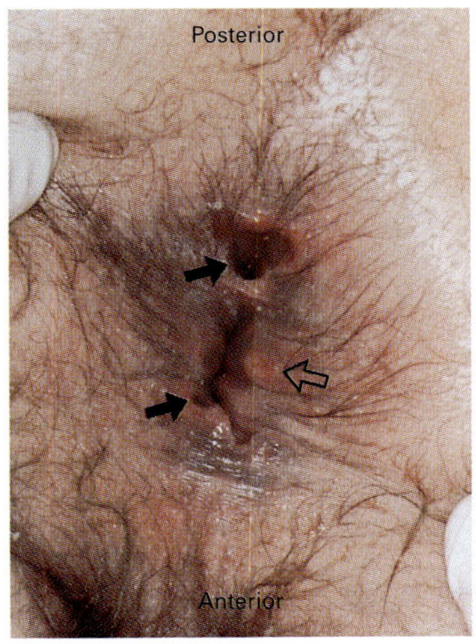

B

Multiple oral and perianal ulcerations were found at presentation in a 48-year-old man with Crohn's disease. The patient had had no diarrhea before the diagnosis but reported having oral and perianal pain for three months and swelling and pain in his right ankle for three days. Examination of his ankle showed acute erythema and edema. Panel A shows aphthous ulcers (arrows) of the palate and uvula (U). The tongue (T) was also involved. SP denotes soft palate. Panel B shows perianal ulcerations (open arrow) and fistulas (solid arrows). Colonoscopy revealed multiple shallow ulcers from the rectum to the cecum, with involvement of the terminal ileum. Microscopical examination of a biopsy specimen from the right colon revealed focal cryptitis without vasculitis. The aphthous ulcers and arthritis improved after a few days of corticosteroid therapy. The fistulas closed after one month of metronidazole therapy.

John M. Carethers, M.D.
W. Michael McDonnell, M.D.

University of Michigan Medical Center
Ann Arbor, MI 48109

June 30, 1994

Membranous Glomerulonephritis

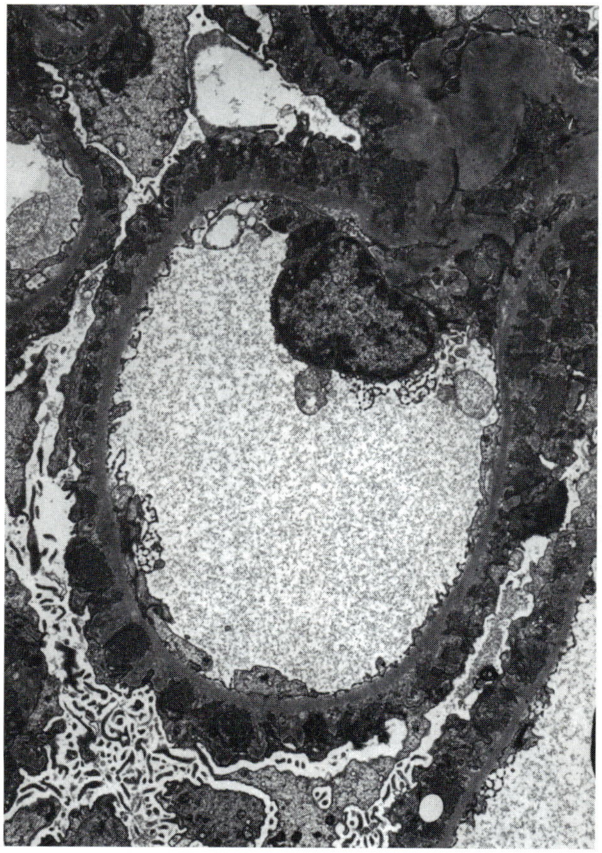

A

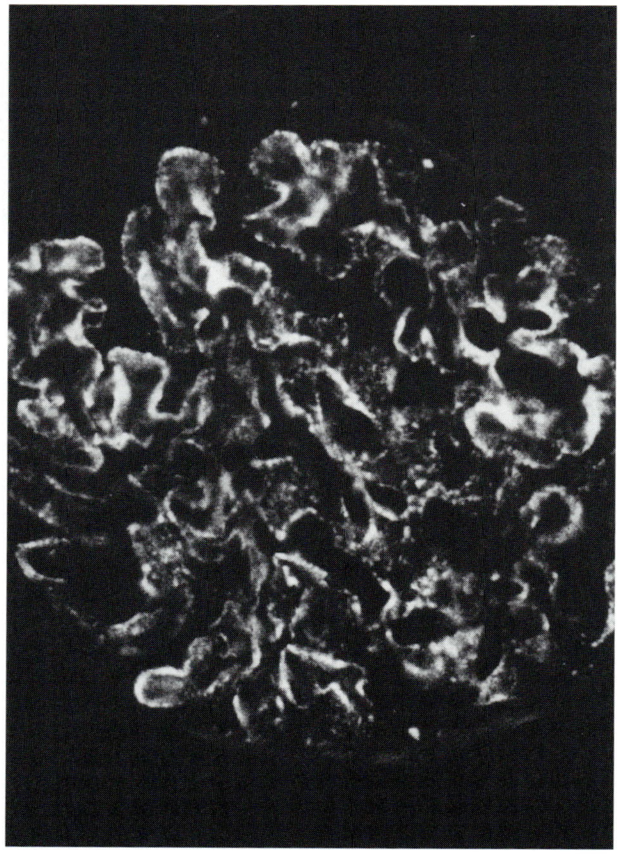

B

A transmission electron micrograph (Panel A) shows a cross section of a glomerular capillary loop with the typical changes of membranous glomerulonephritis (×5300). Large, electron-dense deposits are visible on the outer aspect of the glomerular basement membrane, with interposition of basement-membrane material that forms "spikes." A fluorescence photomicrograph (Panel B) reveals the IgG composition of these immune deposits within the glomerular capillary wall (×72).

Edmund J. Lewis, M.D.
Melvin M. Schwartz, M.D.

Rush–Presbyterian–St. Luke's Medical Center
Chicago, IL 60612

February 18, 1993

Membranoproliferative Glomerulonephritis Type 1

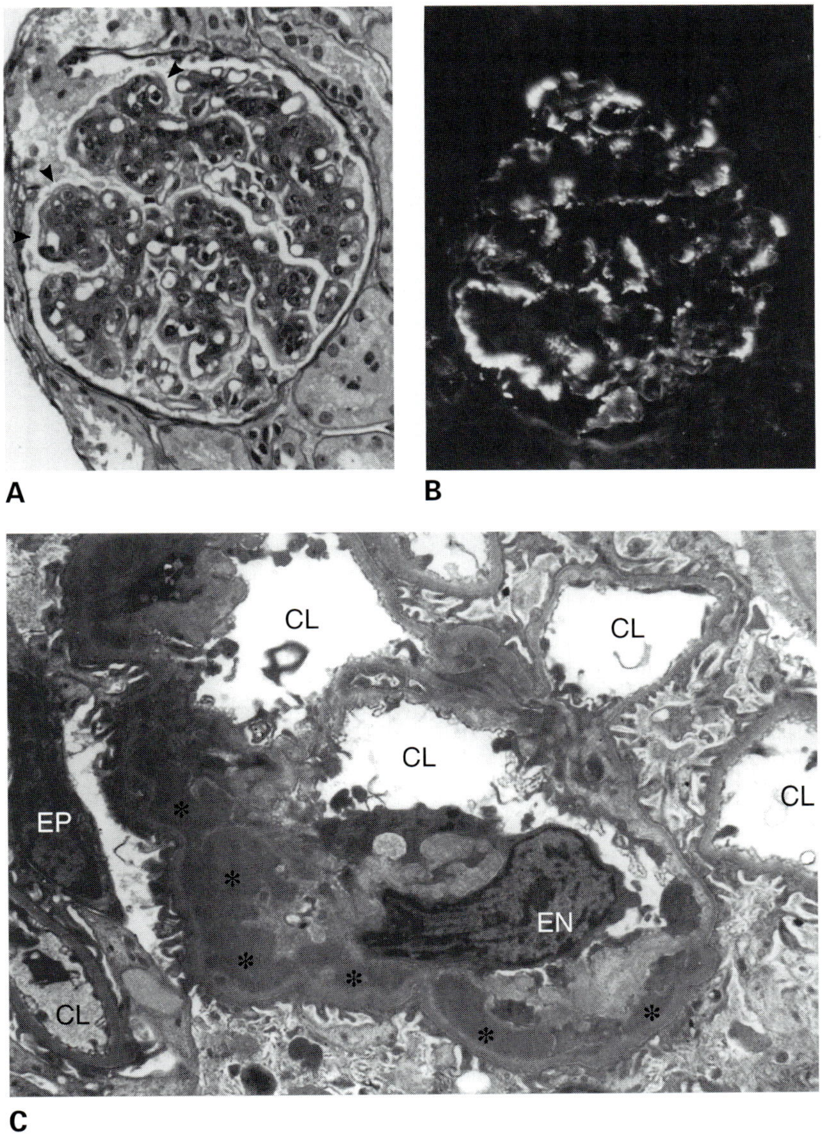

An eight-year-old girl was found to have proteinuria and microscopic hematuria on a routine examination. A photomicrograph (Panel A) shows an enlarged, lobulated glomerulus with irregular thickened glomerular capillary walls, often with a double-contour appearance, so-called tram tracks (arrowheads); moderate mesangial expansion; and moderate hypercellularity (periodic acid–Schiff, ×20). A fluorescence photomicrograph (Panel B) discloses coarse and bulky granular deposits of C3 along the glomerular capillary wall and, to a lesser extent, in mesangial areas (×25). A transmission electron micrograph (Panel C) reveals large, subendothelial, electron-dense deposits (asterisks) and mesangial interposition (×4000). CL denotes capillary lumen, EN endothelial cell, and EP visceral epithelial cell.

Reinold O. Gans, M.D., Ph.D.

State University of New York at Buffalo
Buffalo, NY 14214

Leonard G. Feld, M.D., Ph.D.

Children's Hospital of Buffalo
Buffalo, NY 14222

February 8, 1996

Dysmorphic Urinary Erythrocytes

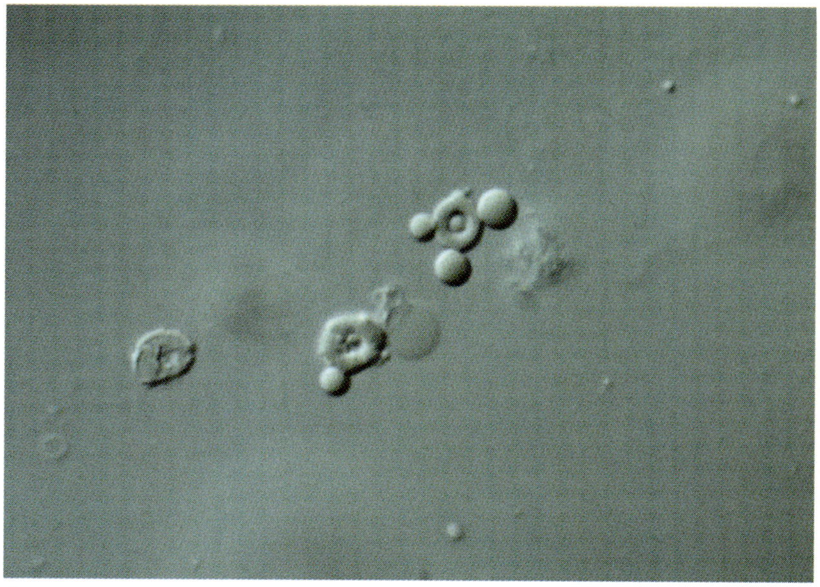

A

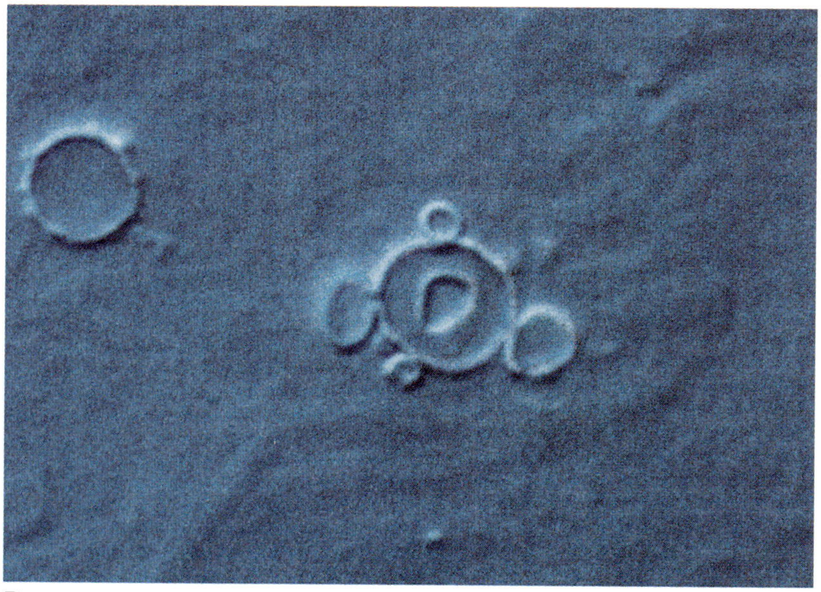

B

A kidney biopsy in a 34-year-old man with IgA nephropathy showed mesangial-cell proliferation and predominant mesangial IgA deposition. At the time of the biopsy, the patient's serum creatinine and blood urea nitrogen levels were 1.3 mg per deciliter (110 μmol per liter) and 13 mg per deciliter (4.6 mmol per liter), respectively. Microscopical examination of the urine revealed many dysmorphic urinary erythrocytes with spheroid surface protrusions (Panel A, ×1450) indicative of glomerular hematuria. A glomerular erythrocyte ghost (Panel B, ×3250) has a small neck at the base of each surface protrusion, demonstrating its connection with the cytoplasm of the cell. Urinary erythrocytes with surface protrusions such as those shown here are present in large numbers only with pathologic glomerular bleeding. (Differential interference contrast microscopy, ×1000).

Theodore F. Saad, M.D.

University of Texas Health Science Center at San Antonio
San Antonio, TX 78284

May 30, 1996

Correspondence

Diagnostic Value of Dysmorphic Urinary Red Cells

October 24, 1996

To the Editor: Dr. Saad's photomicrographs of dysmorphic urinary erythrocytes (Images in Clinical Medicine, May 30 issue),[1] although beautiful, are dangerously misleading. Dysmorphic cells do not represent glomerular bleeding, as the legend implies. They can be produced as a result of kidney biopsies[2] and are therefore not necessarily of glomerular origin. Renal tumors can also be expected to produce dysmorphic hematuria. By assuming that a finding of dysmorphic red cells rules out all causes of hematuria other than glomerulonephritis, one could miss a renal tumor.

Akos Z. Györy, M.D., D.Sc.
Sydney University
Sydney, NSW 2006, Australia

1. Saad TF. Dysmorphic urinary erythrocytes. N Engl J Med 1996;334:1440.
2. Pollock C, Pei-Ling L, Györy AZ, et al. Dysmorphism of urinary red blood cells — value in diagnosis. Kidney Int 1989;36:1045-9.

Dr. Saad replies:

To the Editor: Dr. Györy correctly notes that dysmorphic urinary erythrocytes may have a nonglomerular origin. A wide variety of abnormal-appearing erythrocytes can be seen in the urine, most of them nonspecific with regard to origin. My photomicrographs show erythrocytes with discrete spheroidal protrusions, a morphologic abnormality highly specific for hematuria of glomerular origin.[1,2] These cells were classified as acanthocytes by Köhler et al.[1] with phase-contrast microscopy in a study of 351 patients with hematuria. When cells of this type made up more than 5 percent of urinary erythrocytes, the sensitivity and specificity for glomerular disease were 52 percent and 98 percent, respectively. By contrast, red-cell casts had 24 percent sensitivity and 97 percent specificity for glomerular disease. Two patients with tumor-associated hematuria had urinary acanthocytes whose proportion exceeded 5 percent, but glomerular disease could not be ruled out, because these patients did not undergo kidney biopsy. No other type of dysmorphic erythrocyte was useful in determining the source of the hematuria. Tomita et al.[2] conducted a similar study with interference contrast microscopy. When intact and ghost forms of "doughnut-like cells with one or more blebs" made up more than 1 percent of urinary erythrocytes, the sensitivity and specificity for glomerular disease were 89 percent and 95 percent, respectively. Interference contrast microscopy may improve the sensitivity of these cells in the diagnosis of glomerulonephritis, but they are easily seen with the ordinary bright-field microscopy available to most physicians.

Theodore F. Saad, M.D.
University of Texas Health Science Center at San Antonio
San Antonio, TX 78284

1. Köhler H, Wandel E, Brunck B. Acanthocyturia — a characteristic marker for glomerular bleeding. Kidney Int 1991;40:115-20.
2. Tomita M, Kitamoto Y, Nakayama M, Sato T. A new morphological classification of urinary erythrocytes for differential diagnosis of glomerular hematuria. Clin Nephrol 1992;37:84-9.

Bilateral Nephrocalcinosis

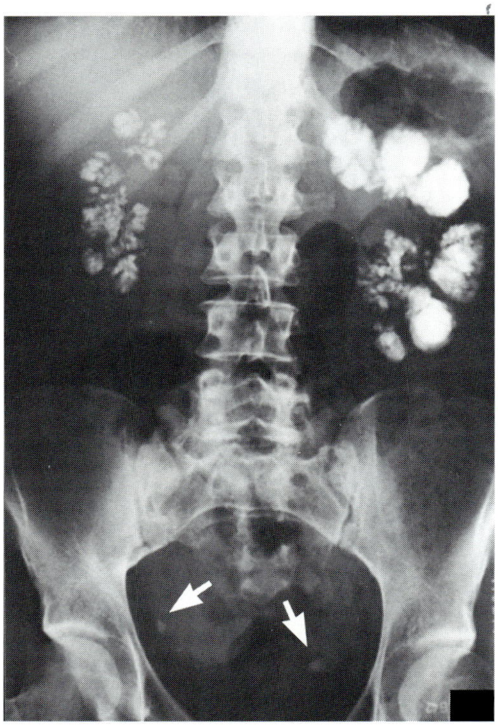

A

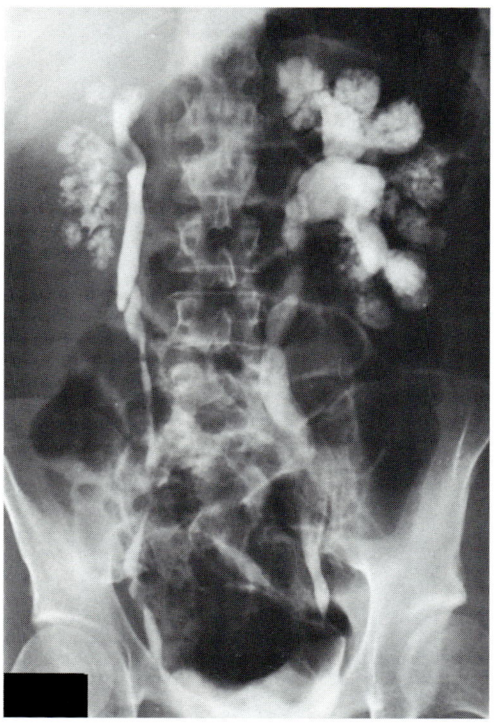

B

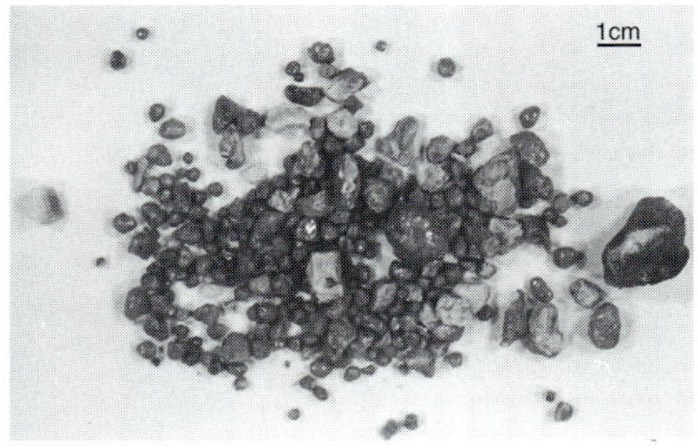

C

A 39-year-old woman presented with a seven-year history of renal calculi. A plain abdominal film obtained when she was 38 (Panel A) showed enlarged kidneys bilaterally with nephrocalcinosis in a papillary distribution and radiopaque calculi in both ureters (arrows). An intravenous urogram done at the same time (Panel B) showed left-sided hydronephrosis. A collection of stones passed by the patient over a two-month period is shown in Panel C. Analysis of the stones showed that the majority were composed of calcium oxalate, with some composed of magnesium ammonium phosphate. Urine cultures showed intermittent coliform infection, with no evidence of urea-splitting organisms. The patient's usual electrolyte values were as follows: serum sodium, 140 mmol per liter; potassium, 4.0 mmol per liter; chloride, 105 mmol per liter; and bicarbonate, 23 mmol per liter. Her 24-hour urinary calcium excretion (290 mg [7.2 mmol] per 24 hr) was at the upper limit of normal for our laboratory. Urinary pH was never below 6, and an ammonium chloride–loading test revealed an acidification defect consistent with the presence of type 1 renal tubular acidosis. Despite a high fluid intake (>3 liters per day) she continues to pass stones intermittently. Fortunately, her serum urea and creatinine concentrations have remained normal.

Jonathan T.C. Kwan, M.D.
Frank P. Marsh, M.A., F.R.C.P.

Royal London Hospital
London E1 1BB, United Kingdom

April 25, 1996

Correspondence

Renal Tubular Acidosis

August 29, 1996

To the Editor: The Image in Clinical Medicine of Drs. Kwan and Marsh (April 25 issue)[1] shows an excellent radiographic example of type 1 (distal) renal tubular acidosis with nephrocalcinosis, but there are some irregularities in the accompanying clinical description. Although the stones passed by this patient were composed mainly of calcium oxalate, most patients with type 1 renal tubular acidosis produce calcium phosphate (brushite) calculi. The patient's plasma bicarbonate concentration was in the low range of normal, so the diagnosis was more likely to be incomplete type 1 renal tubular acidosis.

Despite the absence of systemic acidosis requiring alkalization therapy in such patients, specific medical therapy should be instituted to address intermittent stone passage as well as to prevent worsening of nephrocalcinosis. The most important factor causing calculi formation in patients with type 1 renal tubular acidosis is hypocitraturia, which is due to either a primary defect in citrate transport or intracellular acidosis in the distal tubular cells that prevents citrate excretion into the urine. Citrate is a major inhibitor of stone formation. The pronounced hypocitraturia in type 1 renal tubular acidosis requires therapy with oral citrate preparations at doses of 60 to 90 meq per day. The potassium salt is recommended because serum potassium levels in patients with type 1 renal tubular acidosis, which are already depressed, can drop even further during alkali therapy. The addition of this regimen to a generous fluid intake is more likely to reduce calculi formation than high fluid intake alone.

J. Stuart Wolf, Jr., M.D.
Washington University School of Medicine
St. Louis, MO 63110

1. Kwan JTC, Marsh FP. Bilateral nephrocalcinosis. N Engl J Med 1996;334:1105.

Metastatic Calcification of the Shoulder in Chronic Renal Failure

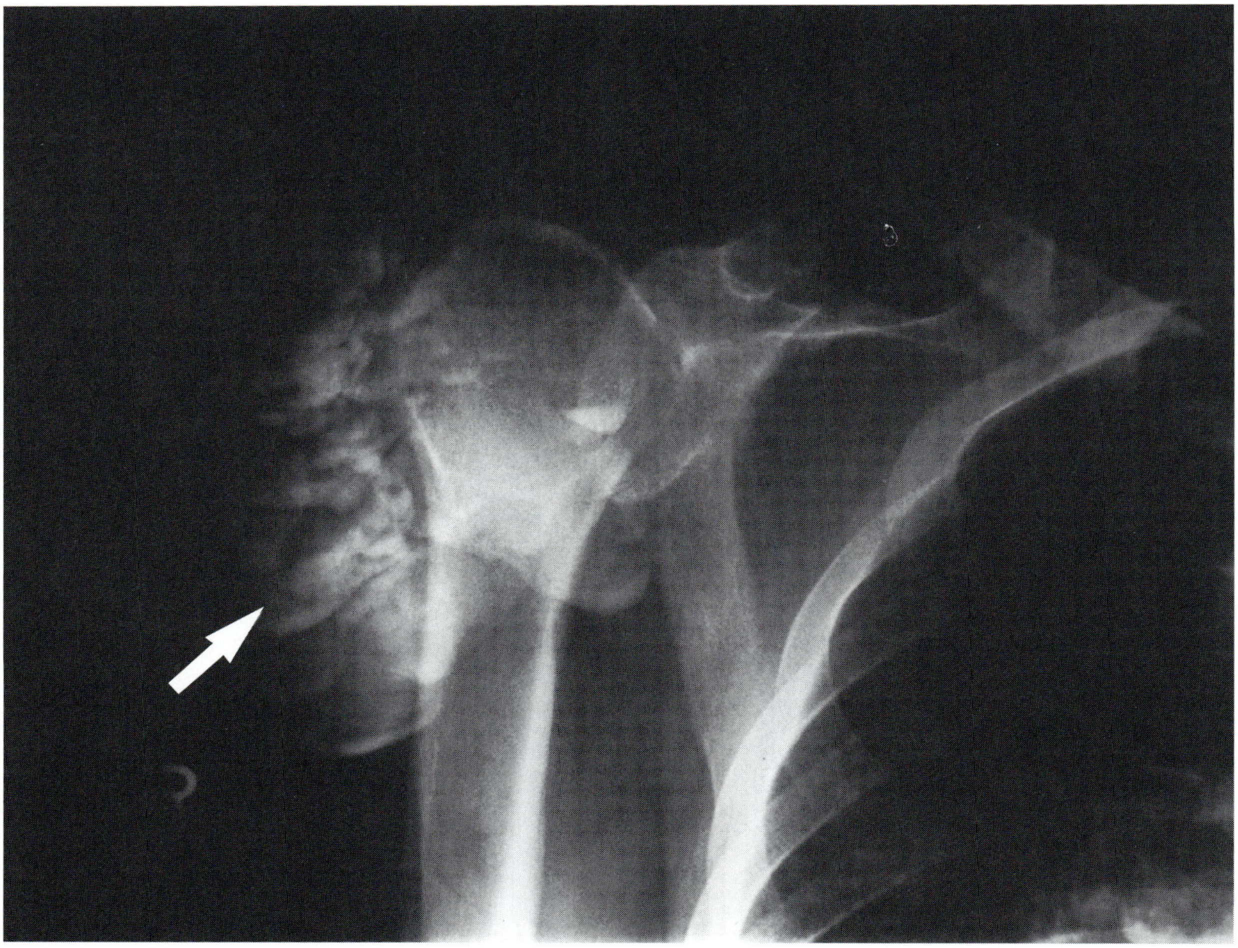

A 32-year-old man with chronic renal failure (from IgA nephropathy) being treated with maintenance hemodialysis began to take his phosphate-binding medications irregularly, and swelling of the right shoulder developed over a period of two months. The calcium–phosphate product (in milligrams per deciliter) was more than 90, and the serum N-terminal parathyroid hormone level was elevated. A biopsy of the shoulder mass (arrow) revealed hydroxyapatite. The patient underwent subtotal parathyroidectomy and was referred for renal transplantation.

Hamid Rabb, M.D.
German Ramirez, M.D.

James A. Haley Veterans Affairs Hospital
Tampa, FL 33612

September 2, 1993

Correspondence

Renal Transplantation in a Noncompliant Patient

February 3, 1994

To the Editor: The Image in Clinical Medicine entitled "Metastatic Calcification of the Shoulder in Chronic Renal Failure" (Sept. 2 issue)[1] leaves readers with the impression that a noncompliant patient who "began to take his phosphate-binding medications irregularly" was an acceptable candidate for transplantation and was therefore "referred for renal transplantation." Nothing could be further from the truth.

One of the chief relative and absolute contraindications to all types of solid-organ transplantation is demonstrated noncompliance. In an era of shrinking resources and with the shortage of available donor organs, transplantation centers have adopted policies that prevent valuable donor organs from being wasted. These policies have been repeatedly upheld by ethics review boards, institutional review boards, and the appellate process of the courts. The caption accompanying the image leaves the impression that anyone can be an organ-transplant recipient without regard to personal responsibility. Patients as well as doctors are responsible for their actions.

Jonathan S. Bromberg, M.D., Ph.D.
P.R. Baliga, M.D.
Medical University of South Carolina
Charleston, SC 29425

1. Rabb H, Ramirez G. Metastatic calcification of the shoulder in chronic renal failure. N Engl J Med 1993;329:695.

The authors reply:

To the Editor: We thank Drs. Bromberg and Baliga for correctly pointing out that a patient who is noncompliant may not be an acceptable candidate for transplantation. Though the patient in question was considered for transplantation at his own request, he did not proceed beyond the initial evaluation. In the legend accompanying the image, we did not elaborate on this point, because we were focusing on the patient's dramatic metastatic calcifications.

Hamid Rabb, M.D.
German Ramirez, M.D.
University of South Florida
Tampa, FL 33612-4745

Macrophages

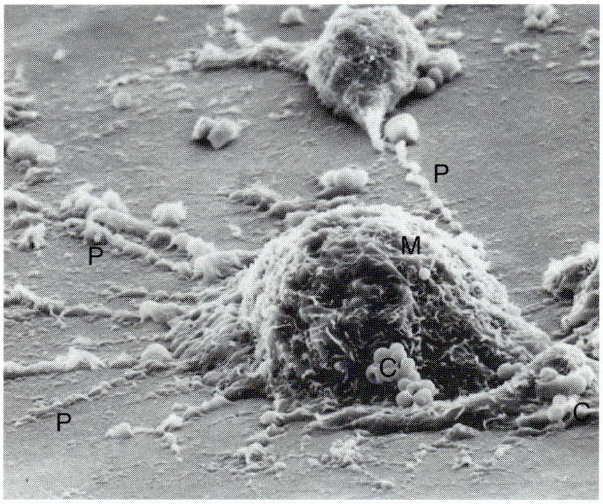

A

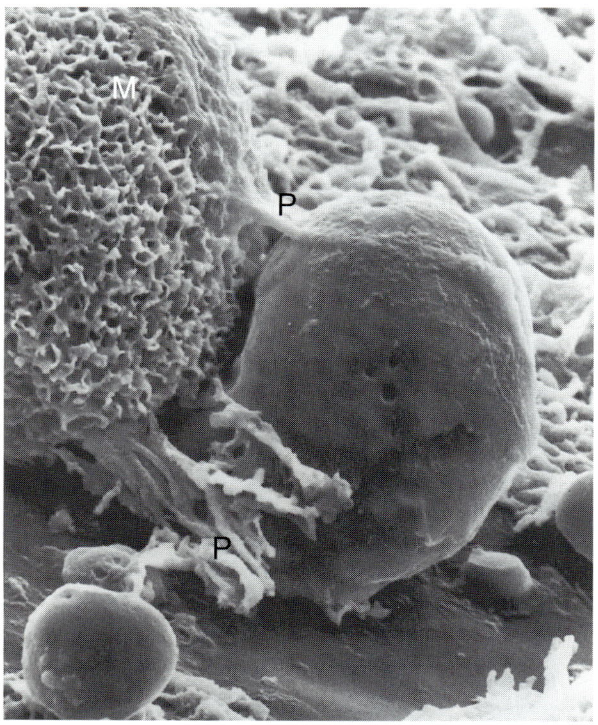

B

Scanning electron micrographs show macrophages on the surface of peritoneal-dialysis catheters after the devices had been removed because of infectious complications. Panel A shows a sessile macrophage (M) with pseudopodia (P) scavenging scattered clumps of coccal forms (C) (×3200). In Panel B another macrophage with pseudopodia is more actively "hugging" an unidentified object (×6400).

Richard Swartz, M.D.

University of Michigan Hospitals
Ann Arbor, MI 48109

Clifford Holmes, Ph.D.

Baxter Healthcare
McGaw Park, IL 60085

December 7, 1995

Nutcracker Phenomenon

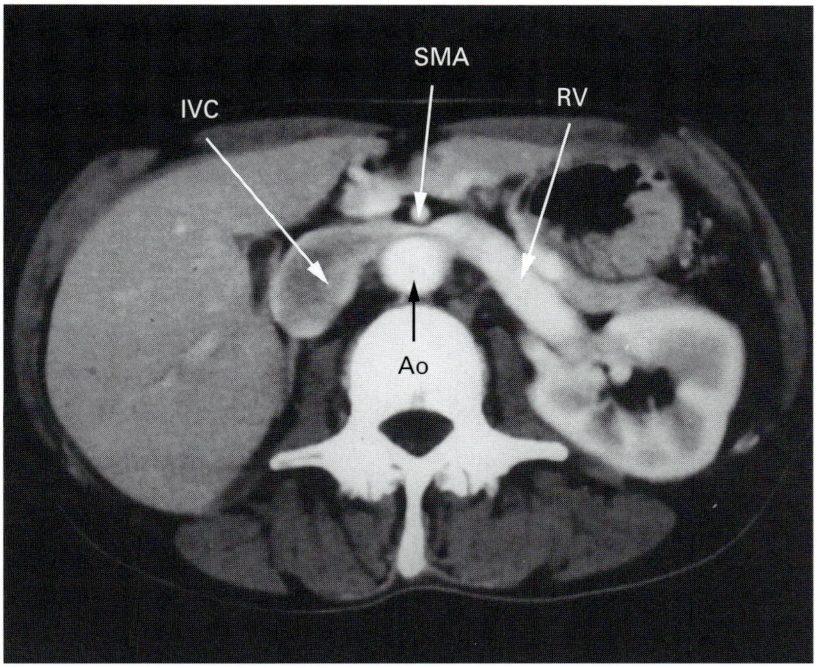

Computed tomography in a 52-year-old woman with mild episodic gross hematuria revealed compression of the left renal vein between the superior mesenteric artery (SMA) and the aorta (Ao) before the vein merges into the inferior vena cava (IVC). This compression caused marked dilatation of the distal part of the renal vein (RV). The renal venous congestion caused hematuria, presumably through the rupture of submucosal veins into the renal pelvis. No treatment was given. Entrapment of the renal vein is a known cause of hematuria.

Kenjiro Kimura, M.D.
Thutomu Araki, M.D.

University of Tokyo
Tokyo, Japan

July 18, 1996

Renal Aneurysms in Hepatitis B–Associated Polyarteritis Nodosa

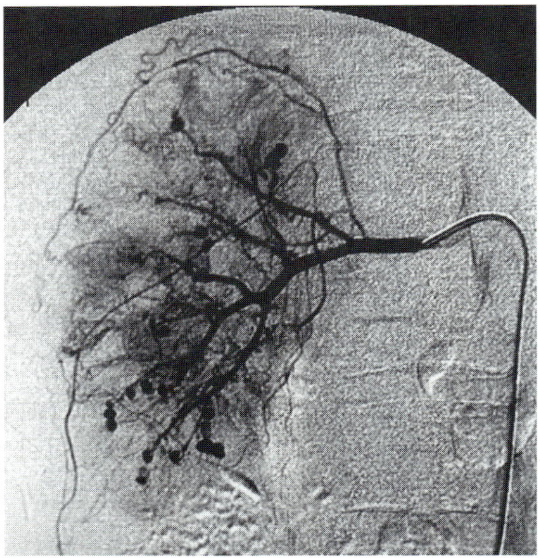

A

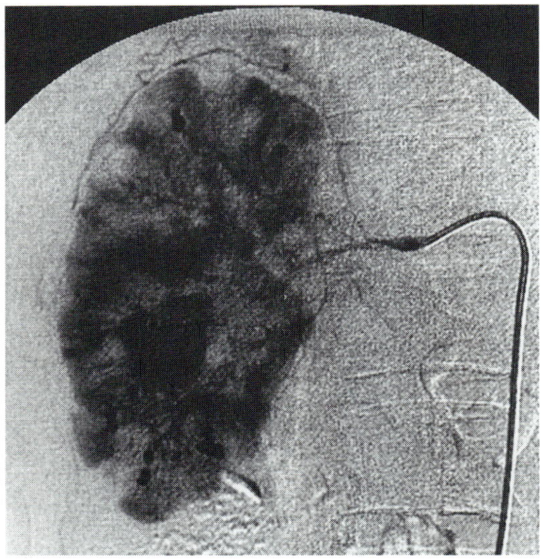

B

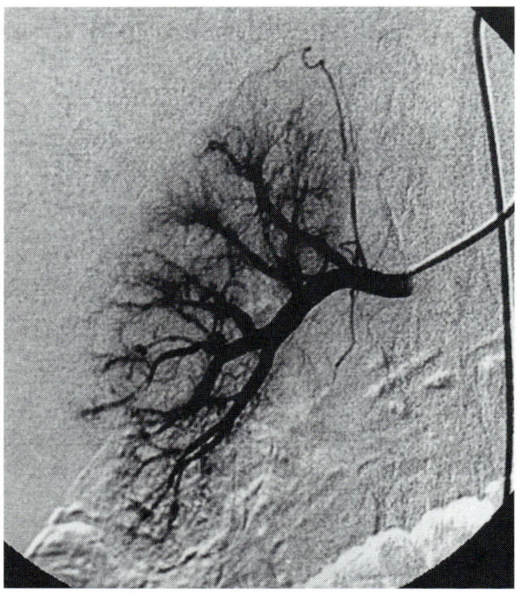

C

Abdominal arteriography was performed in a 21-year-old drug abuser who presented with rapidly progressive renal failure. During the previous two months she had had fever and diffuse abdominal pain and had lost 12 kg in weight. The recent onset of hypertension (blood pressure, 150/120 mm Hg) and cardiac failure was also noted. Tests for hepatitis B surface antigen, hepatitis B virus DNA, and hepatitis C virus antibody were positive, but a test for human immunodeficiency virus antibody was negative. Selective arteriography of the right kidney (Panel A) revealed multiple aneurysms with vessel narrowing and irregularity in medium-sized arteries. The parenchymatous phase (Panel B) revealed large cortical ischemic areas caused by arterial thrombosis. The patient was treated with corticosteroids, plasma exchange, and interferon alfa. Renal failure persisted, and regular hemodialysis was required. Ten weeks later, a second arteriogram showed only a few microaneurysms (Panel C). Tests for hepatitis B surface antigen and hepatitis B virus DNA were still positive. After 16 weeks of hemodialysis, renal function began to improve. Five months after dialysis was discontinued, the patient's serum creatinine concentration was 1.6 mg per deciliter (140 μmol per liter).

Dominique Chauveau, M.D.
Jean-Louis Christophe, M.D.

Hôpital Necker
75015 Paris, France

April 20, 1995

Spontaneous Atheroembolism

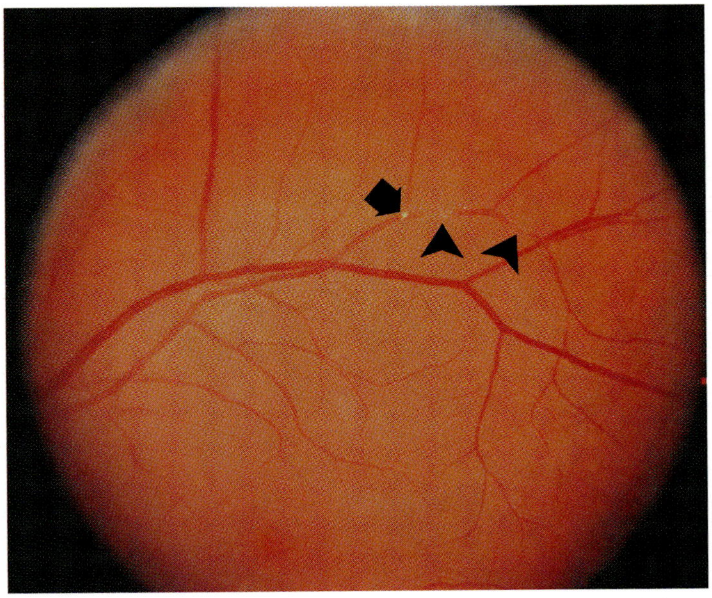

A

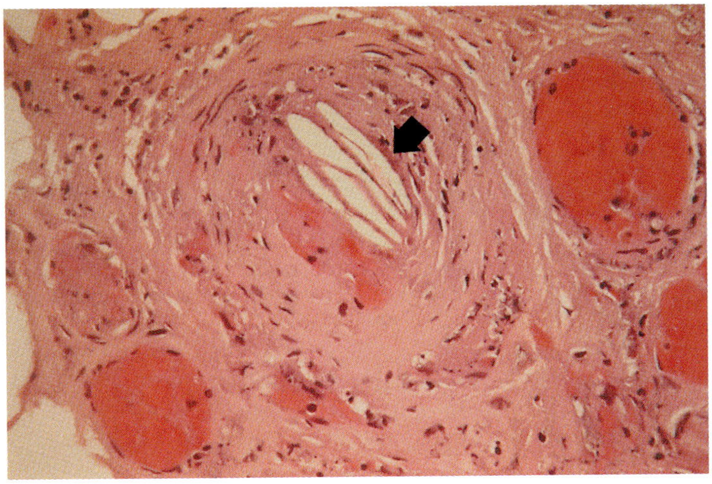

B

A 72-year-old man was admitted to the hospital with delirium, acute renal failure, increasing hypertension, sudden impairment of vision in the left eye, and severe pain in the left foot. Funduscopic examination of the left eye (Panel A) showed a cholesterol embolus, or Hollenhorst plaque (arrow), at the bifurcation of a retinal arteriole and vascular sheathing distal to the occlusion (arrowheads). No other physical findings were present. Distal pulses were palpable, but two toes later turned purple and one required amputation. Histologic examination of the amputated toe (Panel B) revealed an arteriole with characteristic needle-shaped clefts (arrow) resulting from atheroemboli. The patient had undergone no surgical or diagnostic procedures and had not received anticoagulants. Progressive renal failure developed one year later, and the patient died.

Mark Bradley, M.D.

Roseburg Veterans Affairs Medical Center
Roseburg, OR 97470

April 13, 1995

Atheroembolism

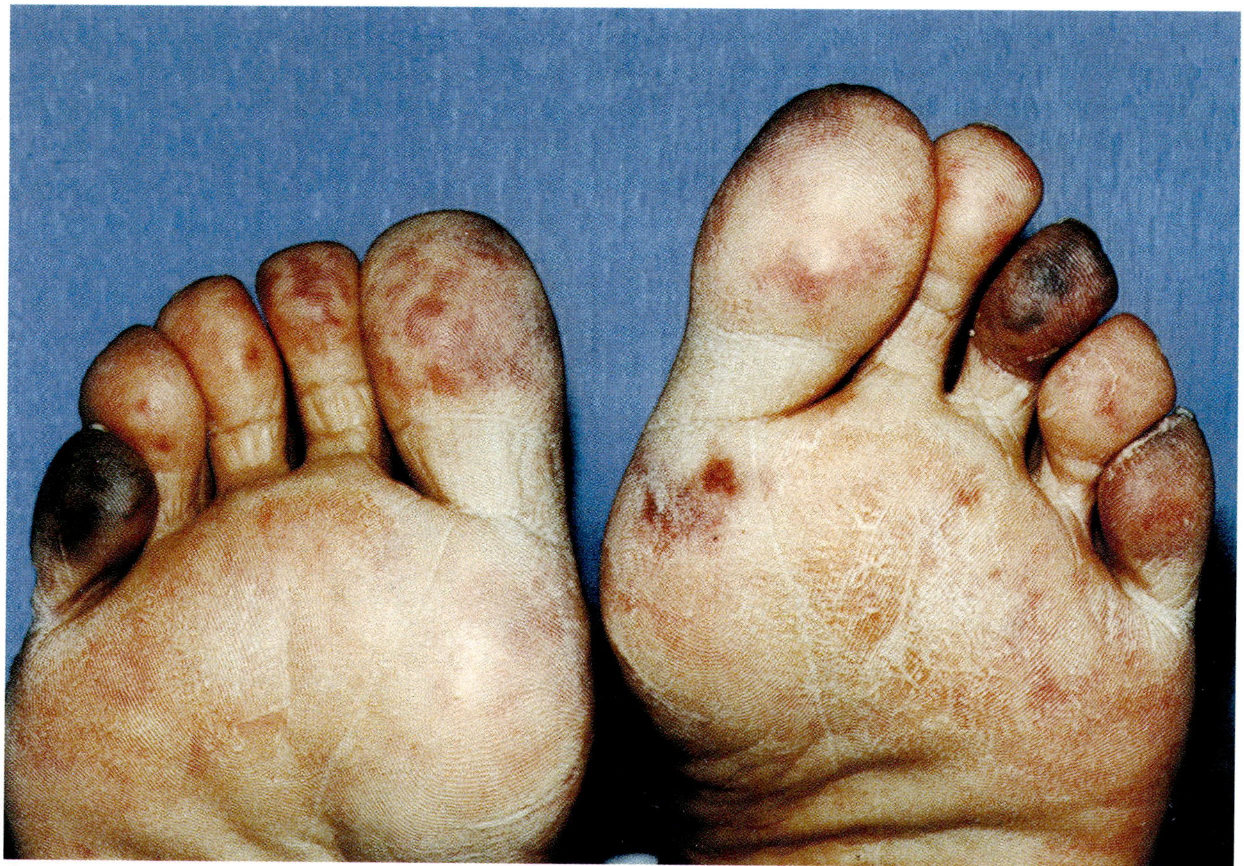

A

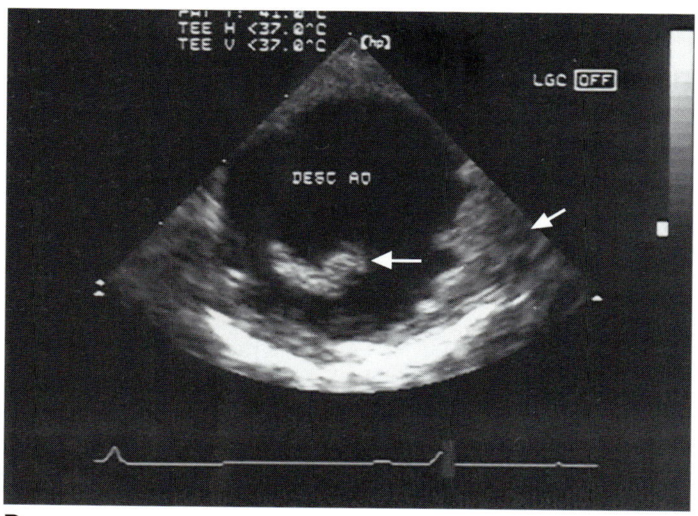

B

Lesions typical of atheroembolism are apparent on the feet (Panel A) of a 65-year-old man who had undergone left heart catheterization through the femoral approach four weeks earlier. Non-oliguric renal failure developed (serum creatinine, 5.5 mg per deciliter [490 μmol per liter]), and livedo reticularis and cutaneous infarcts were present on both feet, with preserved distal pulses. A transesophageal echocardiogram of the descending thoracic aorta showed multiple complex, pedunculated, mobile, protruding lesions presumed to be atheromas (arrows in Panel B), the probable source of embolism.

Ramdas G. Pai, M.D.
J. Thomas Heywood, M.D.

Veterans Affairs Medical Center
Loma Linda, CA 92357

September 28, 1995

Pulmonary Diseases

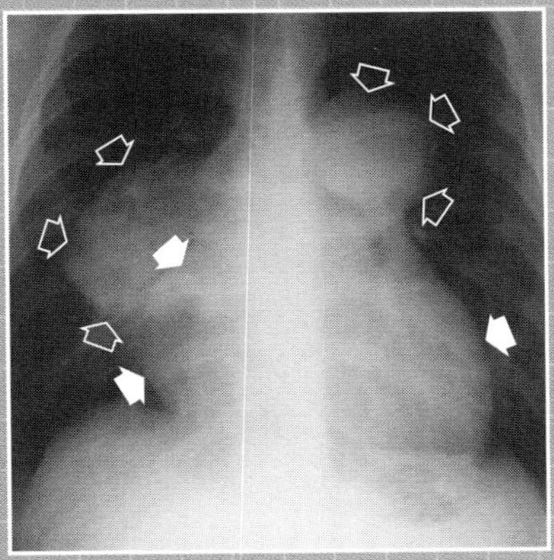

Dilatation of the Pulmonary Arteries in Primary Pulmonary Hypertension

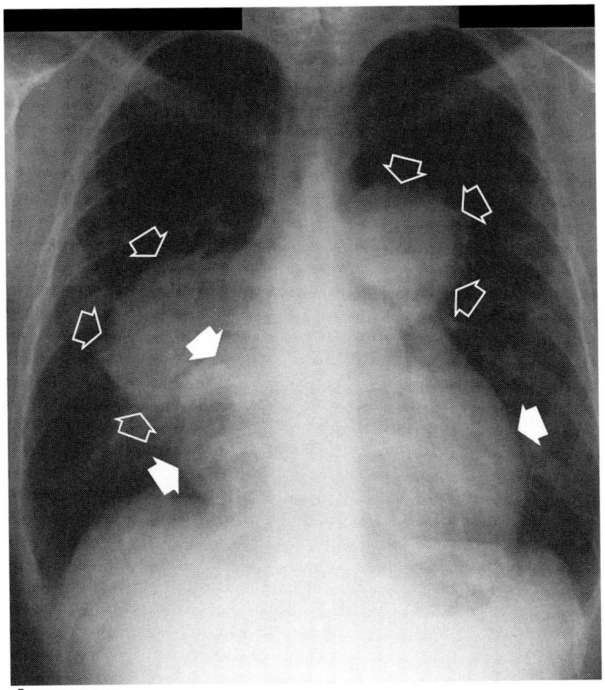

A

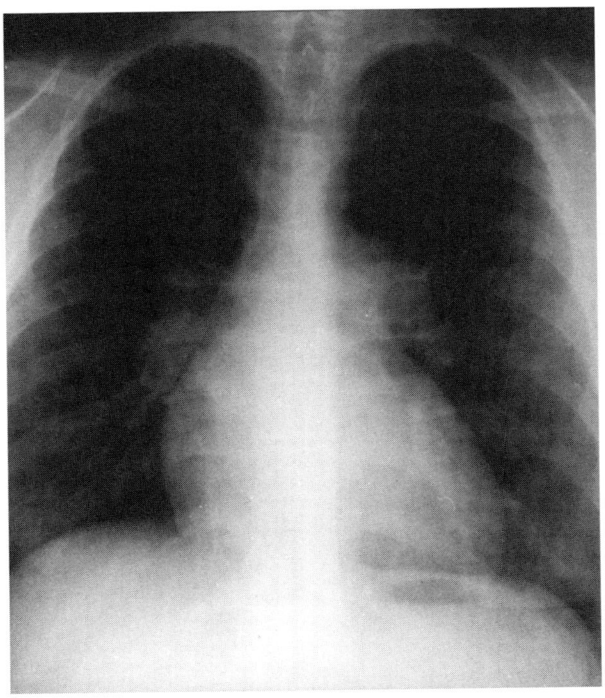

B

A 17-year-old male patient presented with severe pulmonary hypertension of uncertain cause (i.e., primary pulmonary hypertension). A chest x-ray film (Panel A) revealed massive dilatation of the central pulmonary arteries (open arrows) and right ventricular enlargement (solid arrows) that had not been present three years earlier (Panel B). There was no evidence of congenital heart disease. Pulmonary angiography showed no sign of chronic thromboembolic disease or veno-occlusive disease. The pulmonary arterial pressure was 106/58 mm Hg (mean, 76), with a mean right atrial pressure of 9 mm Hg, cardiac output of 5.4 liters per minute, and pulmonary vascular resistance of 17.5 Wood units. Calcium antagonists had no effect on pulmonary hemodynamics. Because of a progressive increase in the pulmonary-artery diameter and recent clinical deterioration with repeated episodes of syncope, a heart–lung transplantation has been recommended.

Irene M. Lang, M.D.
Meinhard P. Kneussl, M.D.

University of Vienna
A-1090 Vienna, Austria

February 1, 1996

Histoplasmosis

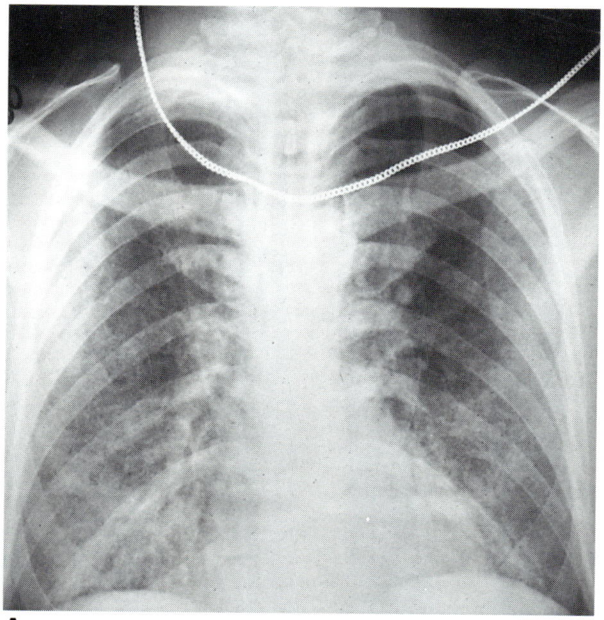

A

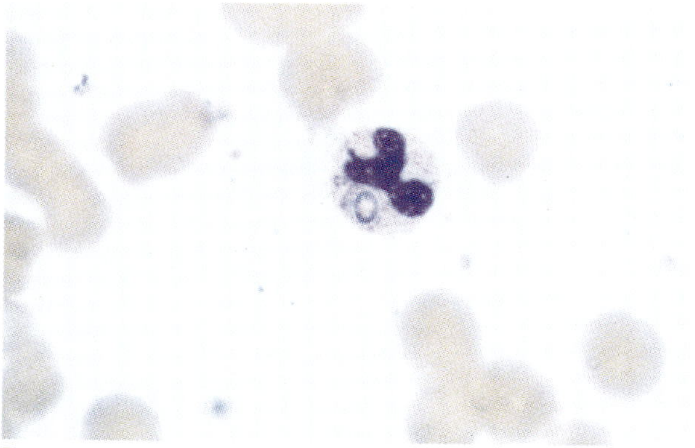

B

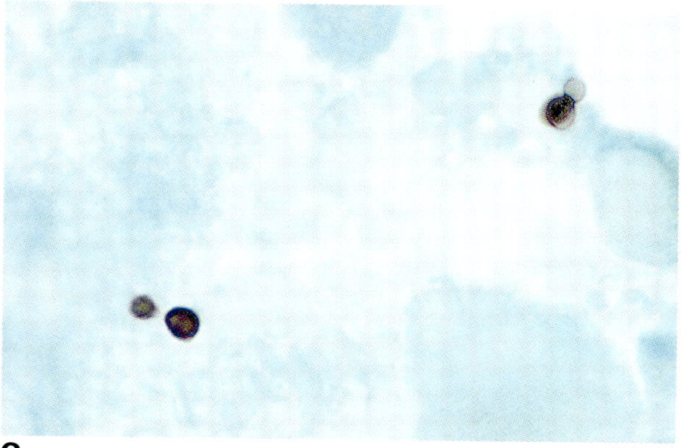

C

A chest x-ray film (Panel A) in a 41-year-old man with human immunodeficiency virus infection who had a four-month history of fever, cough, and worsening dyspnea showed a diffuse, bilateral reticulonodular pattern. A blood smear (Panel B; Wright–Giemsa stain, ×1000) obtained on admission showed intracellular organisms in segmented neutrophils. These yeast-like organisms had a clear halo, suggesting a capsule, and were consistent with histoplasma. The diagnosis was confirmed by bronchoalveolar lavage (Panel C; Grocott's methenamine silver, ×1000), which showed small, budding yeast characteristic of histoplasma (1 to 4 μm in diameter). The patient was intubated and treated with amphotericin B. His fever resolved and he was extubated on the sixth day of treatment, with clearing of the lungs on the chest film. Three days later staphylococcal septicemia developed, and the patient had an acute cerebral event and died.

Philip Daoust, M.D.
Brian Schapiro, M.D.

New England Medical Center Hospitals
Boston, MA 02111

March 14, 1996

Correspondence

A Drumstick?

July 25, 1996

To the Editor: Daoust and Schapiro describe a 41-year-old man with human immunodeficiency virus infection and histoplasmosis in their Image in Clinical Medicine (March 14 issue).[1] Panel B is reported to show a segmented neutrophil with an intracellular, histoplasma-like organism. A drumstick, or Barr body, is easily discernible at the 11 o'clock position in the segmented neutrophil. One can thus conclude that it is either a transfused cell from a female donor or that the male patient had Klinefelter's syndrome. It is also interesting to note that, if transfused, this neutrophil remained viable and functionally capable of phagocytosis.

Leonard Kessler, M.D.
242 Merrick Rd.
Rockville Centre, NY 11570

1. Daoust P, Schapiro B. Histoplasmosis. N Engl J Med 1996;334:700.

The authors reply:

To the Editor: In 1954, Davidson and Smith described a solitary chromatin nodule that becomes separated from the main nuclear lobe in a proportion of neutrophils in females.[1] They termed this nodule a drumstick and defined it as having a solid round head joined to one lobe of the nucleus by a single, fine chromatin strand. We do not concur with Dr. Kessler's identification of the appendage in the neutrophil as a drumstick. The original description of drumsticks notes that they had to be distinguished from "minor lobes," "small clubs," "racket" formation, and sessile nodules,[2] all of which can be observed in male neutrophils. The chromatin condensation seen in Panel B of our image lacks the fine chromatin strand characteristic of a drumstick. Instead, it has a wide base and the features of a sessile nodule.

In addition, even if the appendage were a drumstick, it would not be possible to determine sex on the basis of the single cell in our picture, since at least six drumsticks per 500 neutrophils must be present for the sex to be determined as female.[1] It is possible that the neutrophil in question was infused as part of a blood transfusion from a female blood donor, but we believe that this explanation is highly unlikely, given the short half-life of transfused neutrophils (about seven hours).[3] Drumsticks may be seen in male patients with Klinefelter's syndrome.[3] Our patient, however, had no clinical evidence of this syndrome.

Brian Schapiro, M.D.
Philip Daoust, M.D.
New England Medical Center
Boston, MA 02111

1. Davidson WM, Smith DR. A morphological sex difference in the polymorphonuclear neutrophil leucocytes. BMJ 1954;2:6-7.
2. Sandoz atlas of haematology. 2nd rev. ed. Basel, Switzerland: Sandoz, 1973:Plate 18.
3. Lee GR, Bithell TC, Foerster J, Athens JW, Lukens JN. Wintrobe's clinical hematology. 9th ed. Philadelphia: Lea & Febiger, 1993.

Severe Cryptococcal Pneumonia

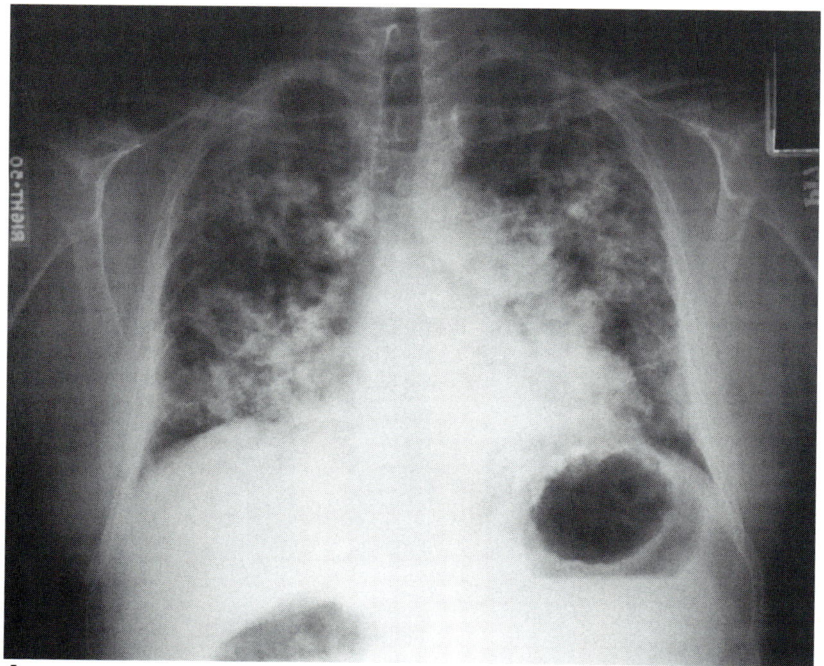

A

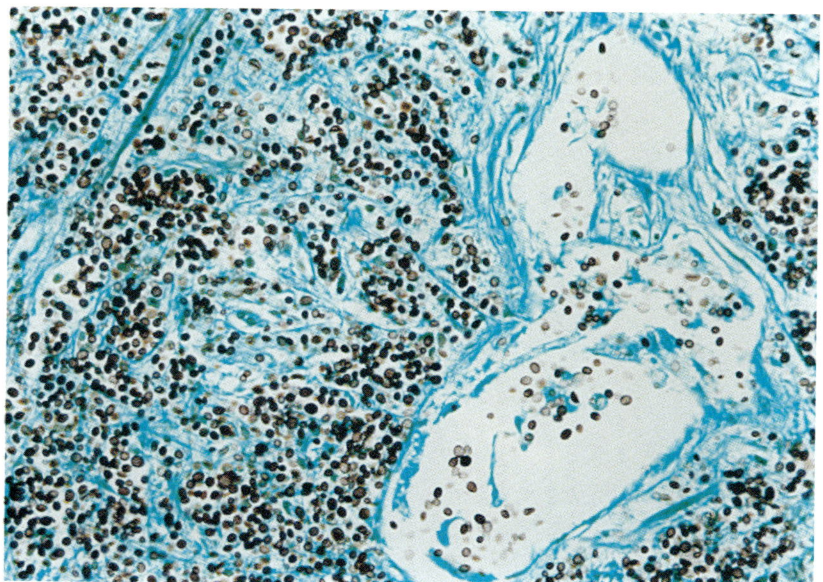

B

A 68-year-old man who had had biopsy-proved cryptococcal pneumonia 19 years earlier after cleaning a pigeon-infested barn was admitted to the hospital with increasing dyspnea, nonproductive cough, reduced exercise tolerance, and fever. His earlier episode of pneumonia had been treated with amphotericin B, but he was able to receive only a total of 1.5 g of the drug, because renal tubular acidosis, azotemia, and electrolyte disorders developed. He had been asymptomatic in the intervening years.

On admission, a chest radiograph showed five-lobe alveolar infiltrates (Panel A). Flexible fiberoptic bronchoscopy revealed cryptococci. Despite treatment with large doses of amphotericin B and fluconazole, the patient died of pneumonia. Panel B shows Gomori's methenamine silver staining of lung tissue obtained at autopsy (×250). The cryptococcal capsules are stained black. Much of the terminal air space is completely filled with the organisms.

The patient had no predisposing conditions, such as immunodeficiency, reticuloendothelial cancer, or hypercortisolism. The cause of the apparent reactivation is unknown.

George R. Robinson II, M.D.

York Hospital
York, PA 17405

June 29, 1995

Lucite-Ball Plombage

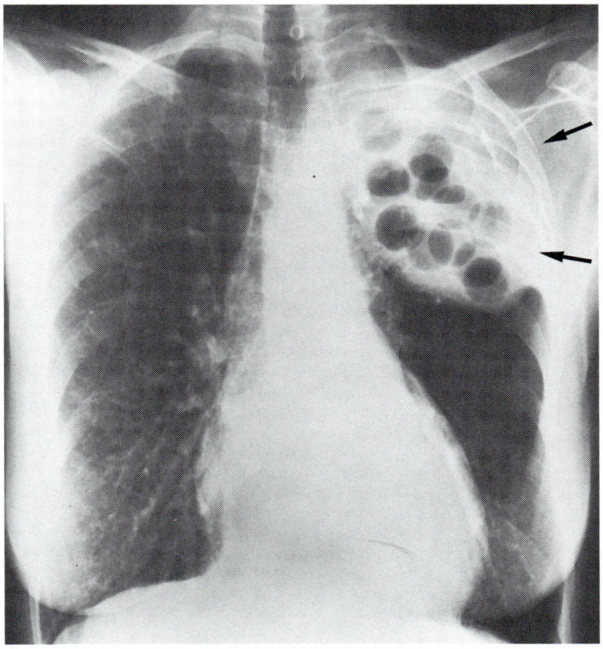

A

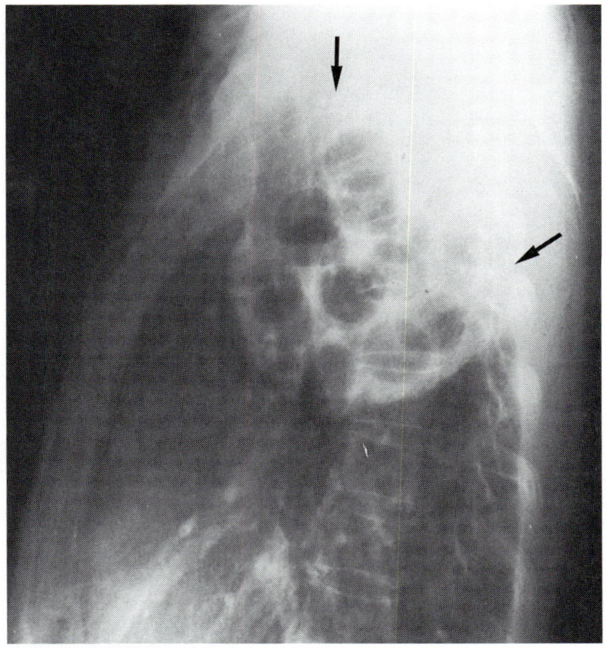

B

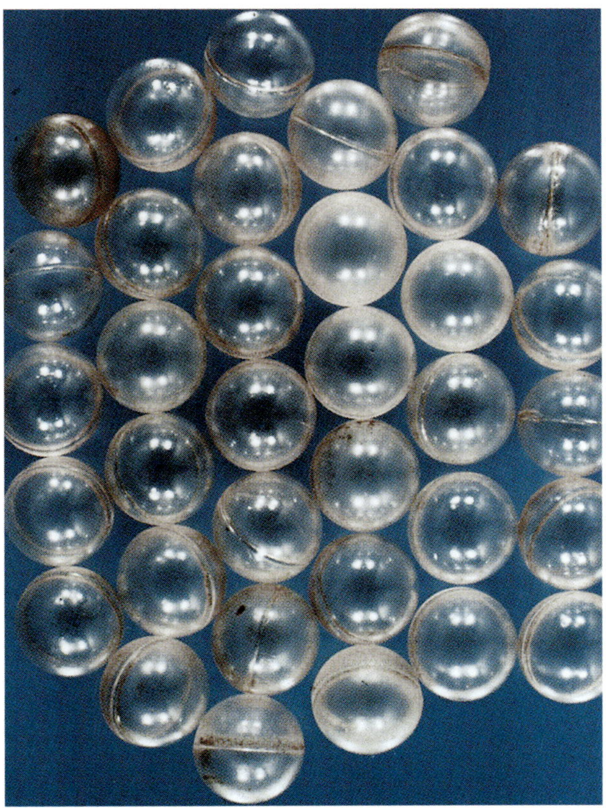

C

Posteroanterior and lateral chest x-ray films (Panels A and B, respectively) were obtained in a 64-year-old woman who was being evaluated for an upper respiratory tract infection. The patient had been treated for tuberculosis 41 years earlier by stripping the parietal pleura from the chest wall and packing the space with inert Lucite balls (arrows). A sample of these balls, each approximately 2.5 cm (1 in.) in diameter (two thirds the size of a Ping-Pong ball), taken post mortem from another patient, is shown in Panel C. The patient has been free of tuberculosis since the plombage was carried out.

David J. Mond, M.D.
Arfa Khan, M.D.

Long Island Jewish Medical Center
New Hyde Park, NY 11042

June 16, 1994

Inflammatory Autobullectomy

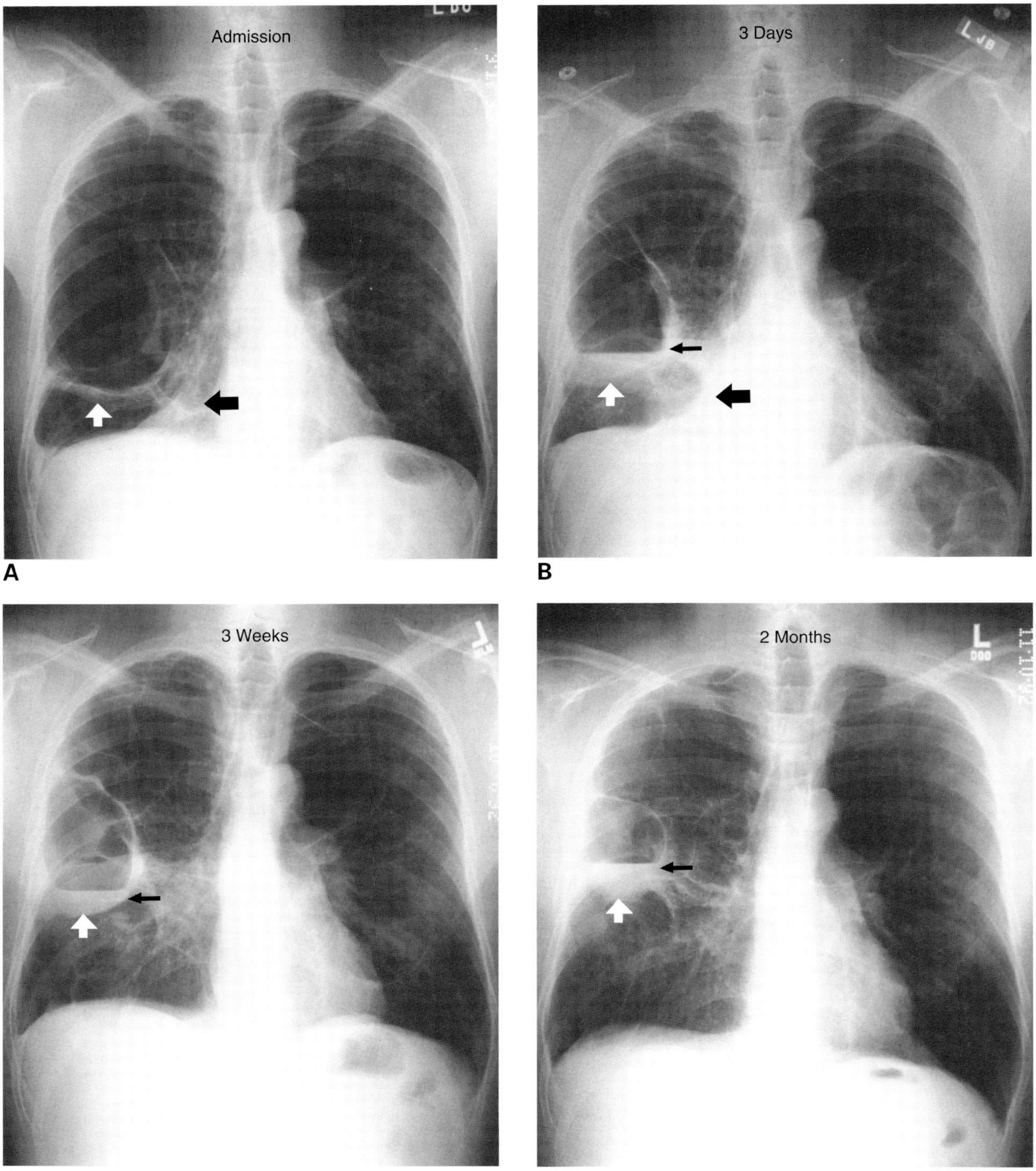

A B C D

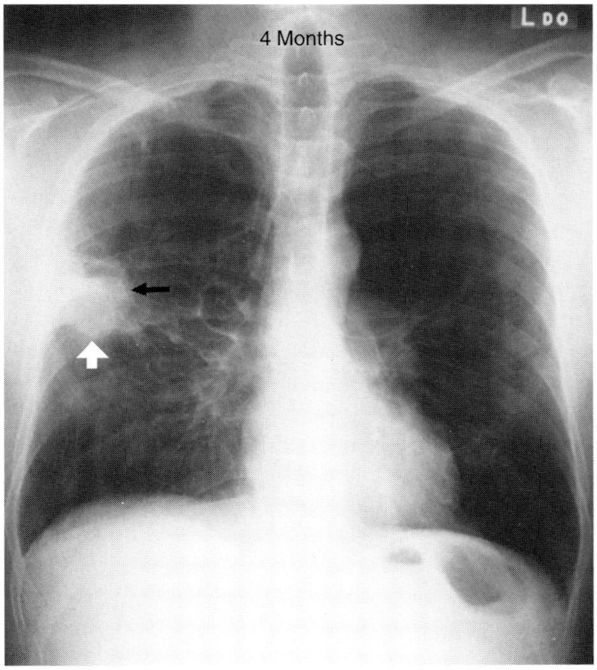

E

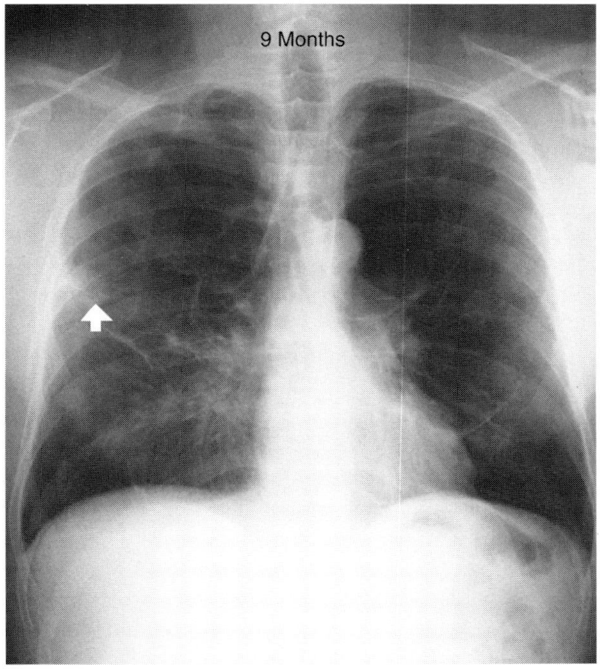

F

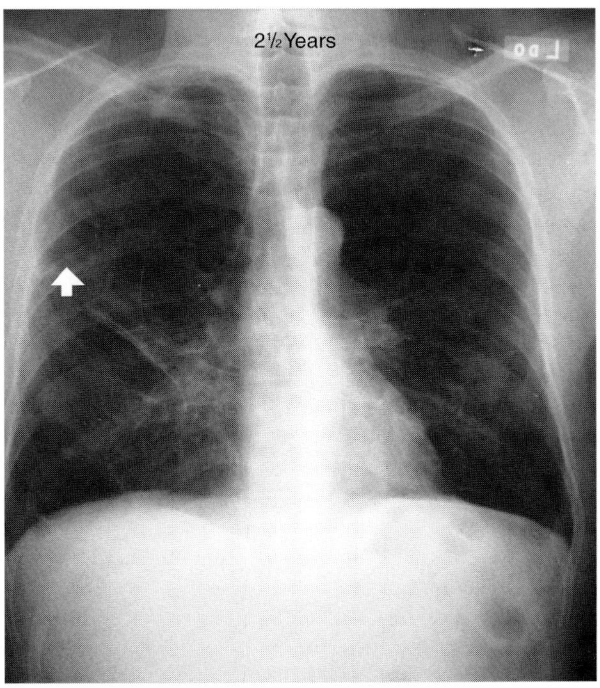

G

A 43-year-old man with bullous emphysema was admitted to the hospital with pneumonia. On admission a chest film (Panel A) showed a bulla (white arrow in Panels A through G), which had also been present 15 months earlier, adjacent to right-lower-lobe pneumonia (thick black arrow in Panels A and B). After three days of antibiotics, an air–fluid level (thin black arrow in Panels B, C, D, and E) developed within the bulla (Panel B). The clinical symptoms and the right-lower-lobe infiltrate resolved (Panel C) during the ensuing six-week course of amoxicillin at a dose of 500 mg orally three times a day, but the air–fluid level persisted (Panels D and E). The patient was followed clinically, with no further antibiotics. Over time, the bulla diminished in size (Panels D, E, and F), finally resulting in only a small, pleural-based scar (Panel G).

This case illustrates the commonly occurring process of a parapneumonic effusion within a bulla adjacent to an area of pneumonia and the rare shrinkage of a bulla, which probably results from the inflammatory process within the bulla and obstruction of the bronchus supplying it.

Richard B. Goodman, M.D.
S. Lakshminarayan, M.D.

Veterans Affairs Medical Center
Seattle, WA 98108

May 23, 1996

Paradoxical Embolus

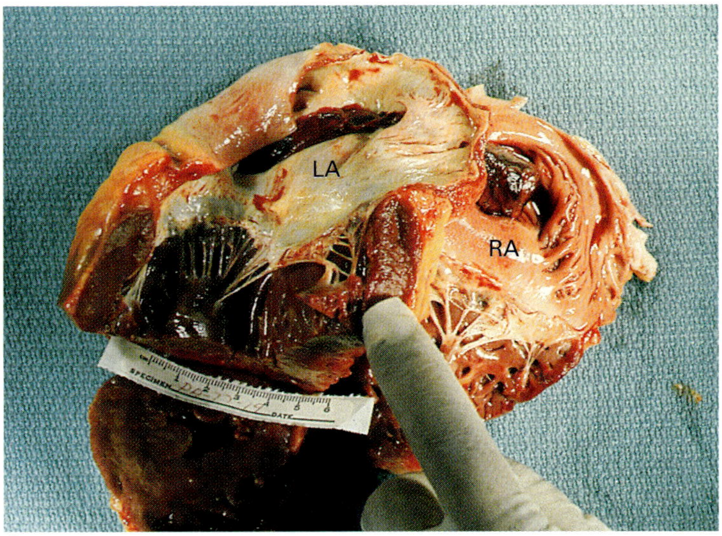

A

A paradoxical embolus was identified in a 64-year-old woman who presented with sudden chest pain and marked dyspnea. Pulmonary embolism was suspected. Soon after admission, she had a massive stroke and died. At autopsy multiple pulmonary emboli were found. The foramen ovale was patent and contained a large, lengthy embolus straddling the atrial septum (Panel A). Panel B shows the embolus trapped in the patent foramen ovale (FO). LA denotes left atrium, and RA right atrium.

Mark E. Silverman, M.D.

Emory University School of Medicine
Atlanta, GA 30309

September 23, 1993

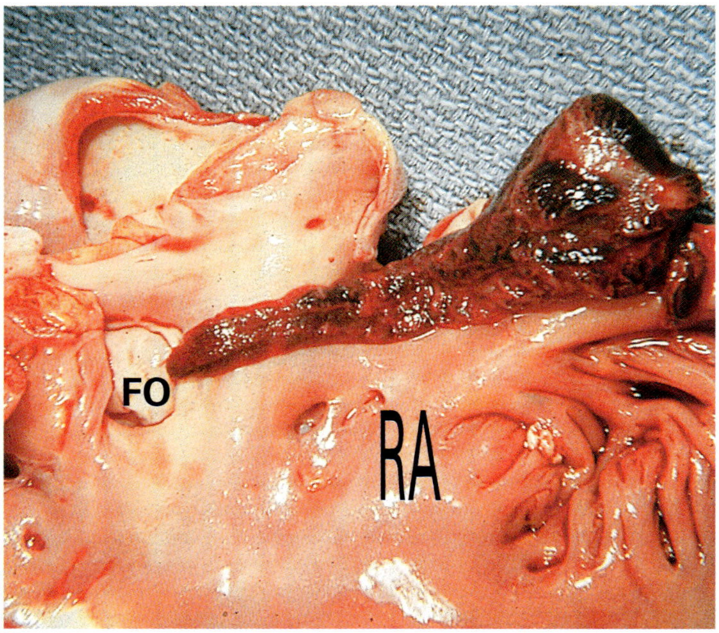

B

Correspondence

Embolism Interruptus

June 16, 1994

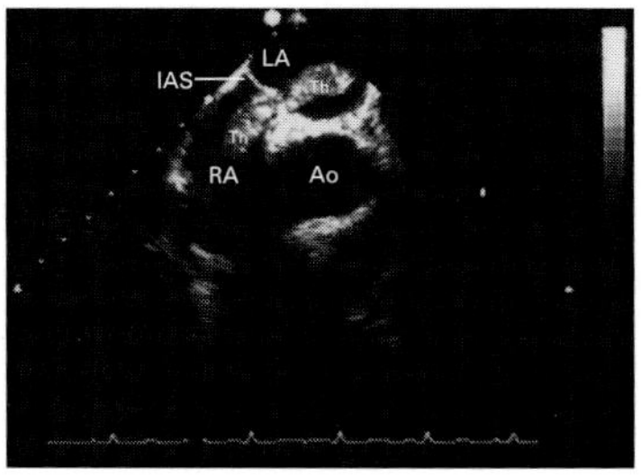

Figure 1. Transesophageal Echocardiogram Showing Thrombus Lodged in the Foramen Ovale.

IAS denotes interatrial septum, LA left atrium, RA right atrium, Ao aorta, and Th thrombus.

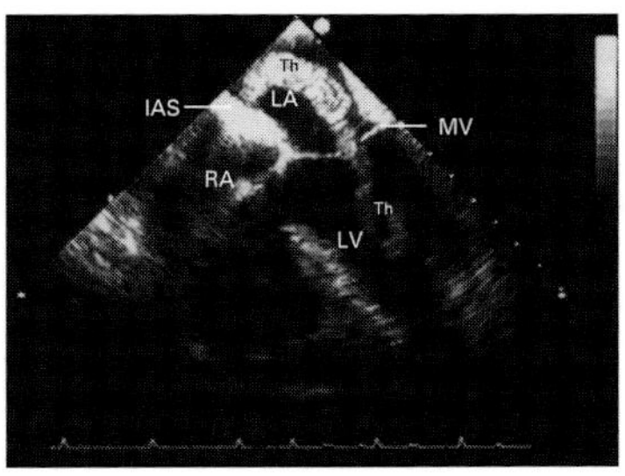

Figure 2. Long-Axis View of the Left Ventricle Showing the Left-Sided Portion of the Thrombus Extending to the Apex of the Left Ventricle.

LV denotes left ventricle, RA right atrium, LA left atrium, MV mitral valve, IAS interatrial septum, and Th thrombus.

To the Editor: The detection of a patent foramen ovale by transesophageal echocardiography in patients with arterial ischemic events is increasingly thought to be associated with a paradoxical embolism.[1] Except for one report of an impending paradoxical embolism detected by transthoracic echocardiography,[2] all diagnoses of paradoxical embolism through a patent foramen ovale have been either presumptive[3] or, as in the image by Silverman (Sept. 23 issue),[4] postmortem. We report a diagnosis of paradoxical embolism made by means of transesophageal echocardiography.

A 51-year-old obese woman was admitted to the hospital with dyspnea, migrating abdominal pain, and bloody diarrhea of five days' duration. A ventilation–perfusion lung scan revealed bilateral perfusion defects, and an abdominal computed tomographic scan revealed areas of attenuation in the spleen that were suggestive of infarcts. Intravenous heparin was started, but on the third hospital day the patient's left arm suddenly became painful, cold, and pulseless. Extensive amounts of thrombus were removed from the left subclavian and axillary arteries by means of an open arteriotomy. Transthoracic echocardiography showed an ill-defined mobile mass in the left ventricle and another possible mass in the right atrium.

Transesophageal echocardiography showed a large, lobulated mass in both atria crossing the inferior interatrial septum (Fig. 1). The left atrial portion prolapsed through the mitral valve into the apex of the left ventricle (Fig. 2). The left-sided mass was 1 cm wide at the septum and 9.5 cm long. The right atrial portion was 1 cm by 4.5 cm.

At surgery, a 15-cm thrombus was removed from a small foramen ovale where it had lodged. The foramen was sutured closed. The patient received anticoagulation therapy with warfarin and recovered, with no further symptoms. A Doppler study of the legs suggested the presence of deep venous thrombosis of the right thigh.

The studies in this patient provided a rare opportunity to observe an embolus originating in the venous circulation in the process of crossing a patent foramen ovale to enter the arterial circulation. Presumably, multiple pulmonary emboli and the accompanying pulmonary hypertension initially caused right-to-left interatrial shunting, forcing a large venous embolus across the patent foramen ovale, where it lodged. The thrombus then gave rise to multiple emboli in the subclavian, mesenteric, and splenic arteries. These findings confirm the hypothesis that large paradoxical emboli can cross a patent foramen ovale.

David Brogno, M.D.
Good Samaritan Hospital, Suffern, NY 10901

Gilead Lancaster, M.D.
Danbury Hospital, Danbury, CT 06810

Marlon Rosenbaum, M.D.
Columbia–Presbyterian Medical Center, New York, NY 10032

1. Movsowitz C, Podolsky LA, Meyerowitz CB, Jacobs LE, Kotler MN. Patent foramen ovale: a nonfunctional embryological remnant or a potential cause of significant pathology? J Am Soc Echocardiogr 1992;5:259-70.
2. Nelson CW, Snow FR, Barnett M, McRoy L, Wechsler AS, Nixon JV. Impending paradoxical embolism: echocardiographic diagnosis of an intracardiac thrombus crossing a patent foramen ovale. Am Heart J 1991;122:859-62.
3. Cheng TO. Echocardiography and paradoxical embolism. Ann Intern Med 1981;95:515.
4. Silverman ME. Paradoxical embolus. N Engl J Med 1993;329:930.

Clubbing and Hypertrophic Osteoarthropathy

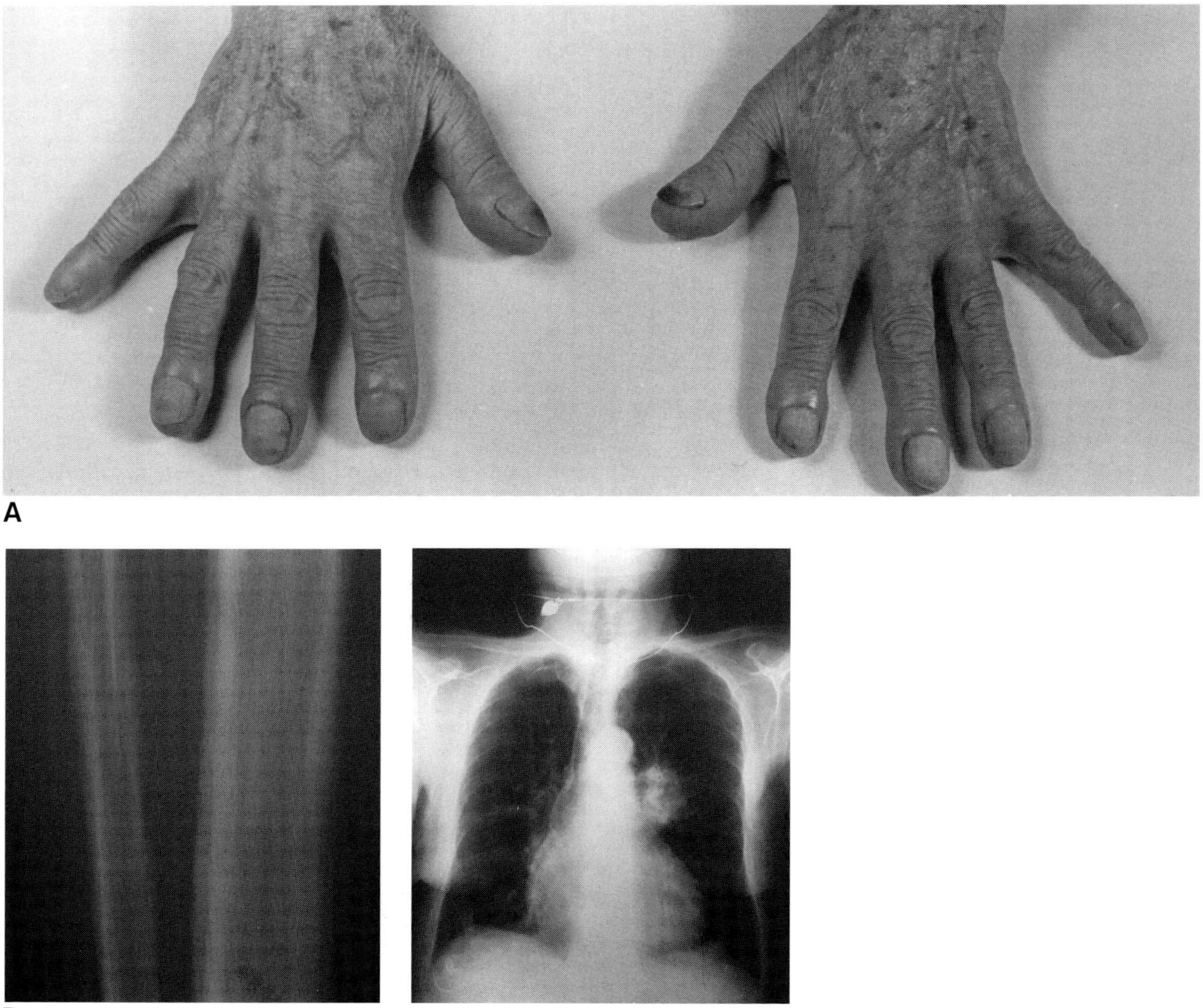

A

B

C

On examination the hands of a 70-year-old woman with worsening cough and pretibial pain show digital clubbing (Panel A). The terminal phalanges are enlarged, and there is loss of the normal nail-to-cuticle angle. A radiograph of the tibia and fibula (Panel B) shows the characteristic periosteal elevation of hypertrophic osteoarthropathy. A chest radiograph (Panel C) shows hyperinflation, borderline cardiac enlargement, and a left hilar mass that proved to be a non–small-cell bronchogenic carcinoma.

Melvin D. Burton, M.D.
John C. Wain, Jr., M.D.

Massachusetts General Hospital
Boston, MA 02114

December 16, 1993

Midtracheal Stricture

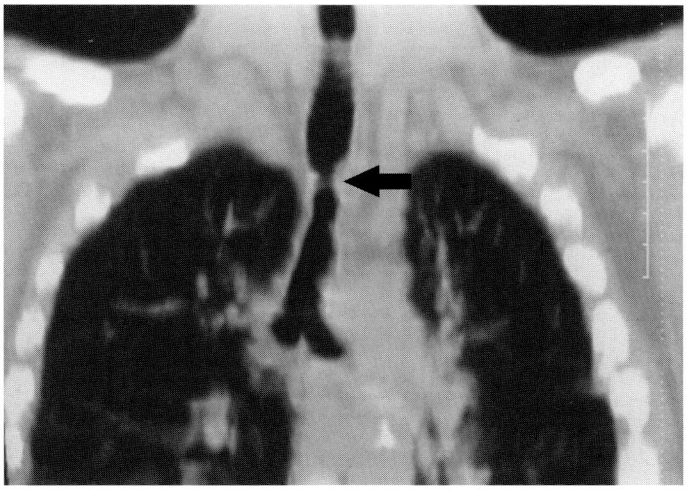

A

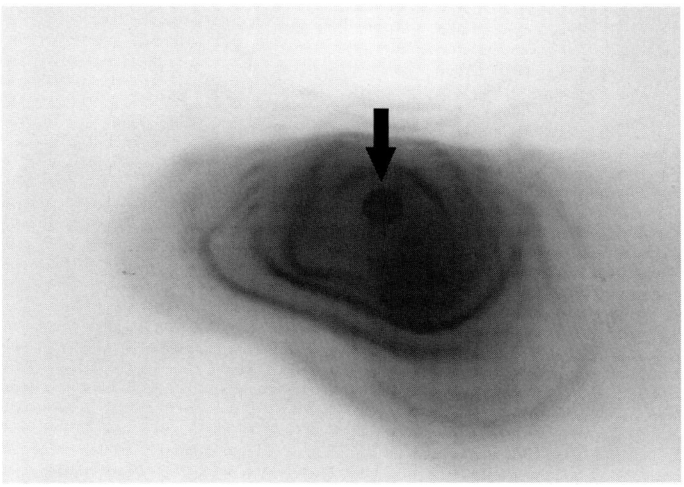

B

A 47-year-old woman presented with dyspnea on exertion and a history of having awoken at night with a sensation of choking twice in the previous week. She had been discharged from the hospital three weeks earlier, after an episode of severe adult respiratory distress syndrome following blunt chest trauma. She had required mechanical ventilation for nearly three months with an endotracheal tube and tracheostomy during that hospitalization. The tracheostomy was performed after 10 days of endotracheal intubation.

On examination the patient had stridorous breath sounds; flexible laryngoscopy showed a normal pharynx. A flow-volume loop demonstrated marked limitation of inspiratory and expiratory flow consistent with the presence of a fixed obstruction of the airway. Helical (spiral) computed tomography in which 5-mm axial sections were obtained every 4 mm from the midportion of the neck through the hila was performed while the patient held her breath. The trachea was then further evaluated with multiplanar coronal reconstructions (Panel A) and internal rendering with a three-dimensional shaded-surface display to simulate the luminal appearance of the trachea as seen from above the carina (Panel B). These images confirmed the presence of a focal stenosis in the midportion of the trachea (arrows in Panels A and B). The stenosis was thought to be caused by hyperinflation of the endotracheal-tube cuff, which in retrospect was evident on a computed tomographic scan obtained on day 7 of the initial hospitalization.

Acute respiratory failure developed approximately 72 hours after admission. After rigid bronchoscopy, the stricture was resected and the trachea was reanastomosed by open thoracotomy. Postoperatively the patient had bilateral dysfunction of the vocal cords and required a tracheostomy but otherwise recovered uneventfully and was sent home on day 27. At follow-up five months later, she continued to have complete paralysis of the right vocal cord and marked weakness of the left.

Martin E. Doerfler, M.D.
David P. Naidich, M.D.

New York University School of Medicine
New York, NY 10016

December 19, 1996

A Ferruginous Body

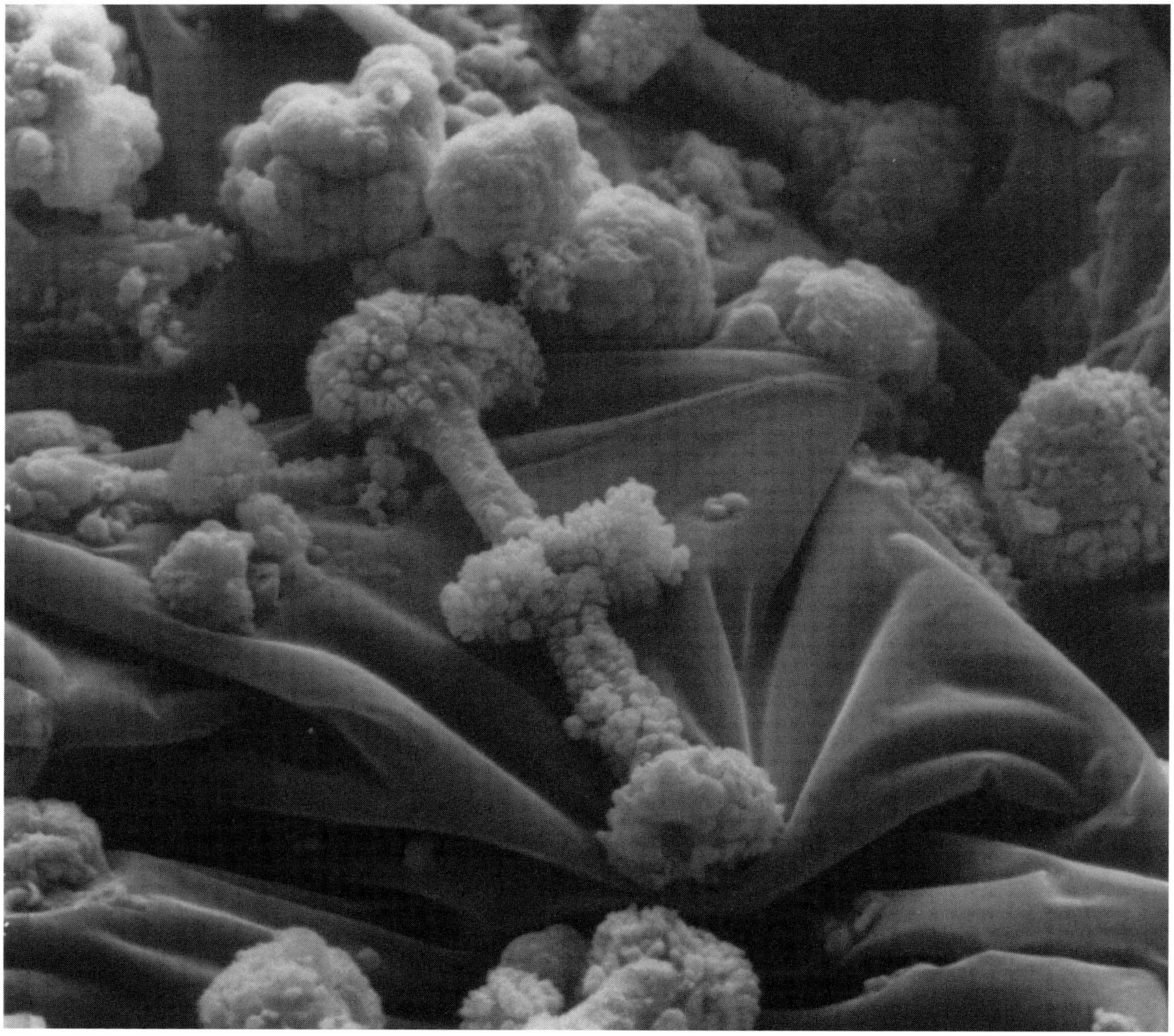

The classic dumbbell-shaped, sometimes beaded appearance of an asbestos fiber, also known as a ferruginous body, is evident in an iron–mucopolysaccharide matrix on scanning electron microscopy (×1595). The fibers were obtained at the postmortem examination of a 58-year-old man with a history of smoking 100 packs of cigarettes per year and long-term exposure to asbestos who died of secondary interstitial pulmonary fibrosis and stage IV non–small-cell bronchogenic carcinoma.

Anne Sorling, B.S./C.T. (A.S.C.P.)
Corey J. Langer, M.D.

Department of Medical Oncology
Fox Chase Cancer Center
Philadelphia, PA 19111

May 13, 1993

Endocrinology, Metabolism, and Nutrition

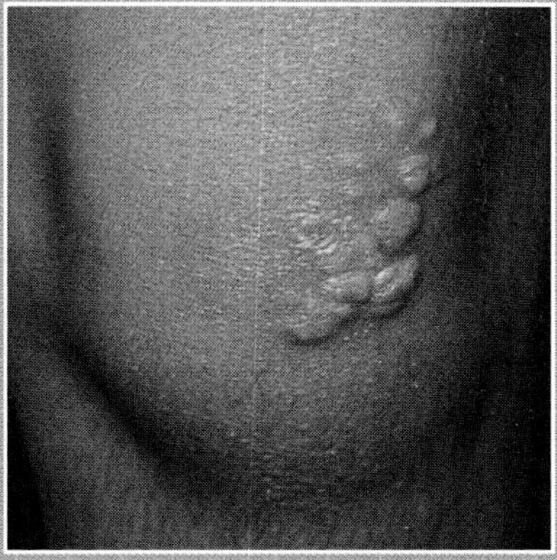

Necrobiosis Lipoidica Diabeticorum

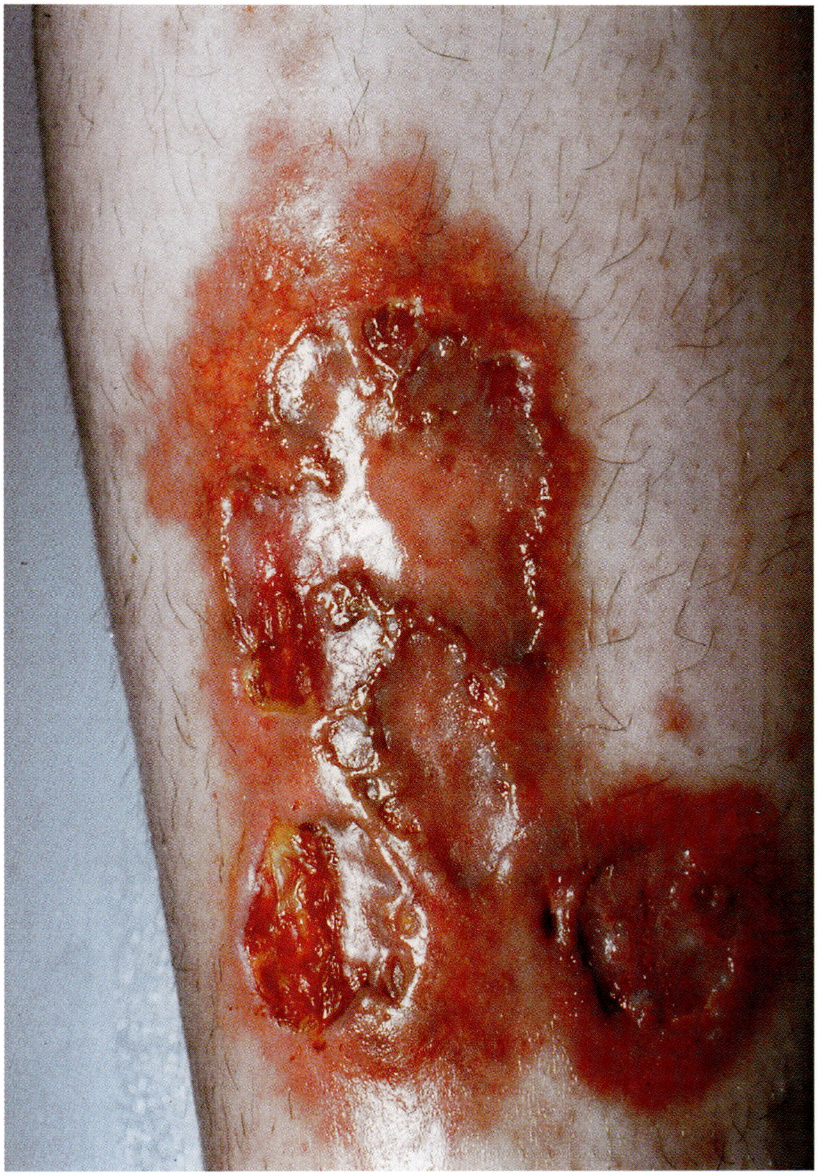

The photograph shows the anterior surface of the lower leg of a 20-year-old woman who had a 10-year history of poorly controlled diabetes mellitus. The lesion measures 9 by 5 cm and has characteristic atrophic, shiny, yellow-brown telangiectatic plaques with ulceration and scarring. Treatment consisted of whirlpool therapy, occlusive dressings, topical steroids, aspirin, and pentoxifylline.

Stephen F. Templeton, M.D.
S. Wright Caughman, M.D.

Department of Dermatology
Emory University School of Medicine
Atlanta, GA 30322

July 29, 1993

Corticosteroid Osteonecrosis

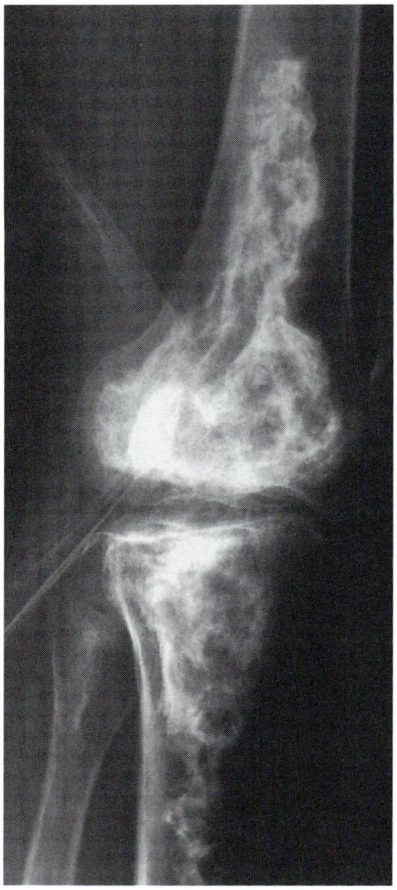

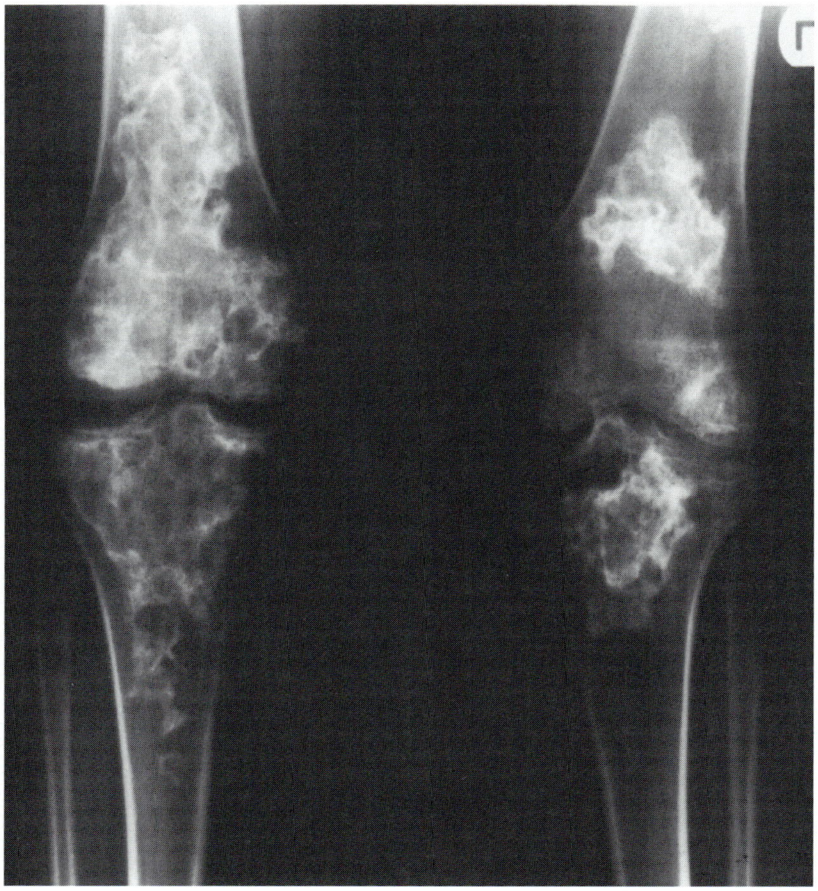

Plain films of the knees of a 50-year-old woman receiving long-term corticosteroid therapy reveal medullary bone infarcts in the distal femurs and proximal tibias. Serpiginous lucencies with peripheral sclerotic rims represent necrotic spongy bone and marrow walled off by calcified collagenous fibrous tissue. Osteonecrosis can also occur with short-term use of corticosteroids.

Cynthia T. Chin, M.D.
Robert C. Sarno, M.D.

New England Medical Center
Boston, MA 02111

February 23, 1995

Correspondence

Corticosteroid Osteonecrosis

July 13, 1995

To the Editor: Chin and Sarno (Feb. 23 issue)[1] state, "Osteonecrosis can also occur with short-term use of corticosteoids." This statement is inexact and incomplete, and it could be used unfairly by lawyers in malpractice suits.

My colleagues and I have reviewed the international literature for any evidence that short-term treatment (less than 2 weeks) with moderate doses of prednisone (starting at 40 mg per day given orally, with the dose reduced over a period ranging from 6 to 14 days) in adults is associated with osteonecrosis. My experience is that this association is not present in a specific subgroup of patients. My colleagues and I are satisfied that in otherwise healthy people with asthma, chronic sinusitis, nasal polyps, or atopic dermatitis, osteonecrosis of bone is not a complication of prednisone treatment as outlined above.

Short-term treatment with corticosteroids may induce osteonecrosis in patients given very high doses, such as patients with head injuries and cerebral edema or those with multiple bone and joint injuries. Osteonecrosis also appears to be more likely among alcoholics and is certainly more likely in patients with collagen disease, such as systemic lupus erythematosus or rheumatoid arthritis.

It is important that this issue be clarified, because doctors may be unfairly judged and punished in courts of law for using a valuable therapeutic regimen in patients with diseases that are debilitating and potentially serious. A short-term regimen of moderate doses of prednisone is used in children as well as adults, also with no evidence of osteonecrosis when the guidelines outlined above are followed.

Allan Knight, M.D.
Sunnybrook Health Science Centre
Toronto, ON M4N 3M5, Canada

1. Chin CT, Sarno RC. Corticosteroid osteonecrosis. N Engl J Med 1995;332:511.

To the Editor: The knee radiographs by Chin and Sarno showing osteonecrosis are excellent teaching aids. However, the term corticosteroid osteonecrosis indicates an unequivocal relation between corticosteroid therapy and osteonecrosis, which oversimplifies the issue. Osteonecrosis had been described by 1888, over 60 years before the era of corticosteroid therapy.[1] Almost 90 percent of patients with nontraumatic osteonecrosis have not received corticosteroids,[2] and osteonecrosis does not develop in most patients who do receive corticosteroids. The risk of osteonecrosis in patients with pulmonary disease or head injuries who receive high-dose corticosteroid therapy has been calculated to be quite low: 0.03 to 1.2 percent.[3-5]

It is important to set the record straight on this point, because the assumption of absolute causation between corticosteroid use and osteonecrosis places an unjustified onus on all physicians who prescribe corticosteroids.

Lawrence N. Parker, M.D.
University of California, Irvine
Long Beach, CA 90822

1. McCarthy EF. Aseptic necrosis of bone: an historic perspective. Clin Orthop 1982;168:216-21.
2. Patterson RJ, Bickel WH, Dahlin DC. Idiopathic avascular necrosis of the head of the femur: a study of fifty-two cases. J Bone Joint Surg Am 1964;46:267-82.
3. Kenzora JE, Glimcher MJ. Accumulative cell stress: the multifactorial etiology of idiopathic osteonecrosis. Orthop Clin North Am 1985;16:669-79.
4. Parker L, Charter R, Wenjen M. A re-examination of the relationship between glucocorticoid therapy and avascular necrosis. Exp Clin Endocrinol 1991;10:59-61.
5. Richards JM, Santiago SM, Klaustermeyer WB. Aseptic necrosis of the femoral head in corticosteroid-treated pulmonary disease. Arch Intern Med 1980;140:1473-5.

Skin Findings in a Patient with Scurvy

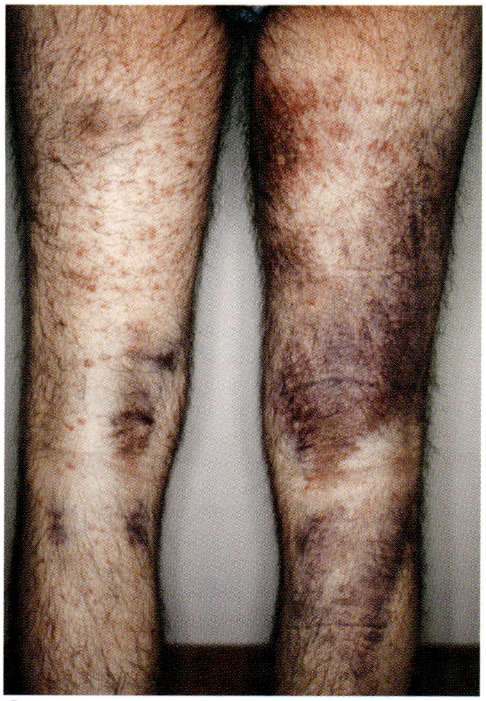

A

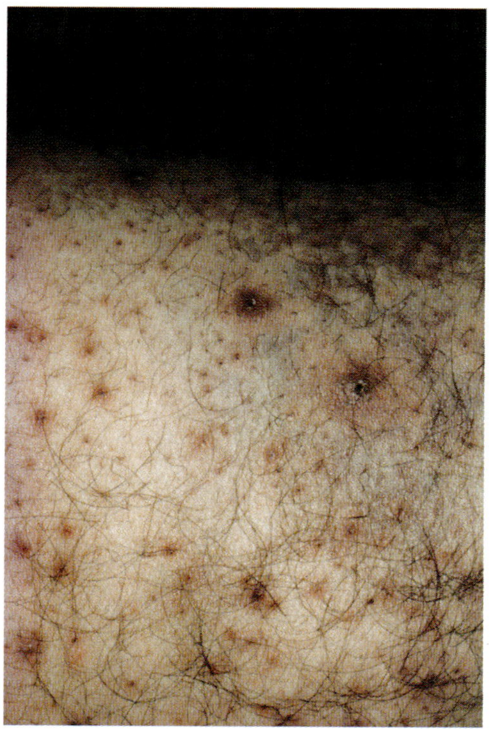

B

The legs of a 46-year-old man with scurvy are shown. The man had a mild mental disorder, and his diet consisted only of bread, pasta, packaged cookies, and water. Large ecchymotic areas extended over the backs of the legs (Panel A). A close-up (Panel B) shows perifollicular hemorrhages and hyperkeratotic papules in which hair is fragmented and buried. The plasma ascorbic acid concentration was 0.11 mg per deciliter (6.25 μmol per liter; normal concentration, >0.62 mg per deciliter [35 μmol per liter]) after three days of a hospital diet. With a normal diet and vitamin C replacement therapy (500 mg orally per day), all findings disappeared within two and a half weeks.

Christoph M. Kronauer, M.D.
Hugo Bühler, M.D.

City Hospital Waid
8037 Zurich, Switzerland

June 15, 1995

Kayser–Fleischer Ring in a Patient with Wilson's Disease

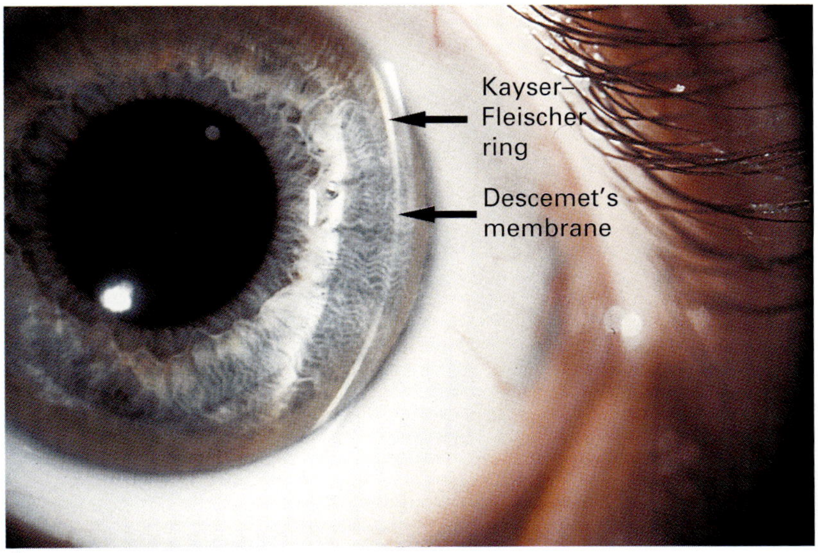

A

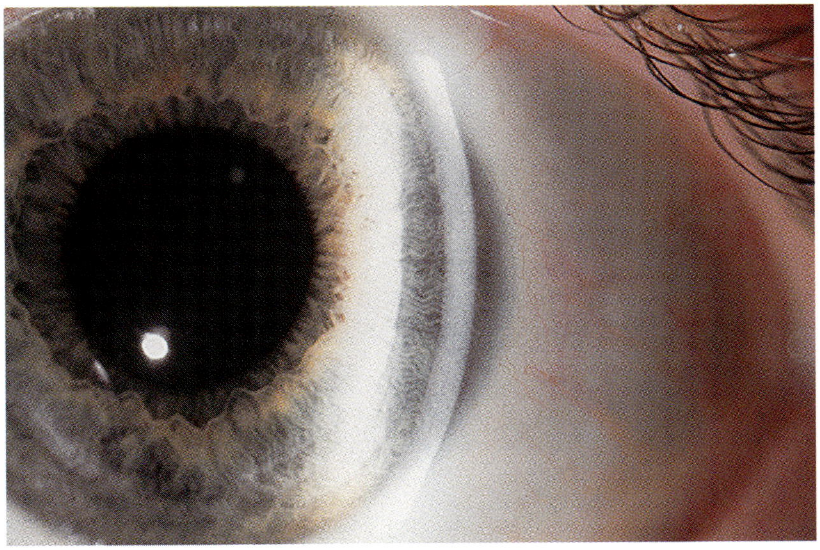

B

Slit-lamp photography shows a dense deposit of copper in Descemet's membrane (a Kayser–Fleischer ring) in a 17-year-old girl with Wilson's disease (Panel A). After eight years of therapy with dimercaprol and penicillamine, the Kayser–Fleischer ring had completely resolved (Panel B). The left eye is shown; the right eye had a similar appearance. (The other line is formed by the beam of the slit lamp.)

Albert W. Biglan, M.D.

University of Pittsburgh
School of Medicine
Pittsburgh, PA 15213

Sharon L. Taylor, M.D.

St. Francis Medical Center
Pittsburgh, PA 15201

June 24, 1993

Cutaneous Xanthomas in Homozygous Familial Hypercholesterolemia

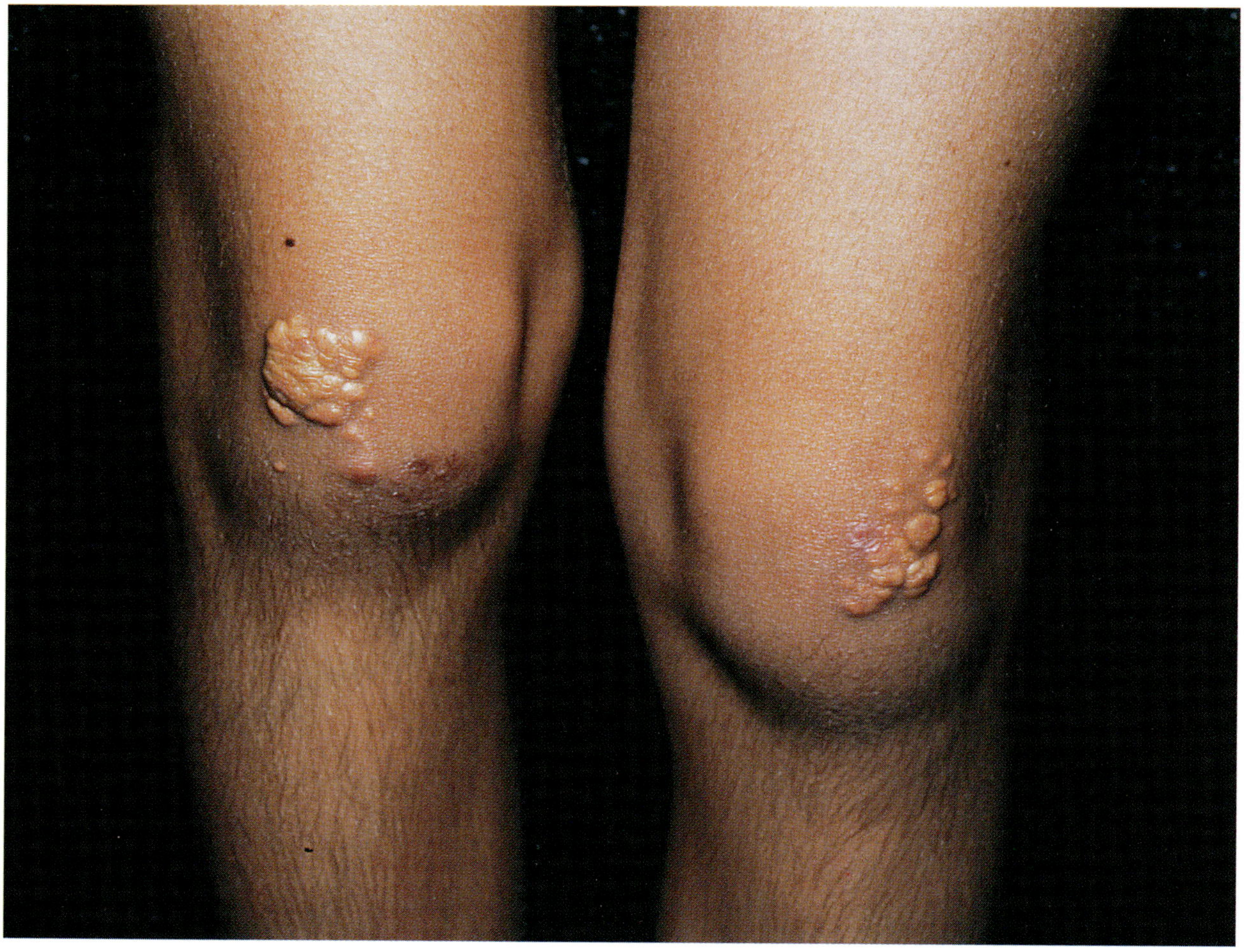

A baby boy was found to have familial hypercholesterolemia at the age of six months. His parents also had hypercholesterolemia. Seven and a half years later, studies of the activity of low-density lipoprotein (LDL) receptors in proliferating lymphocytes indicated that the parents were heterozygous and the child was homozygous for LDL-receptor deficiency. The child's serum cholesterol concentration ranged from 850 to 1000 mg per deciliter (22 to 26 mmol per liter), and he had cutaneous xanthomas on his knees (as shown), elbows, and interdigital folds. Because the hypercholesterolemia was refractory to treatment with lovastatin and cholestyramine, the patient was treated once a week with apheresis to remove the excess LDL cholesterol with an automated dextran sulfate cellulose adsorption system. Just before this treatment was begun, the following lipid concentrations were recorded: total cholesterol, 930 mg per deciliter (24 mmol per liter); total triglycerides, 82 mg per deciliter (1 mmol per liter); LDL cholesterol, 878 mg per deciliter (23 mmol per liter); and high-density lipoprotein (HDL) cholesterol, 38 mg per deciliter (1 mmol per liter). After one year of treatment, the xanthomas disappeared. The mean lipid concentrations during that year were as follows: total cholesterol, 270 mg per deciliter (7 mmol per liter); LDL cholesterol, 200 mg per deciliter (5 mmol per liter); and HDL cholesterol, 58 mg per deciliter (1.5 mmol per liter).

J.L. Teruel, M.D., Ph.D.
M.A. Lasunción, Ph.D.

Hospital Ramón y Cajal
28034 Madrid, Spain

April 27, 1995

Porphyria Cutanea Tarda

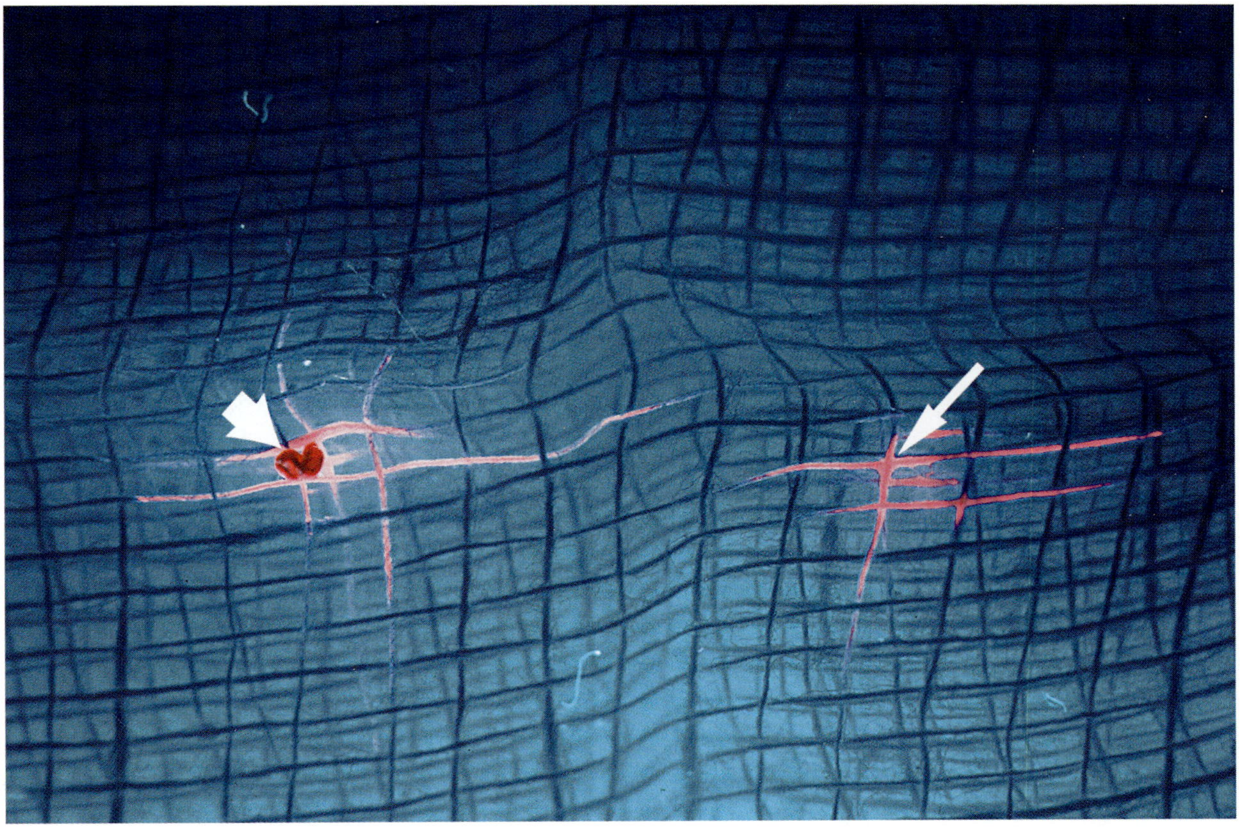

Water-soluble porphyrins from a liver-biopsy specimen from a patient with porphyria cutanea tarda show pink fluorescence under a Wood's light (405 nm). The biopsy specimen (short arrow) was preserved in saline solution to prevent desiccation and then transferred to a piece of gauze. Drops of saline containing fluorescing water-soluble porphyrins, including uroporphyrin (8-carboxylporphyrin) and 7-carboxylporphyrin, stain the gauze pink around the specimen and elsewhere (long arrow).

Marc E. Grossman, M.D.

Columbia–Presbyterian Medical Center
New York, NY 10032

October 13, 1994

Diaper Diagnosis of Porphyria

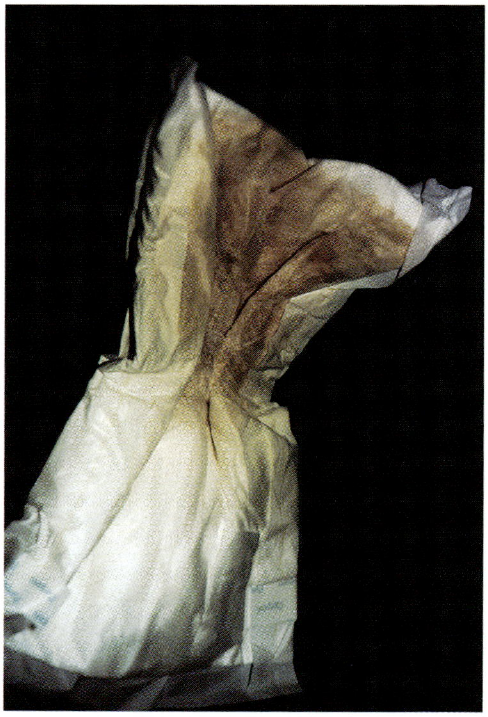

A

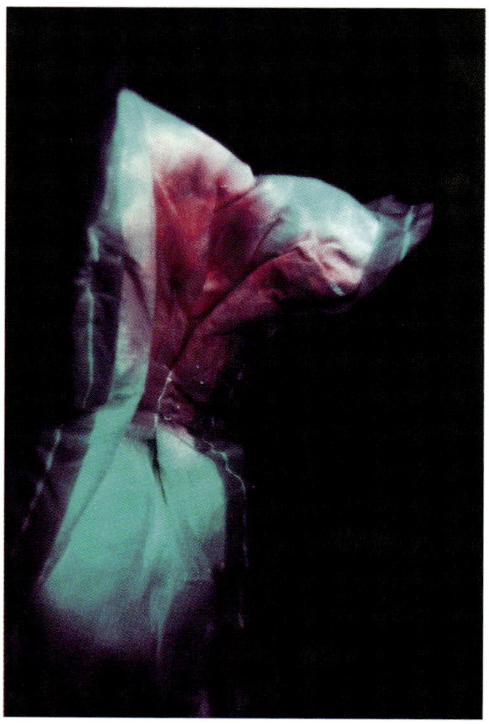

B

A blood- and urine-soaked diaper from a neonate with organomegaly, hemolytic anemia, thrombocytopenia, and cutaneous blisters was photographed under ambient light with a flash apparatus (Panel A) and under Wood's light (320 to 420 nm) (Panel B). The child's parents were first cousins, but the family history was otherwise negative for porphyria. Subsequent investigation showed very high levels of porphyrins in urine, serum, red cells, and stool. Fluorescence of a diaper under Wood's light is an indication that further studies of porphyrin metabolism should be done.

Shoshannah S. Pollack, M.D.

Albert Einstein College of Medicine
Bronx, NY 10461

Mark S. Rosenthal, M.D.

Mount Sinai Hospital
New York, NY 10029

January 13, 1994

Correspondence

A Porphyrin-Soaked Diaper

June 9, 1994

To the Editor: The superb photographs of a diaper soaked with urine containing a high porphyrin level (Jan. 13 issue)[1] warrant additional clarification so as not to mislead readers.[1] No specific diagnosis beyond porphyria is given, and it should be understood that fluorescence of a diaper under Wood's light, as shown in the image, is typically encountered only in congenital erythropoietic porphyria (Günther's disease), which is one of the rarest porphyrias.[2] Since this test or observation is of no value in the other porphyrias, detailed diagnostic tests have to follow the initial suspicion in order to ascertain the specific type of porphyria.

Claus A. Pierach, M.D.
Abbott Northwestern Hospital
Minneapolis, MN 55407

Hellmut Ippen, M.D.
Universitäts-Hautklinik
D-37075 Göttingen, Germany

1. Pollack SS, Rosenthal MS. Diaper diagnosis of porphyria. N Engl J Med 1994;330:114.
2. Boomer JR, Bonkovsky HL. The porphyrias. Dis Mon 1989;35:1-54.

The "Thumb Sign" in Marfan's Syndrome

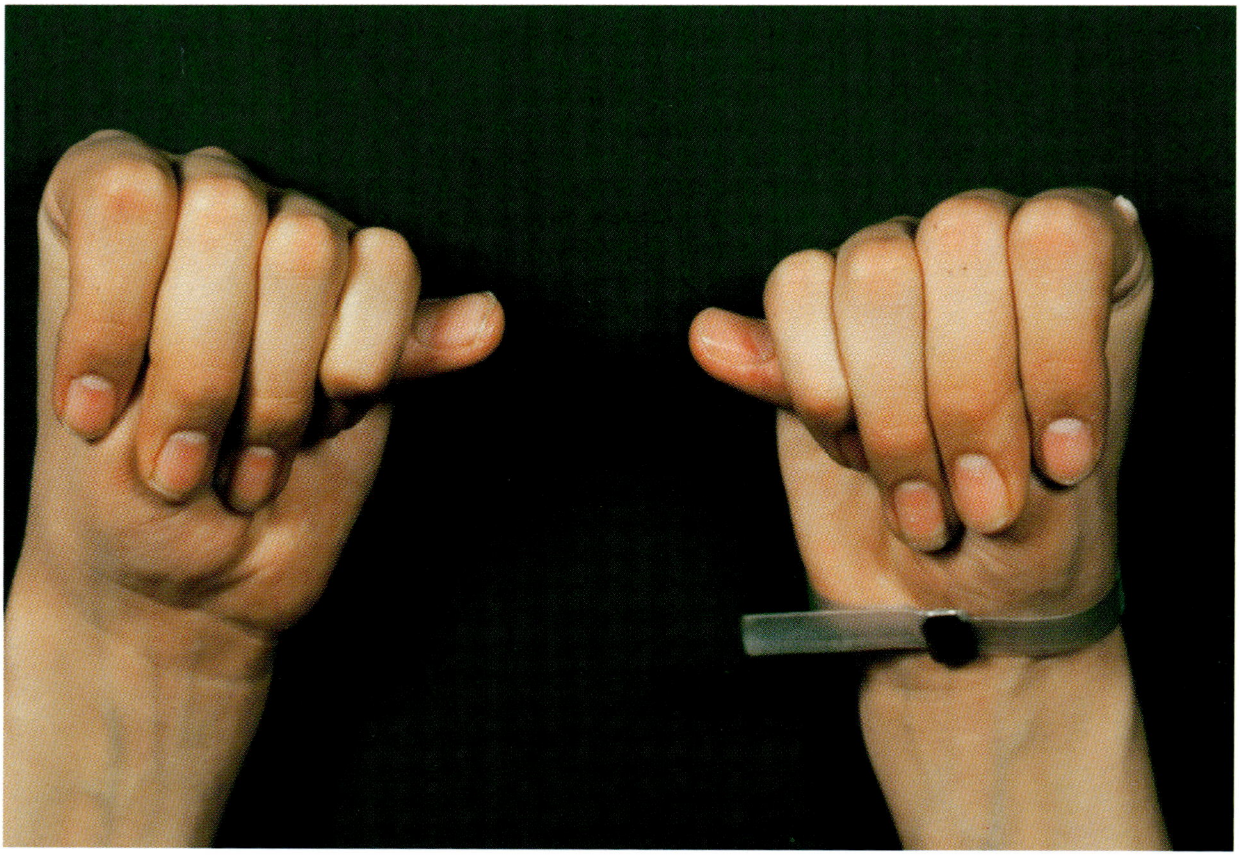

The thumbs protrude from the clenched fists of a 24-year-old man who presented with congestive heart failure due to severe chronic aortic regurgitation and left ventricular dysfunction. Arachnodactyly ("spider finger") and loose joints account for the ability to position the fingers in this way. The patient also had other skeletal features of Marfan's syndrome, including pectus excavatum and a high-arched palate.

Rodney H. Falk, M.D.

Boston University School of Medicine
Boston, MA 02118

August 17, 1995

Tamoxifen-Induced Endometrial Polyp

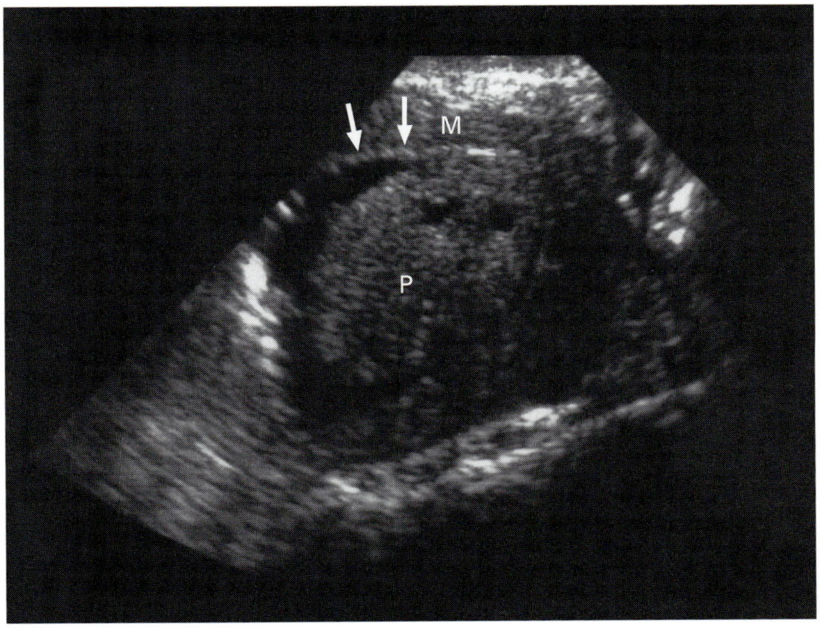

A

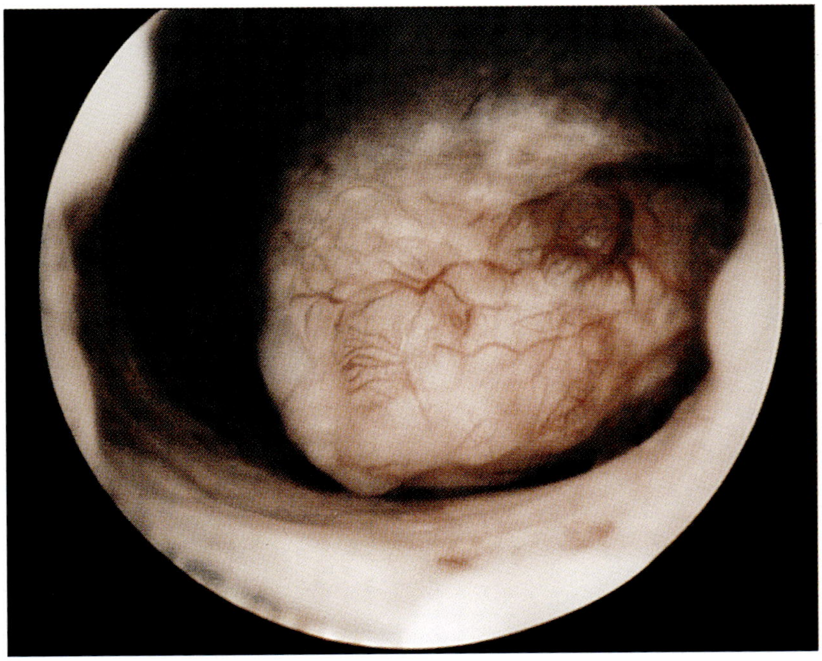

B

A 76-year-old woman with breast cancer who had been receiving adjuvant therapy with tamoxifen (20 mg per day) for 30 months presented with minimal vaginal bleeding. Color Doppler imaging revealed multiple arterial vessels with a very low resistance to flow (pulsatility index, 0.50; resistance index, 0.37) within the endometrium. The presence of a large endometrial polyp was demonstrated by the intrauterine instillation of sterile saline under ultrasonographic control (Panel A). Except for the large floating polyp (P), the endometrium (arrows) was thin and regular. M denotes the surrounding myometrium. The hysteroscopic view of the polyp, which measured 5.5 by 4.0 by 3.8 cm before its removal with a resectoscope, is shown in Panel B. Pathological examination disclosed a benign endometrial glandulocystic polyp without atypical cells. There were multiple small cysts lined with a single layer of epithelium. Tamoxifen was discontinued three weeks postoperatively. The patient stopped bleeding after the polyp was removed, and five months postoperatively, the endometrium had a normal appearance on ultrasonography.

Dirk Timmerman, M.D.
Ignace Vergote, M.D., Ph.D.

University Hospitals Leuven
B-3000 Leuven, Belgium

November 28, 1996

Wounds and Injuries

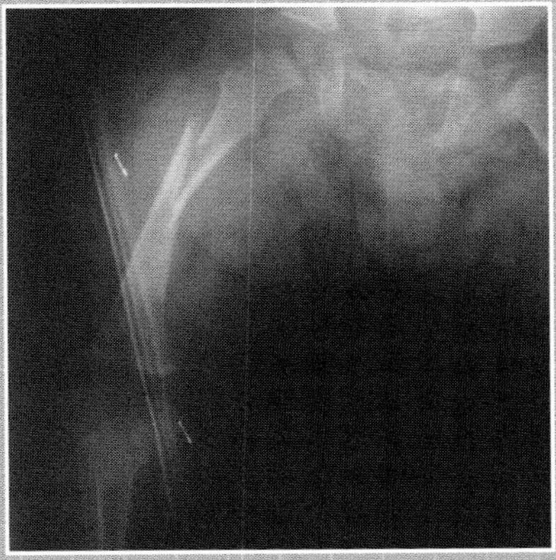

Coining

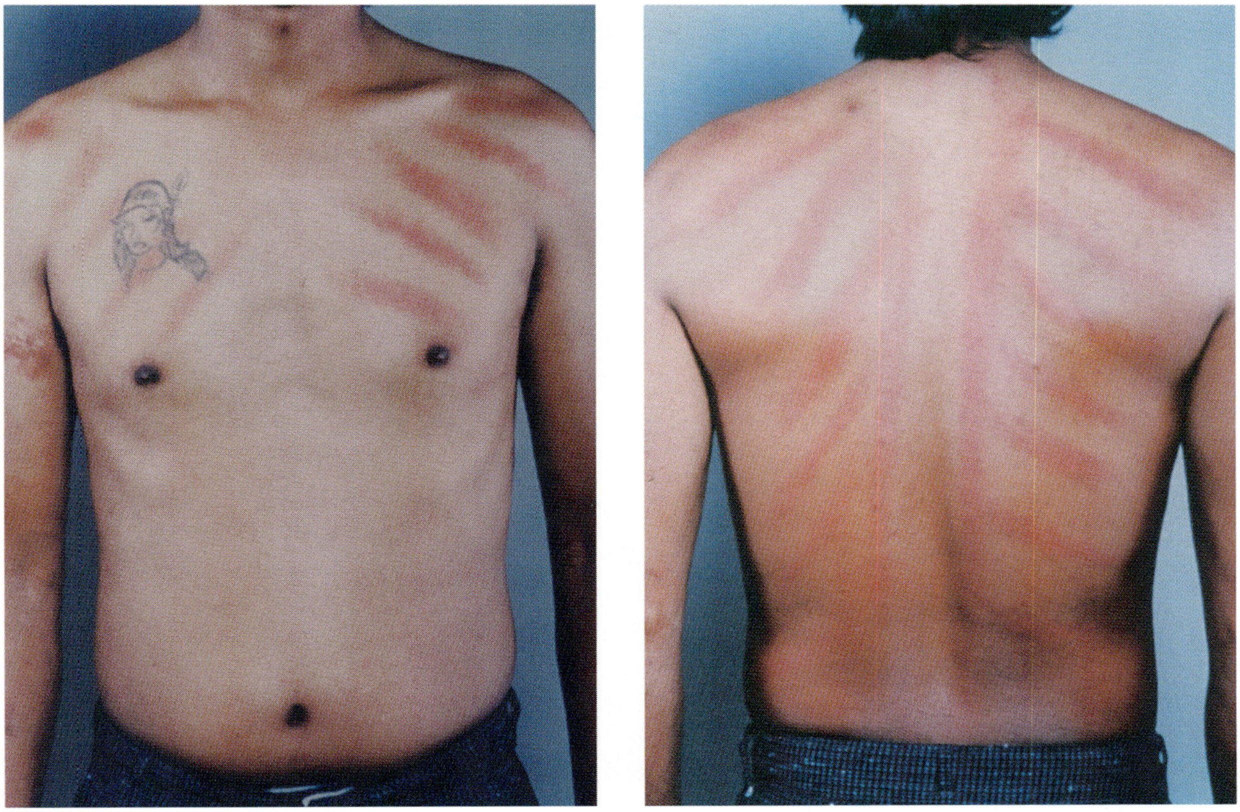

Linear microecchymoses, produced by rubbing the edge of a coin on the skin, are visible on a 33-year-old Vietnamese man who had been using this traditional Southeast Asian treatment unsuccessfully for recurrent migraine headaches. The erythematous stripes usually disappear after one to two weeks, but hyperpigmentation may persist. The lesions from this home remedy should not be mistaken for a manifestation of abuse.

Charles E. Crutchfield, III, M.D.

Gundersen Clinic
La Crosse, WI 54601

Thomas J. Bisig, M.D.

Mayo Clinic
Rochester, MN 55905

June 8, 1995

Consequences of Cupping

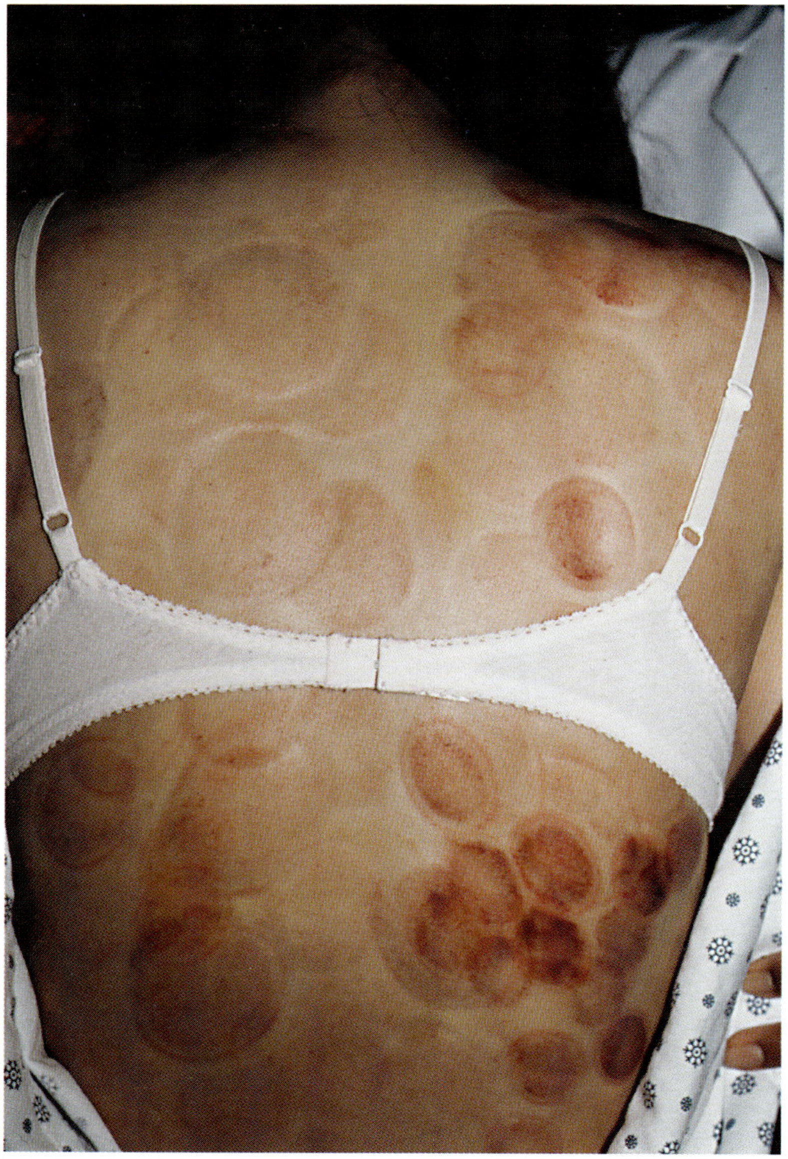

During a routine examination, a 33-year-old Korean woman was incidentally found to have lesions on her back in various stages of healing. The lesions had been created when a friend applied heated cups to the skin to treat back pain. The vacuum created as the cup cools results in erythema, edema, and ecchymoses of the skin, which take several weeks to heal. The patient was unconcerned about these effects of "cupping" and requested no intervention.

Helen Manber, M.D.
Matthew Kanzler, M.D.

Stanford University Hospital
Palo Alto, CA 94304

October 24, 1996

Correspondence

Consequences of Cupping

April 10, 1997

To the Editor: The photograph of the strange East Asian medical technique of cupping (Oct. 24 issue)[1] was wonderful and evocative. I suspect, however, that this bizarre anthropologic "other" is actually a case of the forgotten historical "self." The use of cupping has a long history in the West and was widespread in the United States in the 18th and 19th centuries.[2] The *Journal's* predecessor even published extensive instructions on performing cupping.[3] The importance of cupping was generally acknowledged: "No member of the profession, at this time, can be ignorant of [its] use and importance."[4] As late as 1931, Osler's revered textbook indicated cupping for the treatment of bronchopneumonia and acute myelitis.[5]

Ted J. Kaptchuk, O.M.D.
Beth Israel Deaconess Medical Center, Boston, MA 02215

1. Manber H, Kanzler M. Consequences of cupping. N Engl J Med 1996;335:1281.
2. Ackerknecht EH. Therapeutics from the primitives to the 20th century. New York: Hafner, 1973.
3. Hills M. A treatise on the operation of cupping. Boston Med Surg J 1833;9:261-73.
4. Gillespie WA. Remarks on the operation of cupping, and the instruments best adapted to country practice. Boston Med Surg J 1834;10:27-30.
5. Osler W. The principles and practice of medicine. 11th rev. ed. New York: Appleton, 1931:112, 981.

To the Editor: Manber and Kanzler's interesting photograph shows that cupping is still being used. The photo shows dry cupping. In wet cupping the skin is incised, and therefore more blood may be lost. In some cultures the technique is also used to treat asthma in children. Their backs are used, presumably to avoid creating alarm, but the lesions may be taken for signs of physical abuse[1] when the children come into the orbit of conventional medical practice.

Oliver Dearlove, F.R.C.A.
Royal Manchester Children's Hospital, Manchester M25 2HA, United Kingdom

John Dearlove, M.D.
Yeovil General Hospital, Somerset BA21 4AT, United Kingdom

1. Dearlove J, Verguei AP, Birkin N, Latham P. An anachronistic treatment for asthma. BMJ 1981;283:1684-5.

To the Editor: The photograph of cupping reminded me of what I once saw as a medical student at Kings County Hospital in Brooklyn, New York, back in the late 1940s. I was assigned to work up a patient who had a symmetric line of erythematous lesions in two rows on his back and chest. My resident explained to me that they were the result of improperly applied cupping.

Cupping, or *bahnkes* as it is known in Yiddish, is used in many cultures. The technique is slightly different from that described by Drs. Manber and Kanzler. Small cups are used, such as eyecups or small wine glasses. A small amount of alcohol is put into the cup and ignited, and the cup is immediately pressed tight against the skin. The vacuum is produced by the combustion of the alcohol and the consequent evacuation of oxygen from the cup, not by the cooling of the cup, which would not be expected to produce a vacuum. The theory is that the vacuum then sucks out noxious materials from the body. When the procedure is done properly by an expert in folk medicine, the skin is perhaps slightly reddened but not actually burned.

An interesting sidelight is something I am sure many of your readers have heard. There is an old Yiddish proverb, *Es vet helfen vi a toiten bahnkes,* which translates roughly as "It will help like applying cups to a dead person." In any event, it was fascinating to see this procedure used on a Korean woman, since I had heretofore thought it was primarily an Eastern European phenomenon.

Thank you for your excellent *Journal,* which I still, even after 42 years of practice, find to be a high point of my week.

Noel H. Seicol, M.D., 33 Cedar St., Rye, NY 10580

Acupuncture-Needle Fragments

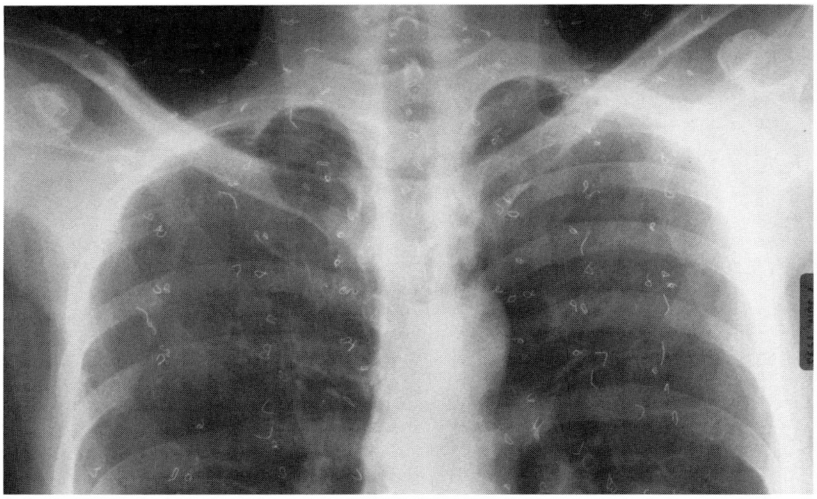

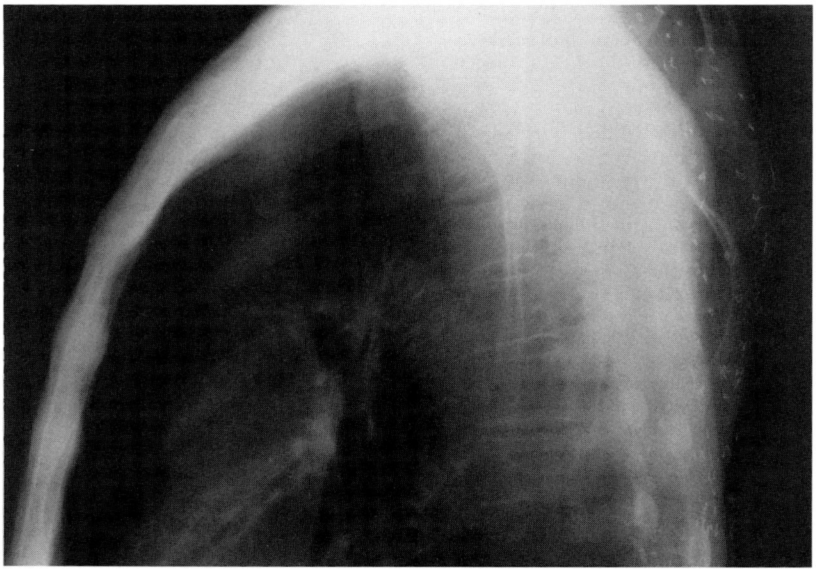

Posteroanterior and lateral chest radiographs of a 42-year-old Japanese man reveal fine metallic opacities in the soft tissues of the back. The opacities represent indwelling gold acupuncture needles aligned along vertical "meridians" of the torso. Four years earlier, the needles had been inserted in the skin by an acupuncturist and then broken off intentionally. The back was normal on physical examination. The patient believes that the needle fragments absorb energy from his surroundings, balance his yin and yang forces, and thereby improve his health. The fragments remain in the subcutaneous tissues permanently.

Ernest S. Chiu, B.A.
John H.M. Austin, M.D.

Columbia University College
of Physicians and Surgeons
New York, NY 10032-3784

February 2, 1995

Correspondence

Acupuncture-Needle Fragments

June 29, 1995

To the Editor: Chiu and Austin (Feb. 2 issue)[1] provide radiographic evidence of multiple, fine, metallic densities in the soft tissue of the back of a Japanese man, representing permanently placed acupuncture needles. We disagree, however, with the statement that the needles remain in the subcutaneous tissue permanently.

This form of acupuncture, known as Hari acupuncture, is undertaken to improve one's general health and specifically to treat pain, paralysis, and skin diseases. The skin is initially prepared with alcohol, and a spring-loaded syringe is used to inject the 1-cm needles along predefined meridians. In a typical session lasting one to two hours, dozens of needles may be placed. Made of gold, silver, or stainless steel, the needles may be placed anywhere in the body.

We studied three Korean patients who had undergone extensive Hari acupuncture in New York City. Ultrasound and computed tomographic (CT) scans were obtained to determine the exact positions of these needles. In one patient the needles had migrated from their initial subcutaneous positions. CT images showed that multiple needles had penetrated the peritoneal cavity, impinging on the anterior aspect of the stomach, the left lobe of the liver, and the transverse colon. Other needles had become embedded in the wall of the urinary bladder.[2] Though this patient has had no ill effects from the acupuncture treatments to date, long-term follow-up is required to determine whether there are sequelae of acupuncture-needle migration.

An unusual radiographic appearance of this sort, usually found incidentally, should alert the clinician to the presence of Hari acupuncture needles and the possible complications that accompany other, more traditional types of acupuncture, such as local infection and transmission of viral hepatitis.[3] Problems associated with permanent subcutaneous placement of needles in Hari acupuncture, such as the migration of the needles from the soft tissue to more distant sites, should always be kept in mind.

Perry S. Gerard, M.D.
Eric Wilck, M.D.
Maimonides Medical Center
Brooklyn, NY 11219

Thomas Schiano, M.D.
Temple University Hospital
Philadelphia, PA 19140

1. Chiu ES, Austin JHM. Acupuncture-needle fragments. N Engl J Med 1995;332:304.
2. Gerard PS, Wilck E, Schiano T. Imaging implications in the evaluation of permanent needle acupuncture. Clin Imaging 1993;17:36-40.
3. Carron H, Epstein BS, Grand B. Complications of acupuncture. JAMA 1974;228:1552-4.

Osborn Waves of Hypothermia

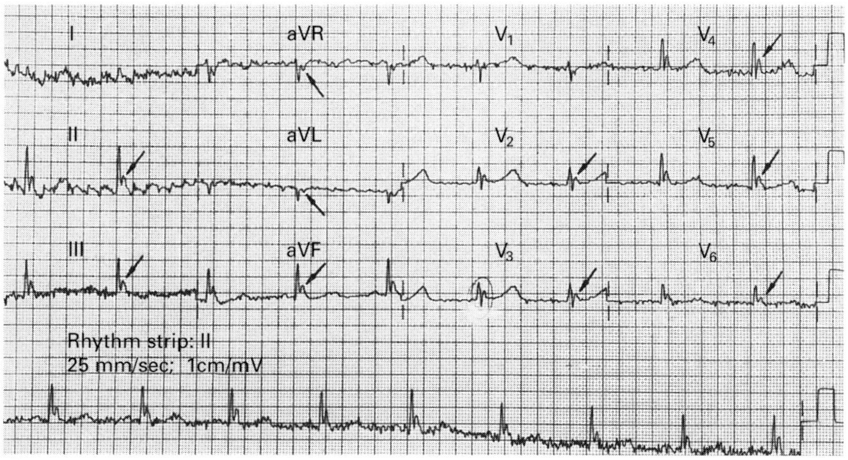

A

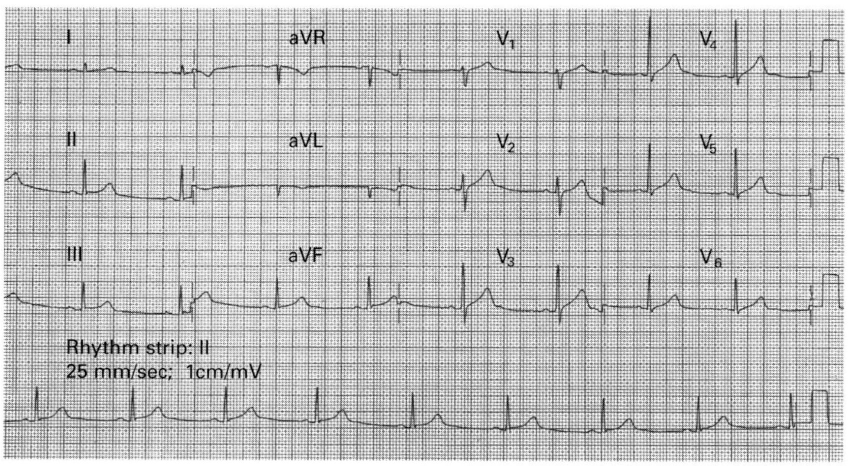

B

A 12-lead electrocardiogram and rhythm strip were obtained in a 40-year-old alcoholic man with a core body temperature of 29°C (84°F) because of accidental exposure to the cold (Panel A). The tracing shows a bradycardic rhythm (probably sinus), prolonged QT intervals, a base-line artifact due to muscle tremors, and distinctive and characteristic Osborn waves (arrows). A second 12-lead electrocardiogram and rhythm strip obtained after the patient was rewarmed to 37.2°C (99°F) show sinus rhythm (Panel B). Both the Osborn waves and base-line artifact are absent. The QT interval is normal for the heart rate.

Archana Patel, M.D.
John Getsos, M.D.

Jersey City Medical Center
Jersey City, NJ 07304

March 10, 1994

Cauliflower Ear

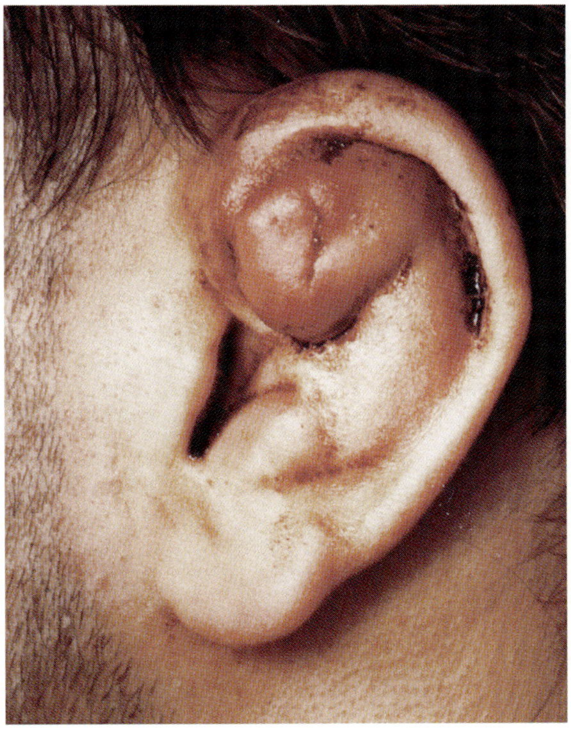

A

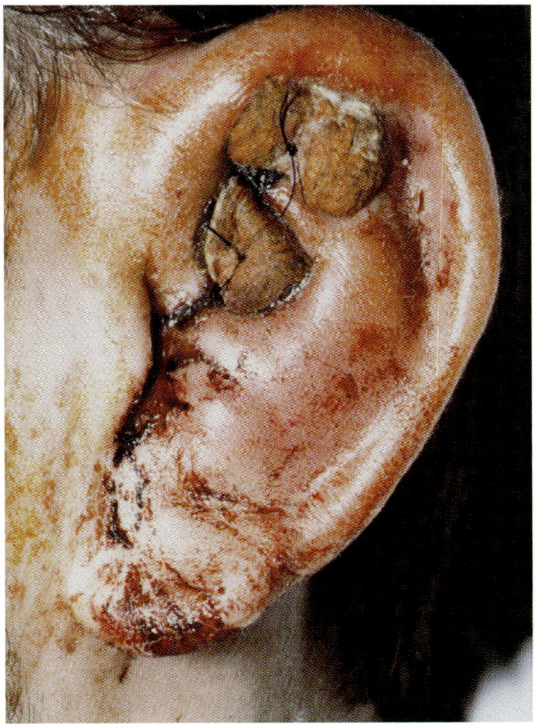

B

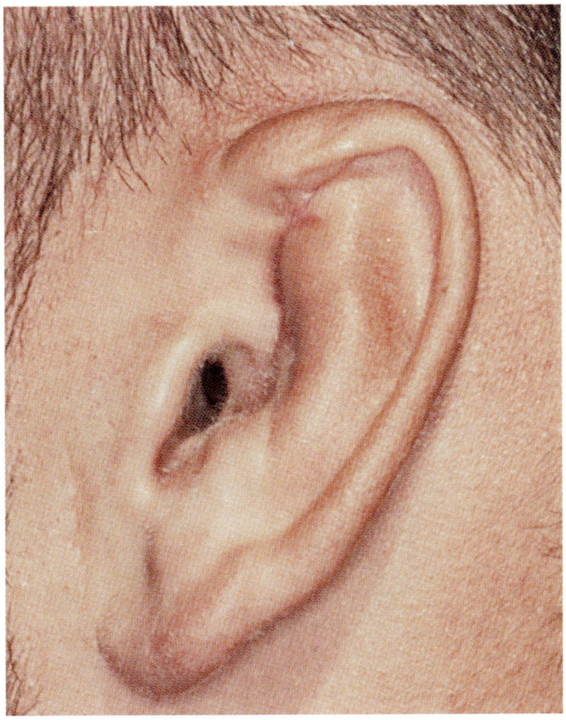

C

A 16-year-old wrestler had thickened neocartilage in his ear as a result of several untreated auricular hematomas. He presented with a recurrent hematoma that had been drained two days earlier in the emergency department. Panel A shows a hematoma in the superior anthelix and triangular fossa. The drainage site is in the center of the hematoma. After more extensive incision and drainage, with resection of the neocartilage, bolsters were placed on the ear to maintain contact between the perichondrium and the underlying cartilage. One day after surgery, infection with *Pseudomonas aeruginosa* developed (Panel B). The patient was treated with parenteral gentamicin for six days and then with topical gentamicin for two weeks. Three months after the completion of therapy, the patient had a cauliflower ear (Panel C). He continued to wrestle, with protective headgear.

Rubia Khalak, M.D.
Jay K. Roberts, M.D.

University of Rochester School of Medicine
Rochester, NY 14621

August 8, 1996

Struck by Lightning

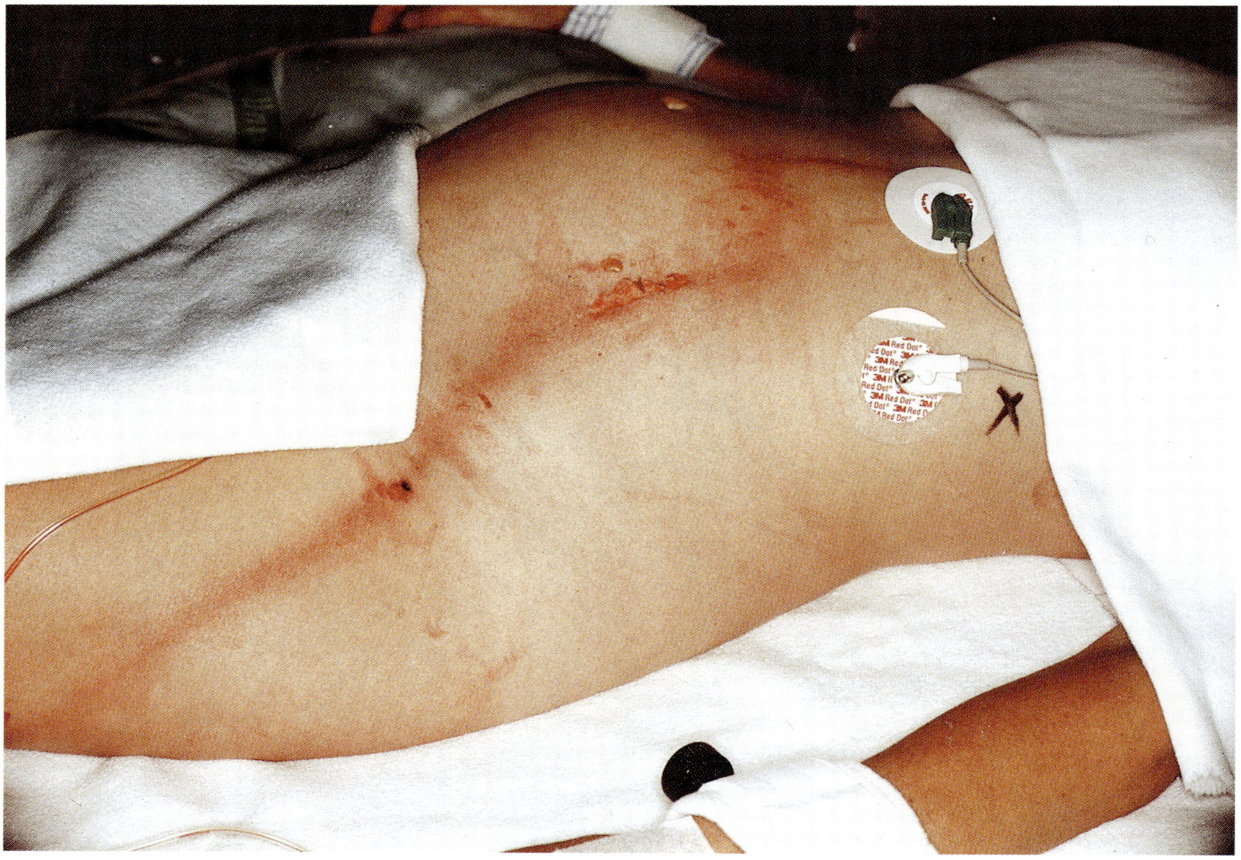

A 41-year-old woman in her 26th week of pregnancy was struck by lightning while standing under a tree during a thunderstorm. The lightning entered her body on the right side of the neck through a necklace, went toward the ground, was deflected by the baby's head, and left the woman's body through the left leg, marking its way by a cutaneous "lightning print." The woman survived, but the baby died.

Manfred Zehender, M.D.

Universitätsklinik Freiburg
79106 Freiburg, Germany

May 26, 1994

Correspondence

Direction of a Lightning Strike

October 6, 1994

To the Editor: The Image in Clinical Medicine entitled "Struck by Lightning" (May 26 issue)[1] was interesting and beautifully presented. However, unless there is a recognized method of distinguishing the entrance and exit wounds caused by lightning, we believe the figure legend misleads the reader. The legend describes the lightning as entering the victim's body by the neck and exiting by her leg. Typically, lightning travels upward, not downward. During thunderstorms an excess negative charge of electrons accumulates in clouds. The earth below is positively charged. When the electromagnetic attraction between the cloud and the earth becomes great enough, electrons stream downward toward the positively charged earth. When this negatively charged leader nears the earth, a positively charged streamer ascends from the earth to meet it. When the descending leader meets the ascending streamer, an intense wave of positive charge, the lightning stroke, travels upward to the cloud. An excellent diagram and simple explanation of this can be found elsewhere.[2]

Denis L. Bourke, M.D.
Charles M. Harrison, M.D.
Juraj Sprung, M.D., Ph.D.
Veterans Affairs Medical Center
Baltimore, MD 21201-1566

1. Zehender M. Struck by lightning. N Engl J Med 1994;330:1492.
2. Williams J. The weather book. New York: Random House, 1992:111-29.

The authors reply:

To the Editor: The description of the physical phenomenon of the discharge of lightning as given by Bourke et al. is correct as far as negatively charged lightning is concerned. In the case of a positive strike, the direction of the lightning will be opposite.

In the case of a negative strike, the partial lightning current through a person next to a tree goes from the leg to the neck, according to the physical definition. Because the polarity of the lightning strike is usually not known, people say colloquially that a partial lightning current "jumps" from the tree to the person in an arc, entering at the neck and leaving the body at the leg.[1]

In some patients, the orientation of the transient, fernlike, superficial skin markings[2] may be helpful in defining the direction of the current better. In our patient[3] these were oriented downward.

Manfred Zehender, M.D.
Universitätsklinik Freiburg
79106 Freiburg, Germany

J. Wiesinger, Ph.D.
Universität der Bundeswehr München
85579 Munich, Germany

1. Uman MA. The lightning discharge. International geophysics series. Vol. 39. Orlando, Fla.: Academic Press, 1987.
2. Bartholome CW, Jacoby WD, Ramchand SC. Cutaneous manifestations of lightning injury. Arch Dermatol 1975;111:1466-8.
3. Zehender M. Struck by lightning. N Engl J Med 1994;330:1492.

Bilateral Femur Fractures

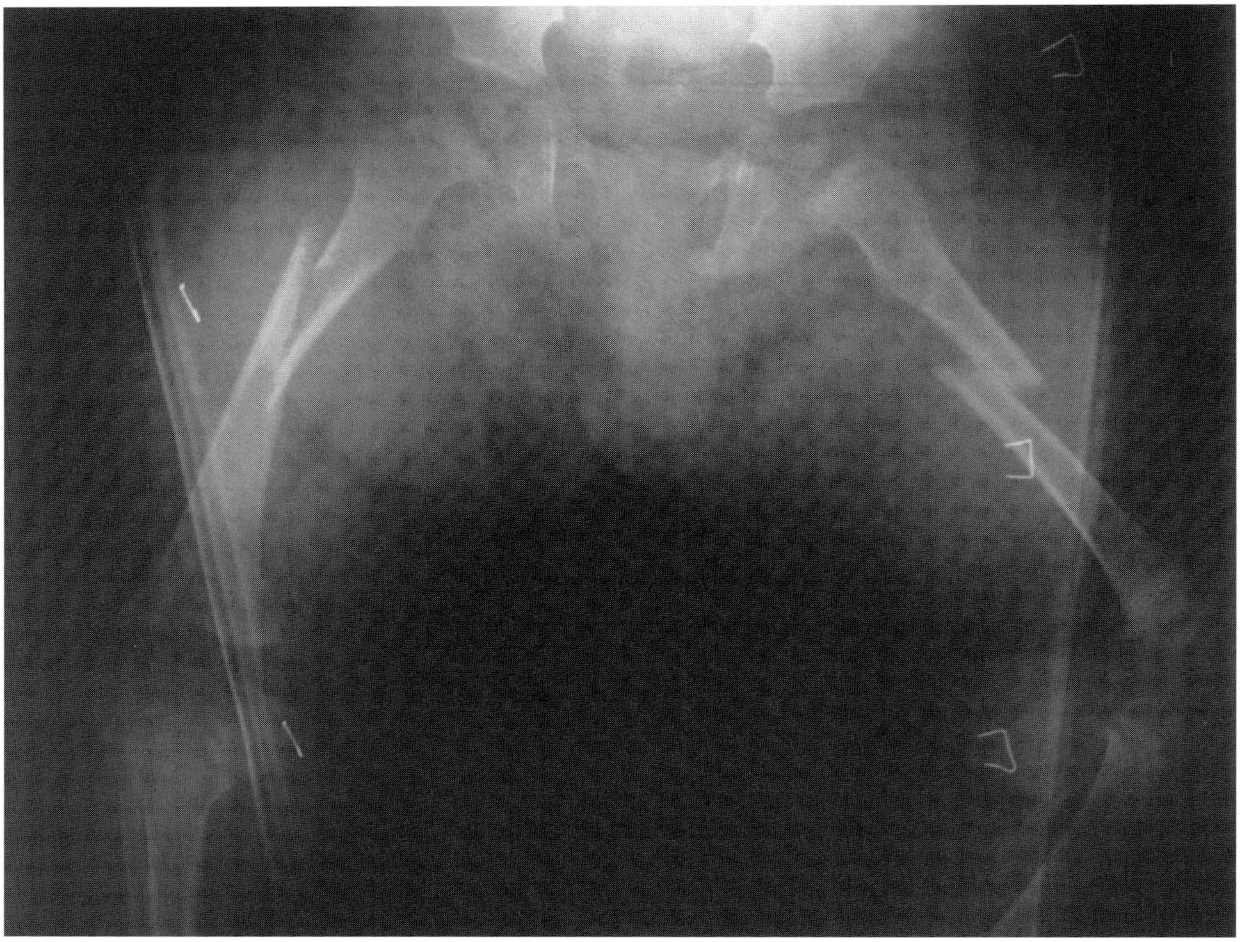

Bilateral femur fractures are visible in a nine-month-old boy who was restrained with only a standard lap belt in the rear seat of an automobile that struck a post at 40 miles (65 km) per hour. The child required hospitalization and a prolonged period in a spica cast. A proper car seat is the only appropriate restraint for a small child.

Gregory P. Conners, M.D.
Daniel W. Ochsenschlager, M.D.

Children's National Medical Center
Washington, DC 20010

August 25, 1994

Allergy, Rheumatology, and Connective Tissue Diseases

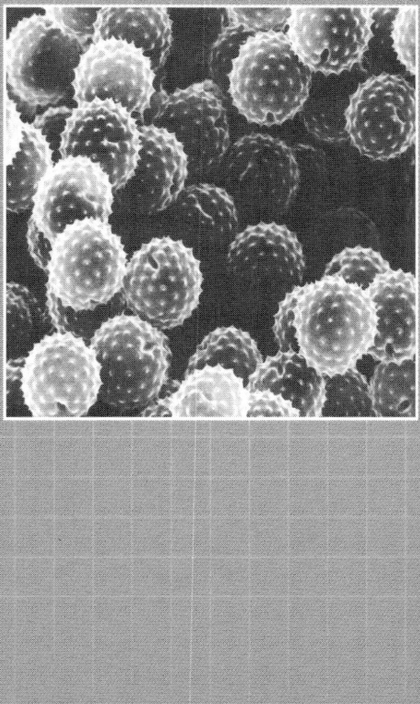

Ragweed Pollen

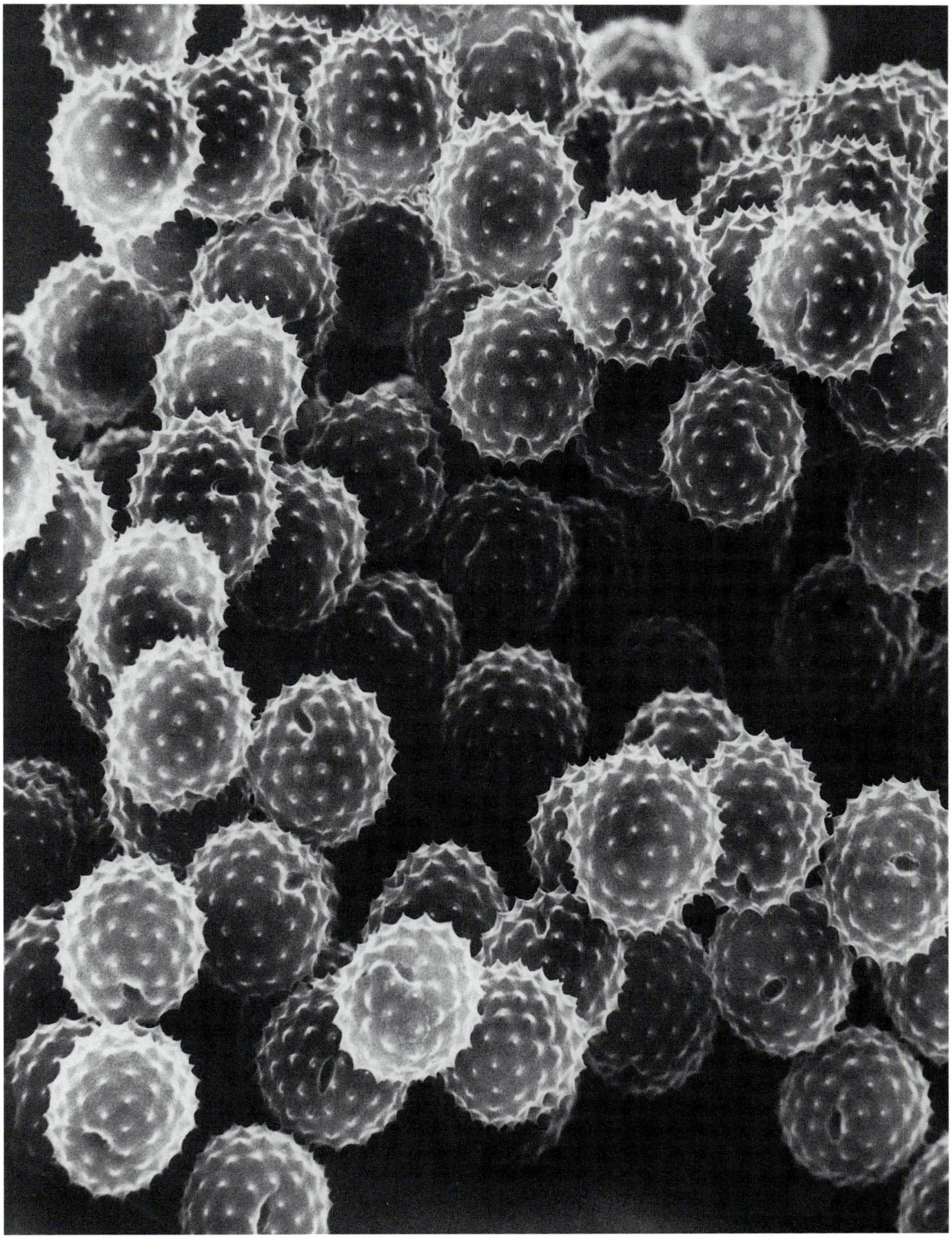

Scanning electron micrograph of ragweed pollen (×5200).

July 16, 1992

David M. Phillips

Center for Biomedical Research
New York, NY 10021

Angioedema of the Intestine

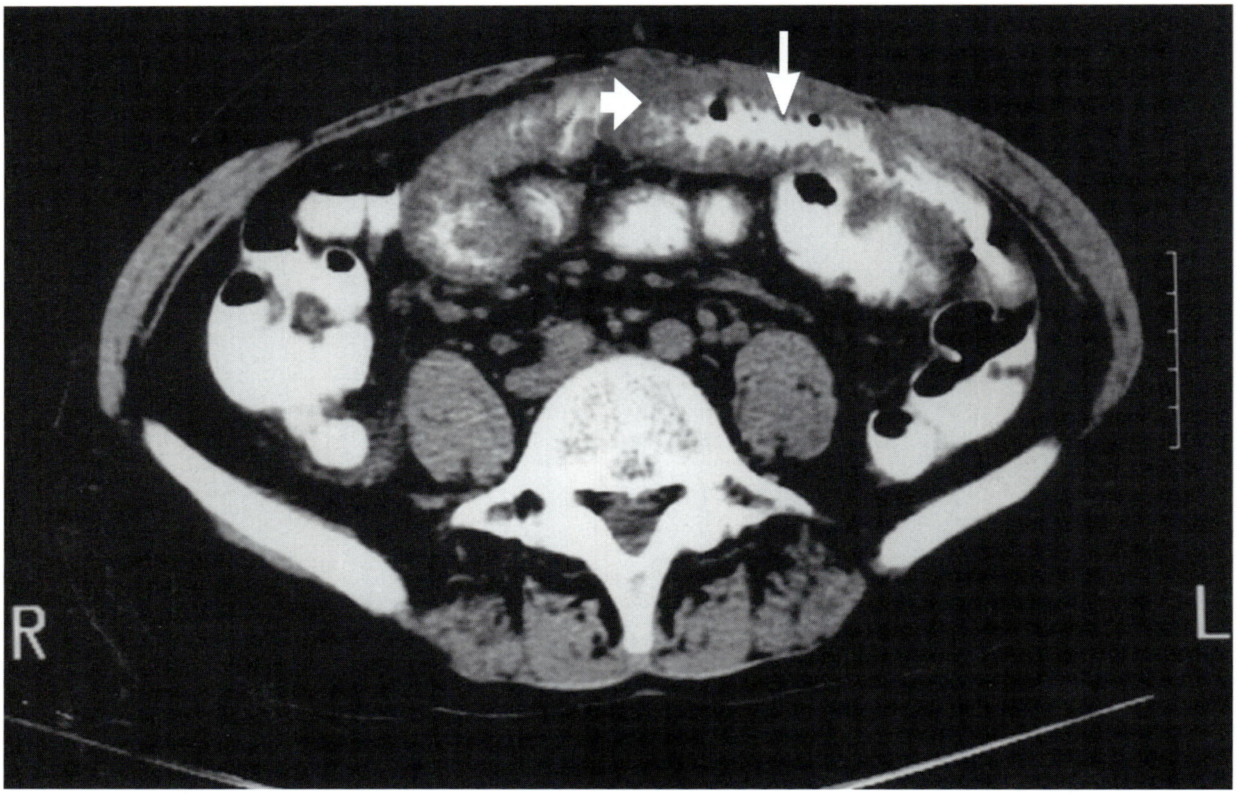

Abdominal computed tomography was performed in a 58-year-old woman with acute abdominal pain, nausea, vomiting, and abdominal distention. The patient had had recurrent swelling of the tongue and pharynx during therapy with lisinopril, but the medication had been continued. On the scan, the mucosa of a loop of small intestine is markedly thickened, and the irregularities within the wall are most consistent with the presence of edema (thick arrow). The valvulae conniventes are prominent and widened (thin arrow), resulting in a severely narrowed lumen. All of the patient's symptoms resolved within 24 hours after the discontinuation of lisinopril.

Kate W.P. Gregory, B.S.
Rufus C. Davis, M.D.

Vanderbilt University
Nashville, TN 37232

June 20, 1996

Correspondence

Angioedema of the Intestine

November 14, 1996

To the Editor: In their image entitled "Angioedema of the Intestine" (June 20 issue),[1] Gregory and Davis did not mention the duration of lisinopril treatment. Since the diagnosis of recurrent swelling of the tongue and pharynx associated with the administration of an angiotensin-converting–enzyme (ACE) inhibitor was missed (lisinopril was continued and angioedema of the intestine developed), I assume that the patient had been treated with lisinopril for a relatively long period.

Although the early onset of the ACE-inhibitor–induced angioedema should not be a diagnostic problem, many physicians are not familiar with late-onset angioedema, and it frequently goes unrecognized.[2-4] The potentiation of the bradykinins is believed to be the pathophysiologic mechanism of this side effect.[5] If this proves to be true, ACE-receptor antagonists may be an alternative therapy for patients who cannot tolerate ACE inhibitors, as implied by Goodfriend et al. (June 20 issue).[6]

Adriana Pavletic, M.D.
University of Nebraska Medical Center
Omaha, NE 68198

1. Gregory KWP, Davis RC. Angioedema of the intestine. N Engl J Med 1996;334:1641.
2. Litman RS, Sher WH, Hausman SA. Life threatening acute airway obstruction due to enalapril induced angioedema. Immunol Allergy Pract 1992;14(5):21-4.
3. Frontera Y, Piecuch JF. Multiple episodes of angioedema associated with lisinopril, an ACE inhibitor. J Am Dent Assoc 1995;126:217-20.
4. Finley CJ, Silverman MA, Nunez AE. Angiotensin-converting enzyme inhibitor-induced angioedema: still unrecognized. Am J Emerg Med 1992;10:550-2.
5. Israili ZH, Hall WD. Cough and angioneurotic edema associated with angiotensin-converting enzyme inhibitor therapy: a review of the literature and pathophysiology. Ann Intern Med 1992;117:234-42.
6. Goodfriend TL, Elliott ME, Catt KJ. Angiotensin receptors and their antagonists. N Engl J Med 1996;334:1649-54.

To the Editor: Gregory and Davis highlight an unusual presentation of angioedema associated with ACE-inhibitor therapy — namely, angioedema of the intestine. It is of interest that the patient had recurrent episodes of swelling of the tongue and pharynx while taking an ACE inhibitor without the treatment's being stopped. These may have been presentations of angioedema that went unrecognized.

The role of ACE inhibitors in patients presenting with angioedema is poorly recognized. This may be because the onset of angioedema can occur after a long period (months to years) of uneventful therapy with ACE inhibitors.[1] In only one of nine cases of ACE-inhibitor–associated angioedema treated at public hospitals was the patient advised to discontinue taking the ACE inhibitor.[2]

Correspondence Continued

Ongoing care of patients with ACE-inhibitor–associated angioedema is a problem. The ACE inhibitor must be stopped to avoid recurrence of this life-threatening event, meaning that alternative therapies must be found. Recently, a new class of drug has become available, the orally effective blockers of angiotensin II receptors (e.g., losartan). These agents provide an alternative means of blocking the renin–angiotensin system. They exert hemodynamic effects similar to those of ACE inhibitors in cardiac failure and are effective antihypertensive drugs.[3] Goodfriend et al. suggested a role for this new class of drug in the treatment of patients unable to tolerate ACE inhibitors.[4] They also state, "It is apparent that these drugs . . . do not have two side effects that can interrupt therapy with ACE inhibitors — cough and angioedema." Angioedema, however, has been reported with losartan.[5]

Genevieve M. Gabb, M.B., B.S.(Hons.)
Australian Medicines Handbook
Adelaide SA 5000, Australia

1. Pigman EC, Scott JL. Angioedema in the emergency department: the impact of angiotensin-converting enzyme inhibitors. Am J Emerg Med 1993;11:350-4.
2. Weiner JM. Failure to recognise the association of life-threatening angio-oedema and angiotensin-converting enzyme inhibitor therapy. Aust N Z J Med 1995;25:241-2.
3. Johnston CI. Angiotensin receptor antagonists: focus on losartan. Lancet 1995;346:1403-7.
4. Goodfriend TL, Elliott ME, Catt KJ. Angiotensin receptors and their antagonists. N Engl J Med 1996;334:1649-54.
5. Acker CG, Greenberg A. Angioedema induced by the angiotensin II blocker losartan. N Engl J Med 1995;333:1572.

To the Editor: The image submitted by Gregory and Davis is a computed tomographic (CT) scan showing angioedema of the small intestine due to lisinopril. It would have been interesting, as well as clinically relevant, if the authors had included amylase or lipase values as well as an image of the pancreas, since lisinopril has been associated with acute pancreatitis.[1-3] The authors note that the patient presented with abdominal pain, nausea, vomiting, and distention, which are consistent with the presence of acute pancreatitis.

ACE inhibitors have recently been implicated as a potential cause of acute pancreatitis, with reports of cases associated with lisinopril, captopril, and enalapril.[1,2] Cases of lisinopril-associated pancreatitis have been reported to occur from two weeks to two years after therapy is begun.[1] A fatal case of acute pancreatitis associated with lisinopril was recently reported.[2]

Angioedema of the upper aerodigestive tract is a well-known adverse effect of ACE inhibitors and may be due to altered bradykinin metabolism.[1,4] Angioedema of pancreatic tissue may result in obstruction of the ductal system and lead to pancreatitis.[3,4] Clinicians should consider acute pancreatitis in any patient in whom abdominal pain develops who is taking lisinopril or another ACE inhibitor.

Mark A. Marinella, M.D.
University of Michigan Medical Center
Ann Arbor, MI 48109

1. Marinella MA, Billi JE. Lisinopril therapy associated with acute pancreatitis. West J Med 1995;163:77-8.
2. Standridge JB. Fulminant pancreatitis associated with lisinopril therapy. South Med J 1994; 87:179-81.
3. Dabaghi S. ACE inhibitors and pancreatitis. Ann Intern Med 1991;115:330-1.
4. Marinella MA. Angio-oedema induced by ACE inhibitors. J Intern Med 1996;239:371-2.

Correspondence Continued

To the Editor: I found the abdominal CT scan submitted by Gregory and Davis interesting in a way that went beyond the pathologic process it demonstrated. In the case presented, a patient taking an ACE inhibitor who had angioedema of the upper airway was proved on CT scanning to have angioedema of the bowel wall as well. At a cost of approximately $500 per case at our institution, the CT has proved what clinical judgment could have deduced earlier. This patient was exposed to the risk associated with continued lisinopril therapy and was subjected to a procedure that might have been indicated had her condition not improved on withdrawal of the offending medication.

The need of physicians to visualize and prove with certainty what good clinical judgment suggests to be likely continues to be a problem that we must all come to terms with. Cumulatively, the costs to the system and at times to our patients are great.

Daniel C. Smith, M.D.
Baystate Medical Center
Springfield, MA 01199

Drs. Gregory and Davis reply:

To the Editor: We appreciate the interest in our image expressed by Drs. Pavletic, Gabb, Marinella, and Smith.

In response to Dr. Smith: this patient presented with no known history of ACE-inhibitor–induced angioedema, and she reported having no past difficulties with these drugs. She reported four episodes of a "food allergy" involving swelling of the lips and tongue that had occurred approximately one year previously. That she was taking an ACE inhibitor was established only in retrospect. Several days before her presentation, she was given another prescription for lisinopril by a physician who was unaware of her previous angioedema. Thus, our patient presented with severe abdominal pain, nausea, and vomiting of unclear cause. Except for the recent use of lisinopril, the patient's history and the examination of the oropharynx were normal. Abdominal radiographs revealed only minor, nonspecific bowel dilation; routine laboratory tests were remarkable only for leukocytosis; and an abdominal ultrasound study was nondiagnostic. Because of the severity of the symptoms, we think abdominal CT scanning was appropriate and indicated.

Marinella describes the important association between ACE inhibitors and pancreatitis and notes the similarities between the presenting symptoms in our patient and those seen in acute pancreatitis. In our patient, CT images of the pancreas were unremarkable, and her amylase level was normal.

Kate W.P. Gregory, M.D.
Rufus C. Davis, M.D.
Vanderbilt University
Nashville, TN 37232

Tophaceous Gout

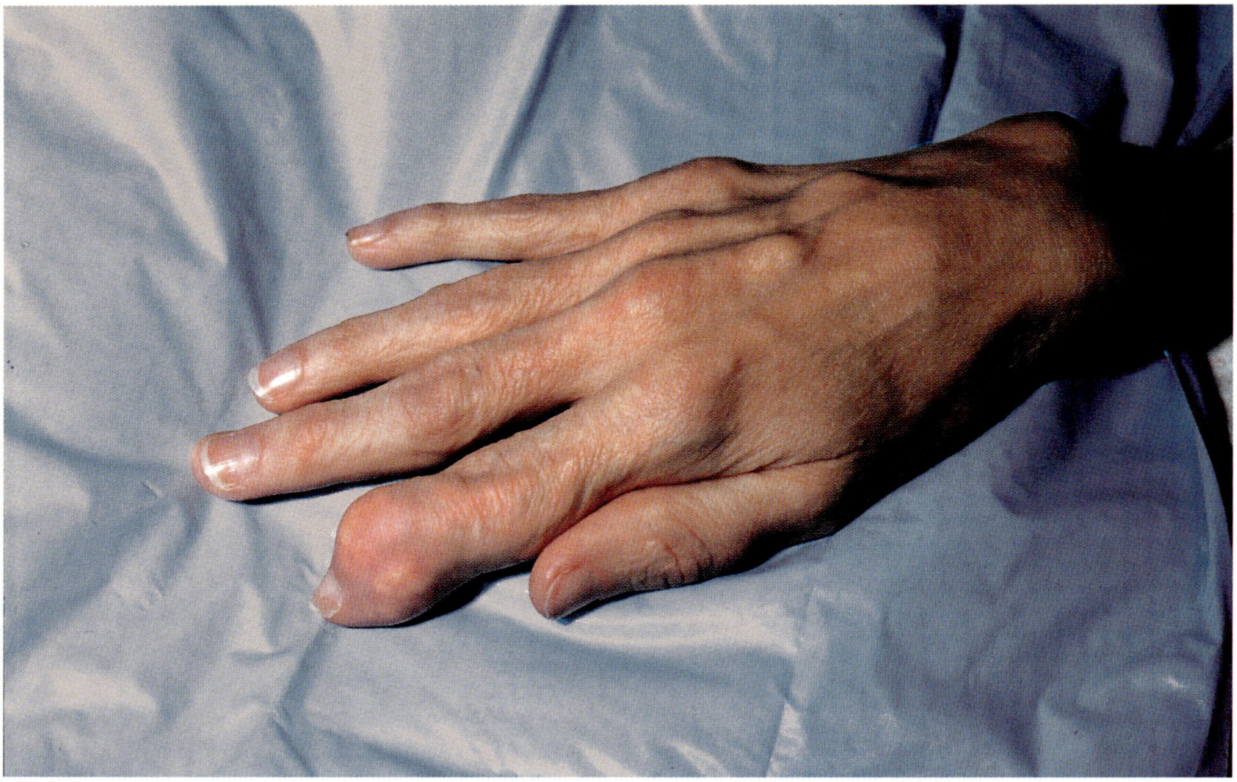

Deforming gouty arthritis is evident in a 39-year-old woman who has had anorexia nervosa since the age of 15. Attacks of acute arthritis began at the age of 23; crystals of monosodium urate monohydrate were found in the joints during those attacks. The multiple cutaneous nodules on the distal aspect of the index finger are tophaceous deposits of monosodium urate crystals. Tophi first appeared when the patient was 24.

Daniel A. Wuthrich, M.D.

University of Washington
Seattle, WA 98195

Arthur L. Lebowitz, M.D.

Boston University Medical Center
Boston, MA 02118

March 9, 1995

Cholesterol Crystals

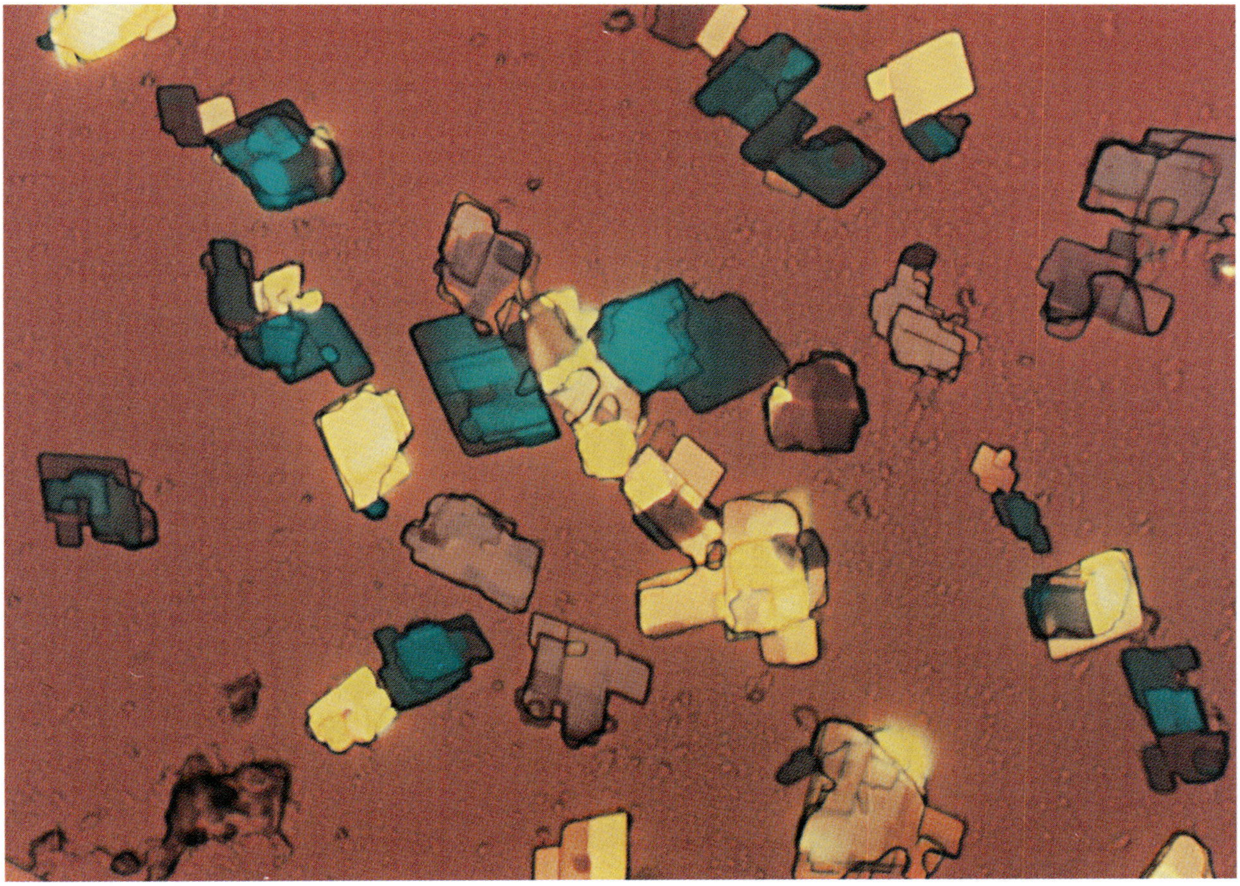

A 70-year-old man presented with a history of rheumatoid arthritis, insulin-dependent diabetes mellitus, chronic renal insufficiency, and hypertension. He had had rheumatoid arthritis for 17 years, was seropositive for rheumatoid factor, and had destructive arthritis documented by plain radiographs of the hands. His olecranon bursa was chronically swollen but had never been injected with a corticosteroid preparation.

The aspirate of an effusion from the olecranon bursa reveals cholesterol crystals (×400). These crystals are characterized by broad plates with a notched corner, created by their propensity to adhere to one another's surfaces. They are variably and mildly birefringent. The differing colors are due to the rotation of light by the crystals under compensated polarized light microscopy.

Paul J. DeMarco, M.D.
Richard M. Keating, M.D.

Naval Medical Center
San Diego, CA 92134

November 16, 1995

Psoriatic Arthritis

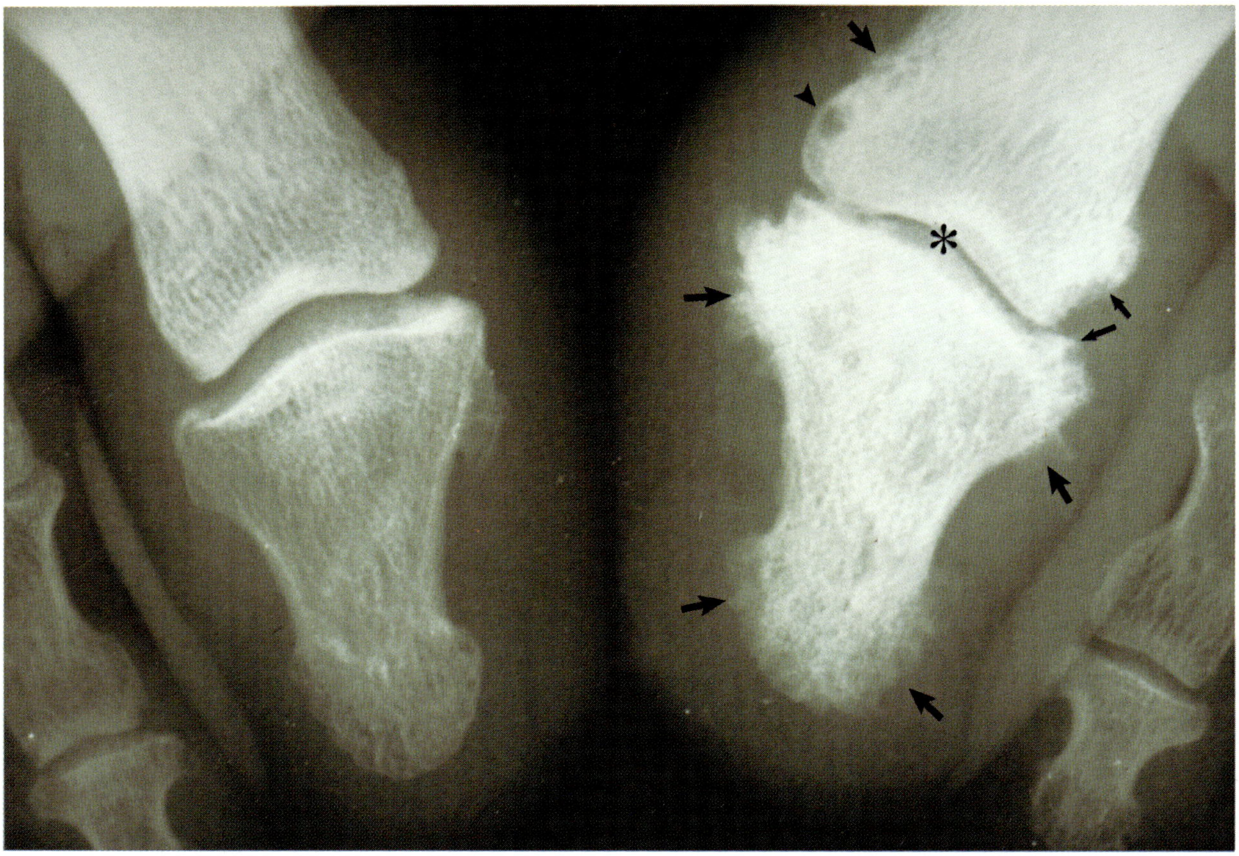

An anteroposterior radiograph of the great toes of a 41-year-old man with psoriatic arthritis shows that the toe on the left is normal. On the right there is soft-tissue swelling that is not confined to the distribution of the joint. The interphalangeal joint space is narrowed (asterisk), and there are subchondral cysts (arrowhead) and marginal erosions (thin arrows). There is new periosteal bone formation (thick arrows) and endosteal bone formation (the so-called ivory phalanx). These findings and the asymmetric distribution are typical of psoriatic arthritis.

Domenico Biasi, M.D.

Istituto di Patologia Speciale Medica
37134 Verona, Italy

Paola Caramaschi, M.D.

Istituto di Clinica Medica
37134 Verona, Italy

August 3, 1995

Calcifications in Dermatomyositis

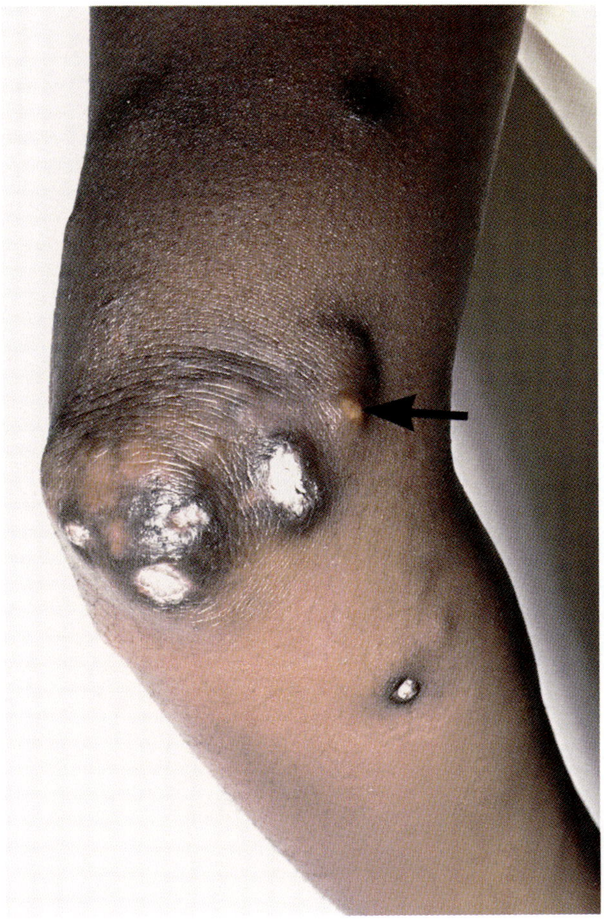

A

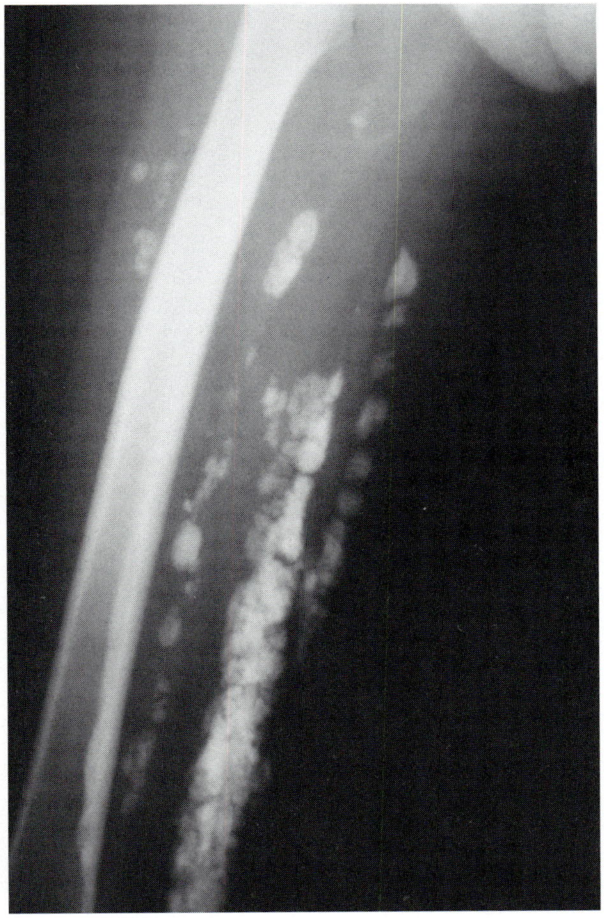

B

The elbow (Panel A) of a 33-year-old woman who had had dermatomyositis since childhood shows subcutaneous calcifications extruding through the skin. A focus of purulent inflammation within a calcium deposit is evident (arrow).

An x-ray film of the patient's thigh (Panel B) shows calcifications beneath the skin and within the muscle tissue. Some lesions on the skin in this area were palpable, and others were not visible. Deposition of calcium continued in this patient despite therapy with prednisone, azathioprine, and diphosphonates.

Marinos C. Dalakas, M.D.

National Institute of Neurological Disorders and Stroke
Bethesda, MD 20892

October 12, 1995

Pseudoxanthoma Elasticum

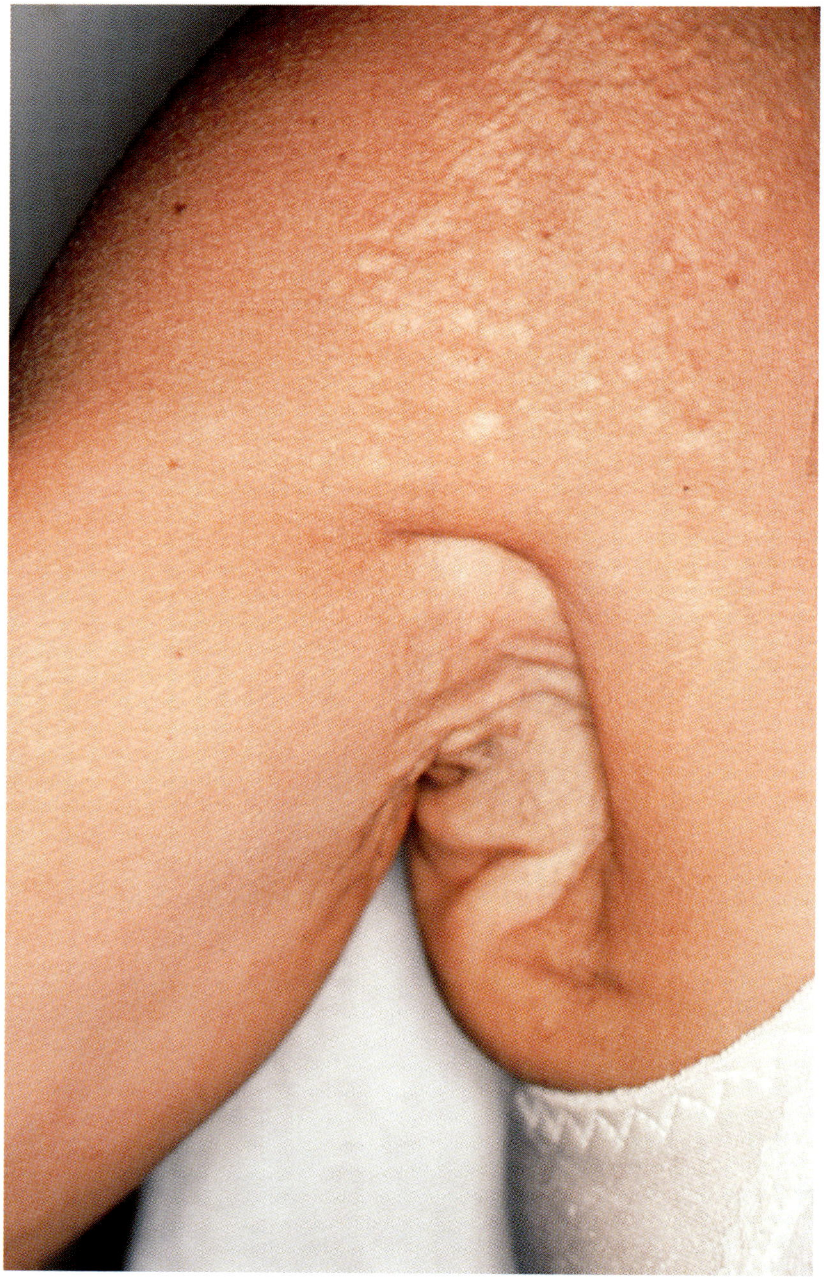

Characteristic skin lesions can be seen in the axilla and anterior to the axilla in a patient with pseudoxanthoma elasticum, an inherited disorder of connective tissue. The lesions are yellow, xanthoma-like papules that have become confluent to form plaques, and there are redundant folds of skin in the axilla. In general, the skin lesions of pseudoxanthoma elasticum occur in flexural sites such as the neck, axillae (as in this patient), antecubital and popliteal fossae, and groin, and are said to resemble "plucked chicken skin." Typically, patients with this disease also have angioid streaks on retinal examination and are at risk for premature cardiovascular disease.

Mark Lebwohl, M.D.

Mount Sinai Medical Center
New York, NY 10029

October 21, 1993

Hypopyon

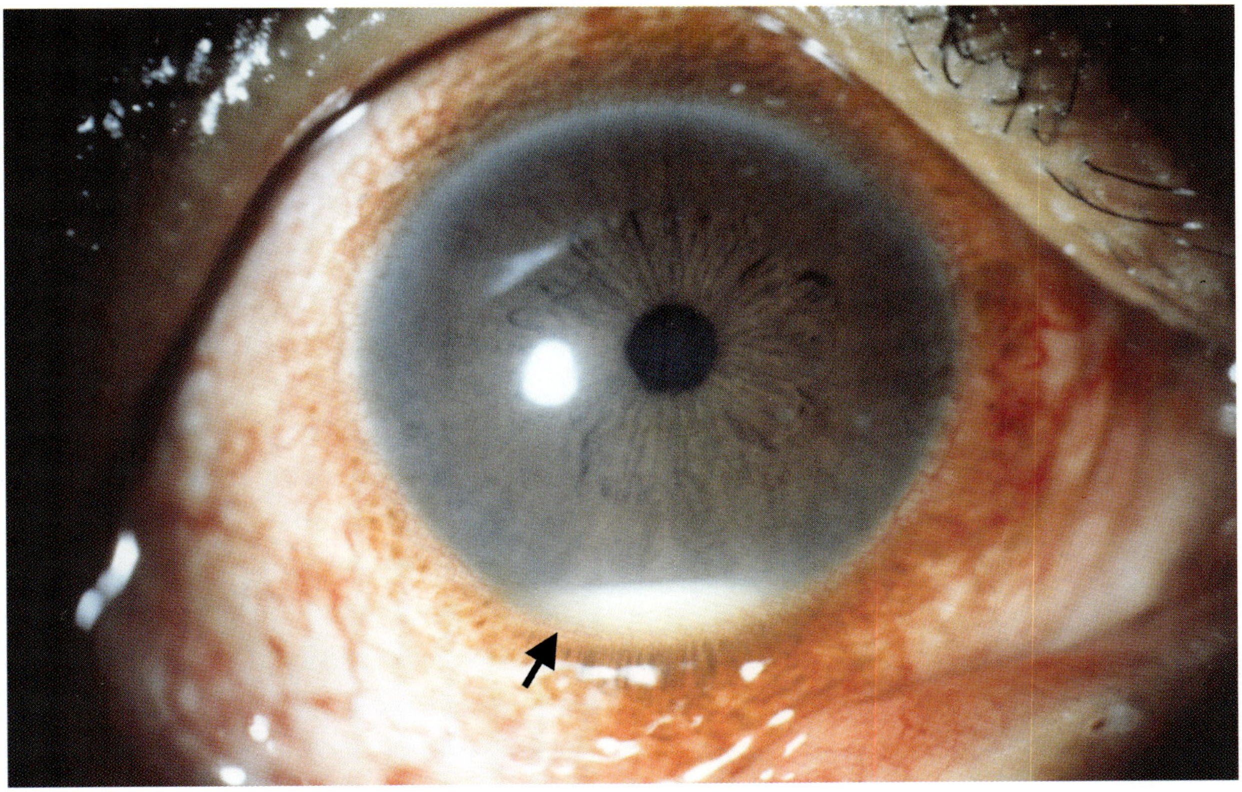

A 36-year-old man had painless, intermittent loss of vision. In this photograph, a hypopyon, or leukocytic exudate, is seen in the anterior chamber (arrow) of the eye, and the conjunctiva and the underlying episclera appear injected. These findings, with the accompanying severe retinopathy, were caused by Behçet's disease. Treatment with chlorambucil and prednisone eye drops, and later with cyclosporine, failed to improve the patient's vision.

Stephen Soloway, M.D.

2791 South Delsea Dr.
Vineland, NJ 08360

David Weissgold, M.D.

Philadelphia Veterans Affairs Medical Center
Philadelphia, PA 19104

June 6, 1996

Relapsing Polychondritis

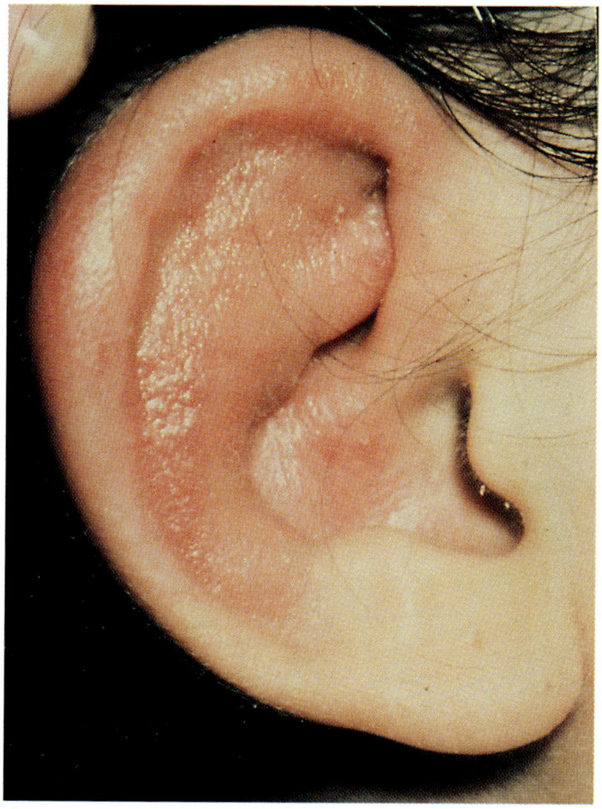

A

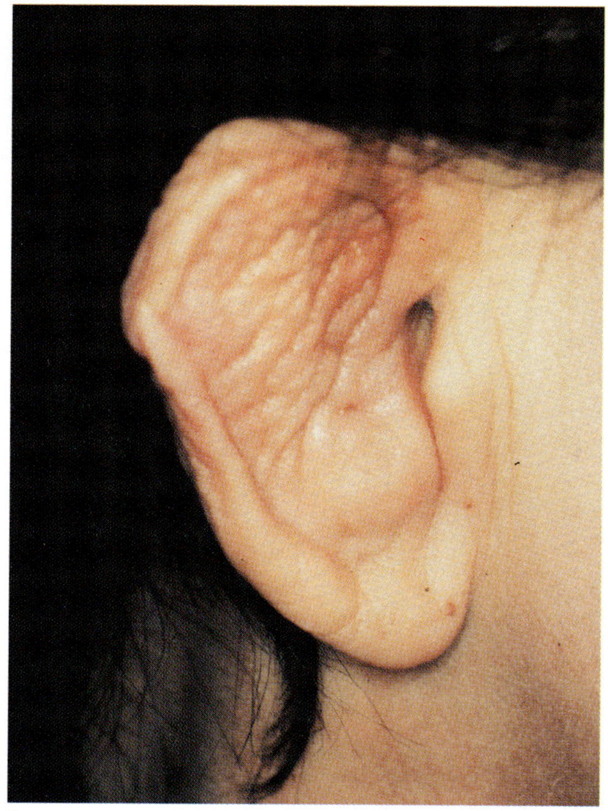

B

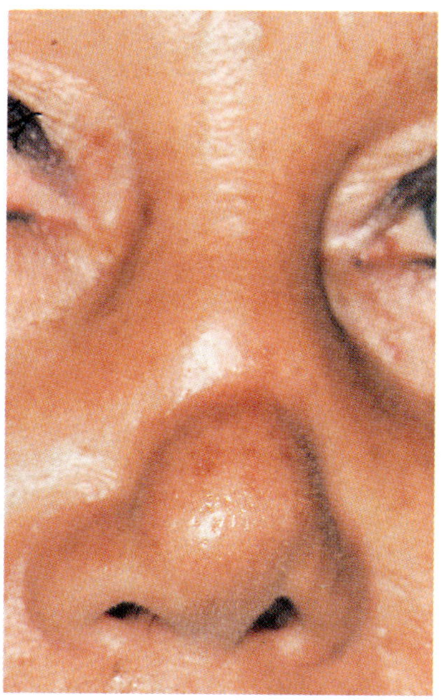

C

The typical characteristics of relapsing polychondritis are shown in three patients: acute auricular chondritis with marked redness, swelling, warmth, and tenderness of the pinna (Panel A); a deformity of the ear that followed recurrent acute attacks (Panel B); and saddle nose, which usually follows repeated, painful nasal chondritis (Panel C).

Jean-Charles Piette, M.D.
Camille Frances, M.D.

Pitié–Salpêtrière Hospital
75651 CEDEX 13 Paris, France

March 2, 1995

Correspondence

Saddle Nose

August 24, 1995

To the Editor: Three photographs of patients with relapsing polychondritis were recently published in the *Journal's* Images in Clinical Medicine series (March 2 issue),[1] including a photograph of a patient with saddle nose. As shown in Figure 1, saddle nose can also be part of the clinical spectrum of Wegener's granulomatosis. In fact, the two diseases may have similar features of nasal and subglottic cartilaginous inflammation and collapse.[2] When other clinical characteristics are not helpful in the differential diagnosis, it may be useful to search for serum antineutrophil cytoplasmic antibodies, which are quite specific markers for Wegener's granulomatosis.[3]

Guido Valesini, M.D.
Roberta Priori, M.D.
Fabrizio Conti, M.D.
Università "La Sapienza"
00161 Rome, Italy

1. Piette J-C, Frances C. Relapsing polychondritis. N Engl J Med 1995;332:580.
2. Michet CJ. Vasculitis and relapsing polychondritis. Rheum Dis Clin North Am 1990; 16:441-4.
3. Gross WL, Schmitt WH, Csernok E. ANCA and associated diseases: immunodiagnostic and pathogenetic aspects. Clin Exp Immunol 1993;91:1-12.

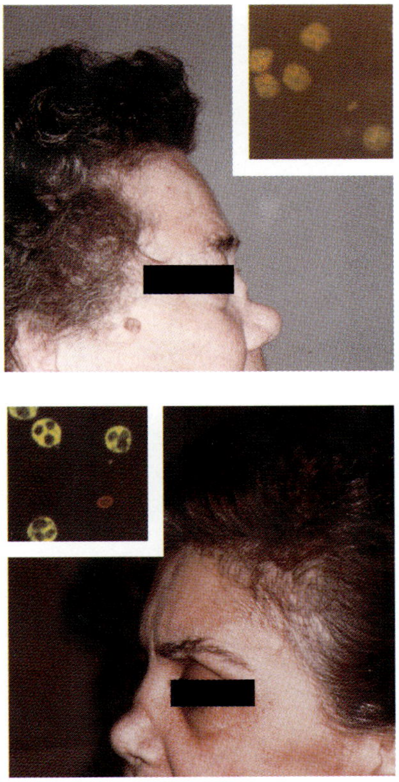

Figure 1. Two Patients, Both with Saddle Nose, but Each with a Different Disease.

The upper panel shows a 70-year-old patient with relapsing polychondritis, and the lower panel a 54-year-old patient with Wegener's granulomatosis. An indirect immunofluorescence assay of alcohol-fixed neutrophils showed that the patient with relapsing polychondritis did not have serum antineutrophil cytoplasmic antibodies, whereas the patient with Wegener's granulomatosis tested positive for such antibodies.

Paget's Disease of Bone

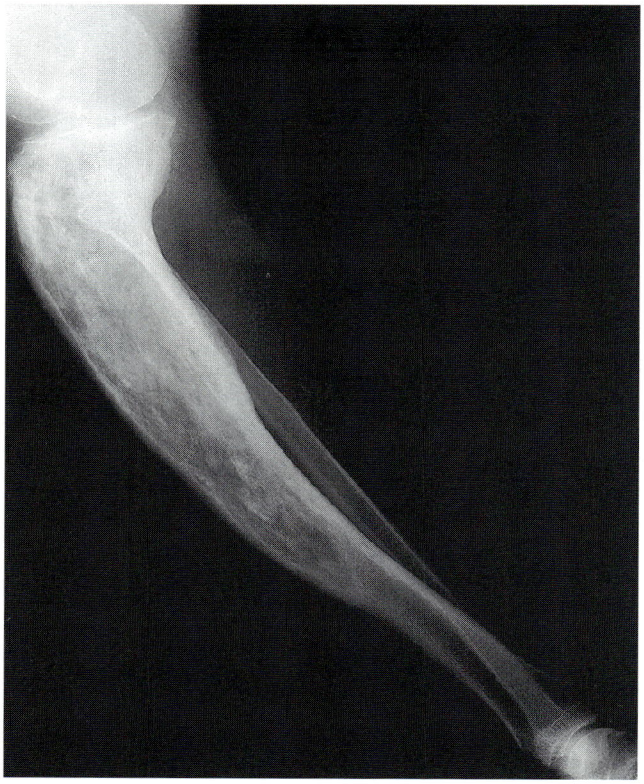

A

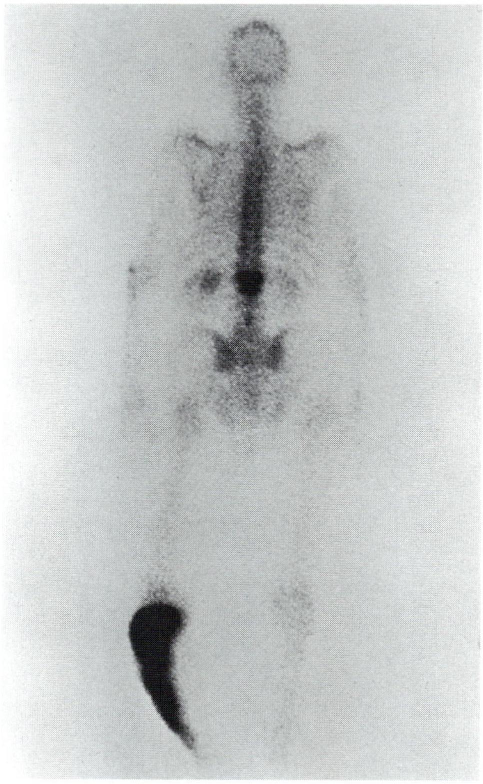

B

A 67-year-old man had Paget's disease involving the right tibia and the first lumbar vertebrae. The patient initially presented with bone pain and bowing of his right lower leg, but the vertebral lesion was not symptomatic. An x-ray film of the right tibia (Panel A) and a bone scan obtained after the administration of technetium-99m–labeled methylene diphosphonate (Panel B) show a marked expansion of bone and a bowing deformity in the right tibia. In addition, the x-ray film shows mixed lytic and sclerotic changes typical of chronic Paget's disease. The accumulation of radionuclide in the right kidney on the bone scan was caused by a large renal cyst.

Kenneth J. Simcic, M.D.
Albert J. Moreno, M.D.

William Beaumont Army Medical Center
El Paso, TX 79920

January 18, 1996

Paget's Disease of Bone

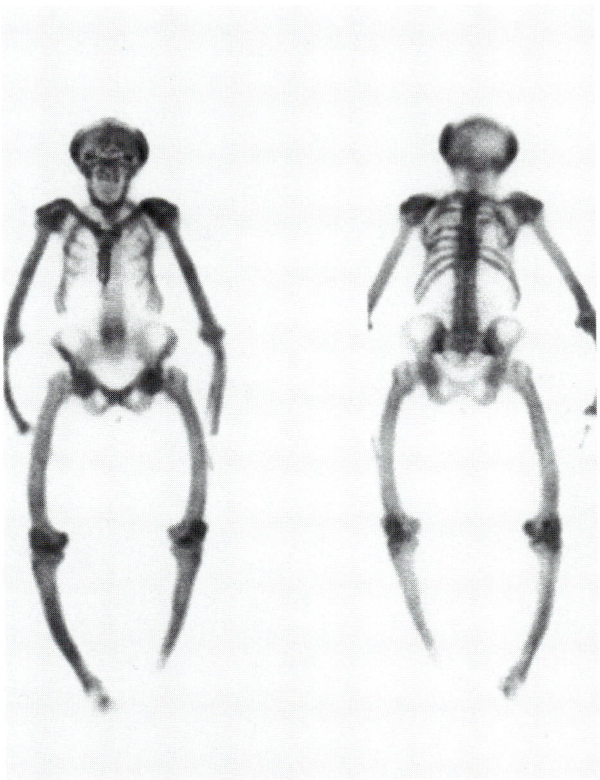

A

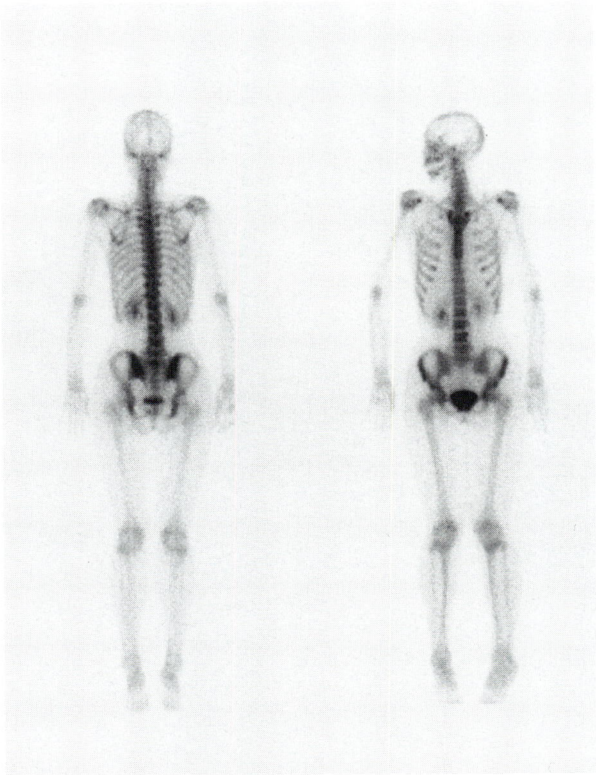

B

A 67-year-old woman had a 20-year history of Paget's disease of bone, resulting in conductive hearing loss, bone and joint pains, pathologic fractures, limb deformities, and difficulty walking. Treatment with calcitonin and etidronate had been unsuccessful. Panel A shows anterior and posterior images from a bone scan obtained after the administration of technetium-99m–labeled methylene diphosphonate. The markedly increased accumulation of radionuclide in almost the entire skeleton, sparing only the distal extremities, reflects the increased bone turnover in Paget's disease. The bowing deformity of the long bones is typical of the disease. Panel B shows a normal bone scan for comparison.

Paul Thomas, B.Med.
Douglas Howarth, B.Med.

John Hunter Hospital
Newcastle, NSW 2310, Australia

January 18, 1996

An Amyloid Deposit in the Shoulder

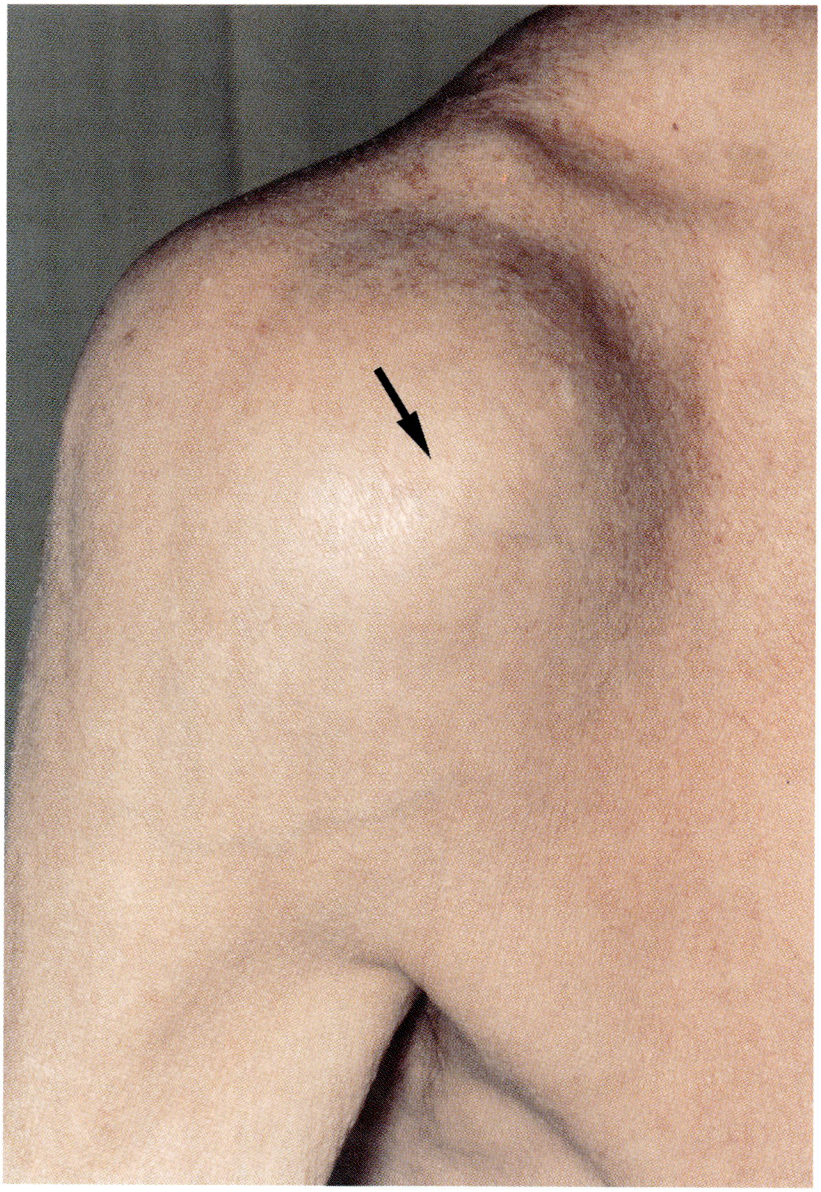

A subcutaneous amyloid deposit is shown (arrow) in a patient with a three-month history of weight loss and multiple subcutaneous masses.

V. Alin Botoman, M.D.

Allegheny General Hospital
Pittsburgh, PA 15212

April 15, 1993

Sarcoidosis

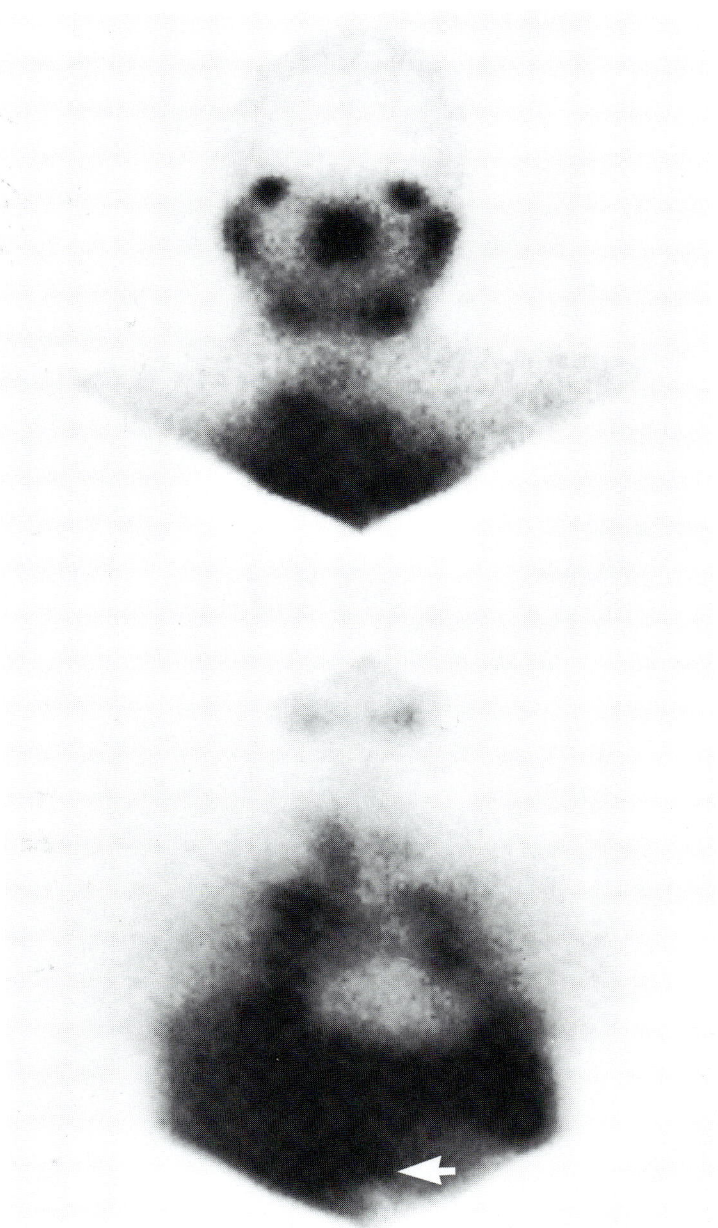

This image was obtained by scanning with gallium citrate Ga 67 in a 24-year-old woman with uveitis and iritis, fatigue, night sweats, myalgia, arthralgia, and a nonproductive cough. The study shows intense localization of the tracer in the lacrimal and salivary glands and in several nodal groups, including the paratracheal nodes, hilar nodes, and celiac nodes (arrow); the diffuse pulmonary uptake signals parenchymal involvement. This scintigraphic pattern — with the "panda" appearance of the face — is typical of sarcoidosis.

Elizabeth Oates, M.D.
Jeanne Metherall, C.N.M.T.

New England Medical Center
Boston, MA 02111

November 4, 1993

Surgery

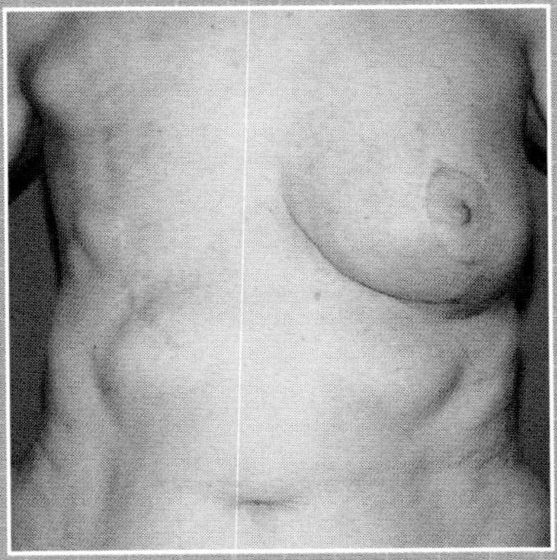

Breast Reconstruction

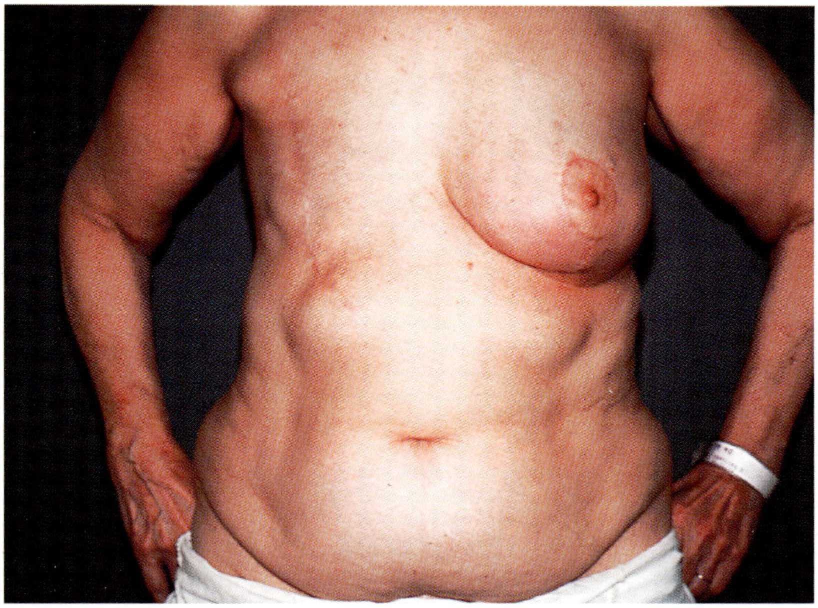

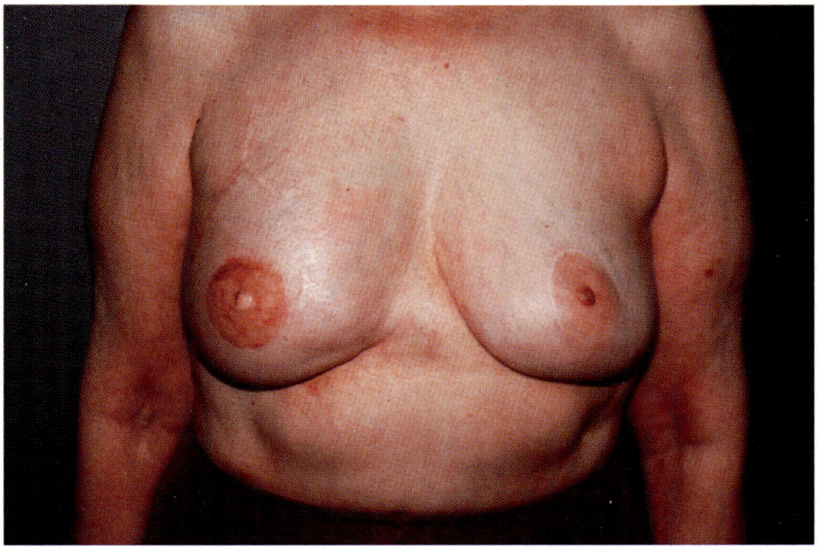

A 65-year-old patient underwent the removal of her right breast because of an infiltrating ductal carcinoma (upper panel). Reconstruction of the breast (lower panel) was accomplished by moving redundant tissues from the lower abdomen to the position of the right breast, with blood supply based on the left rectus abdominis muscle.

James W. May, Jr., M.D.

Massachusetts General Hospital
Boston, MA 02114

September 17, 1992

Transfer of a Toe to the Hand

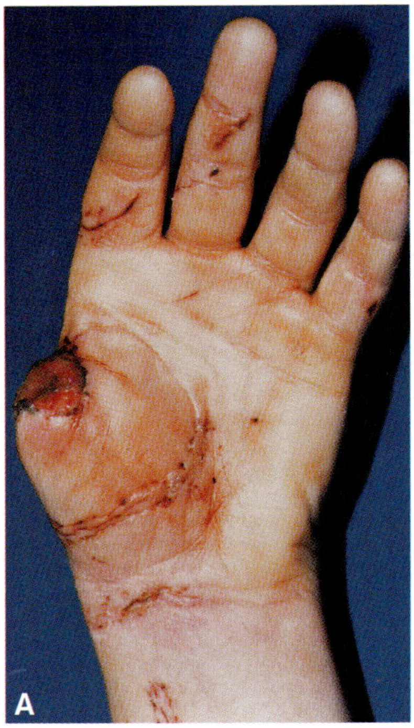

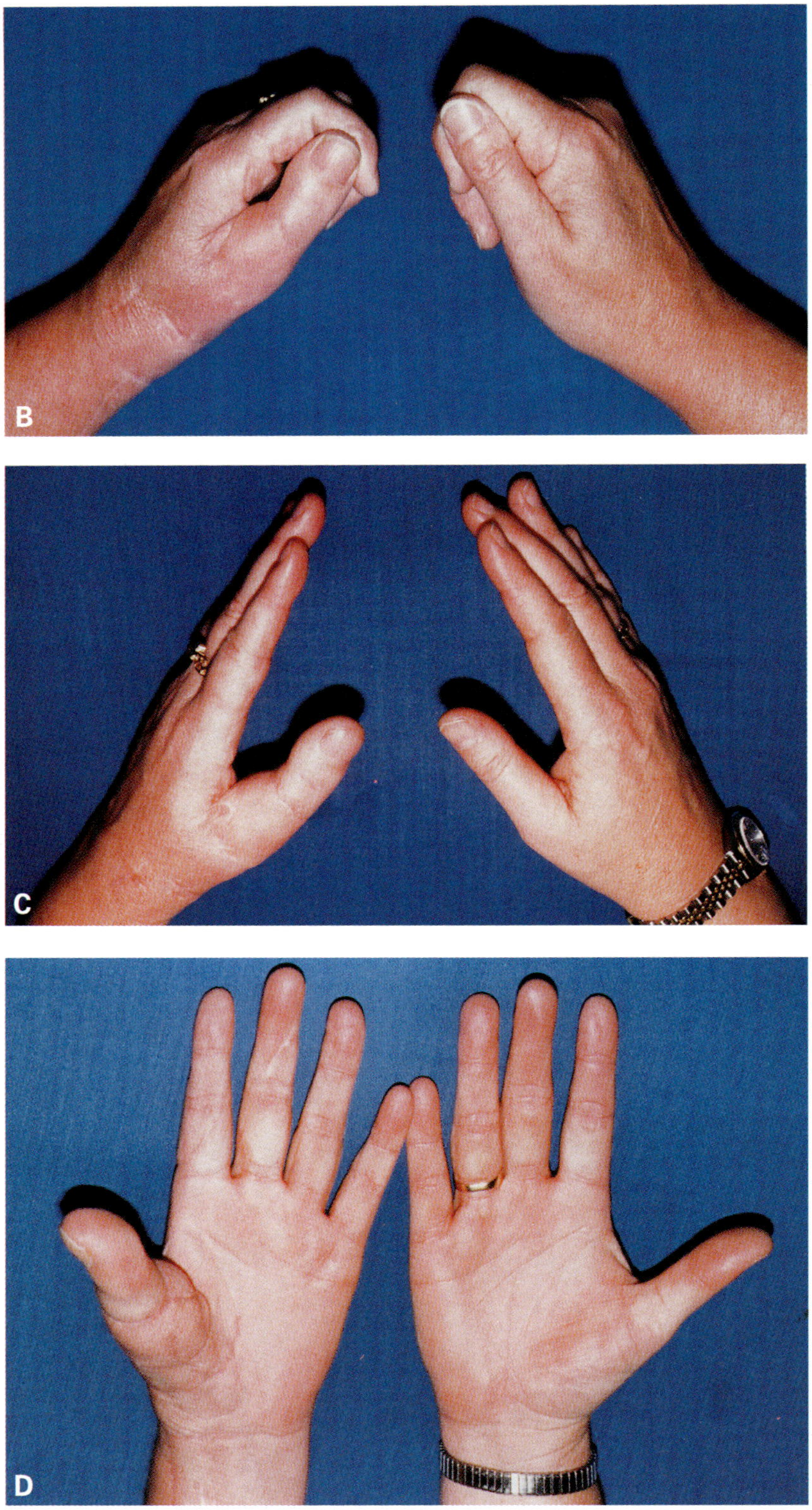

A 38-year-old woman's left thumb was amputated by a boat propeller while she was scuba diving, and it was not retrieved. Panel A shows her left hand three weeks after the accident. Four months after the accident skin from the groin was attached to the thumb stump and web area, and three months later a toe was transferred microsurgically. Panels B, C, and D show the result five years after the reconstructive surgery. By that time the new thumb had adequate sensibility (two-point discrimination of 15 mm) and 50 percent of the adduction power of the thumb on her other hand. She had adequate range of motion at the left metatarsophalangeal joint and interphalangeal joint and full extension of the thumb. Despite the loss of her toe, she was able to walk without difficulty.

James W. May, Jr., M.D.

Massachusetts General Hospital
Boston, MA 02114

March 23, 1995

Endoscopic Laser Third Ventriculostomy

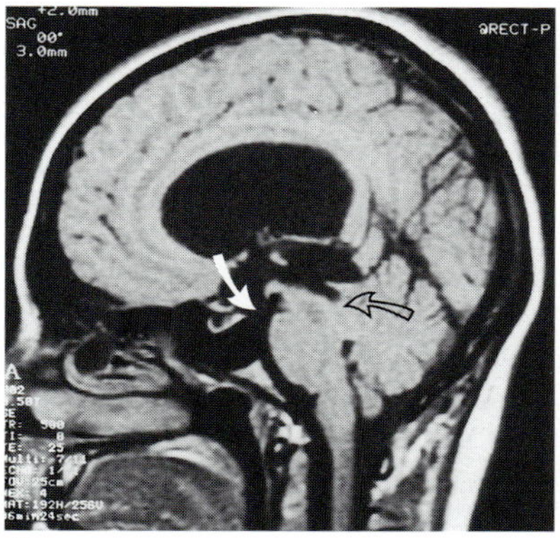

A

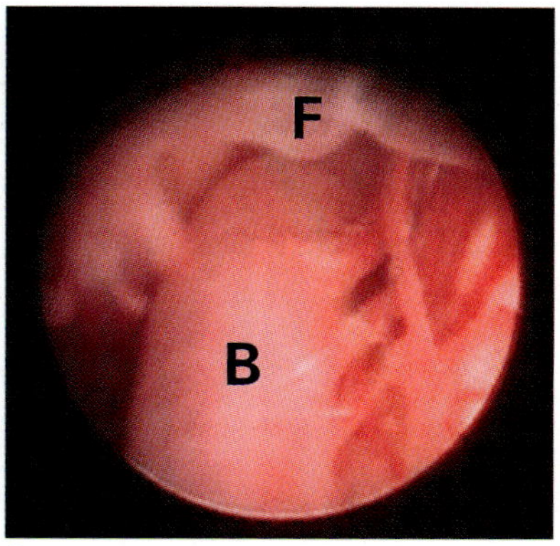

C

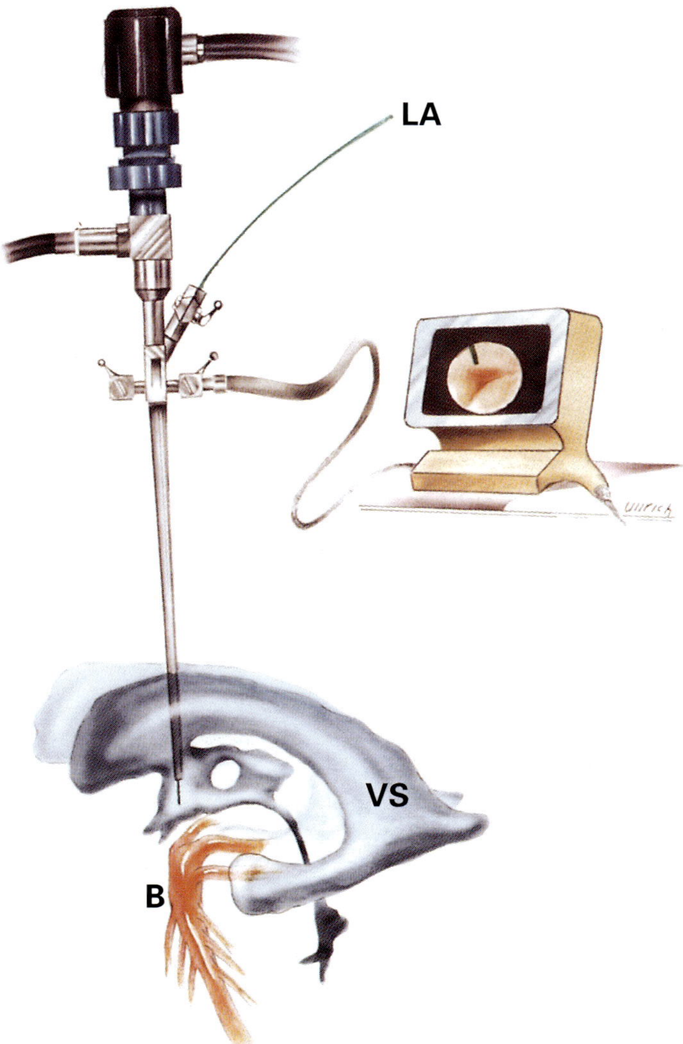

B

A 37-year-old woman was admitted to the hospital because she had had headaches for two years. A neurologic examination was remarkable for the absence of retinal venous pulsations.

Magnetic resonance imaging of the brain (Panel A) showed noncommunicating hydrocephalus due to stenosis of the caudal aqueduct of Sylvius (open arrow), with enlargement of the third ventricle and attenuation of its floor (solid arrow).

Endoscopic laser third ventriculostomy (Panel B) was performed in an effort to control hydrocephalus without the use of a ventricular shunt. The right lateral ventricle was cannulated through a coronal burr hole, and an endoscope was inserted through the foramen of Monro into the third ventricle. A fiberoptic neodymium:yttrium–aluminum–garnet laser was used to fenestrate the floor of the third ventricle anterior to the mamillary bodies, allowing cerebrospinal fluid to escape into the subarachnoid space and bypass the obstruction at the aqueduct. B denotes basilar artery, VS ventricular system, and LA laser.

The endoscope was then passed through the third ventriculostomy (Panel C), and the basilar artery and its pontine perforating branches were visualized in the prepontine cistern. F indicates the edge of the hole created by the laser in the third ventricular floor.

The patient's headaches resolved, and the ventricular size decreased on follow-up magnetic resonance imaging.

Alan R. Cohen, M.D.

New England Medical Center
Boston, MA 02111

February 25, 1993

Colloid Cyst of the Third Ventricle

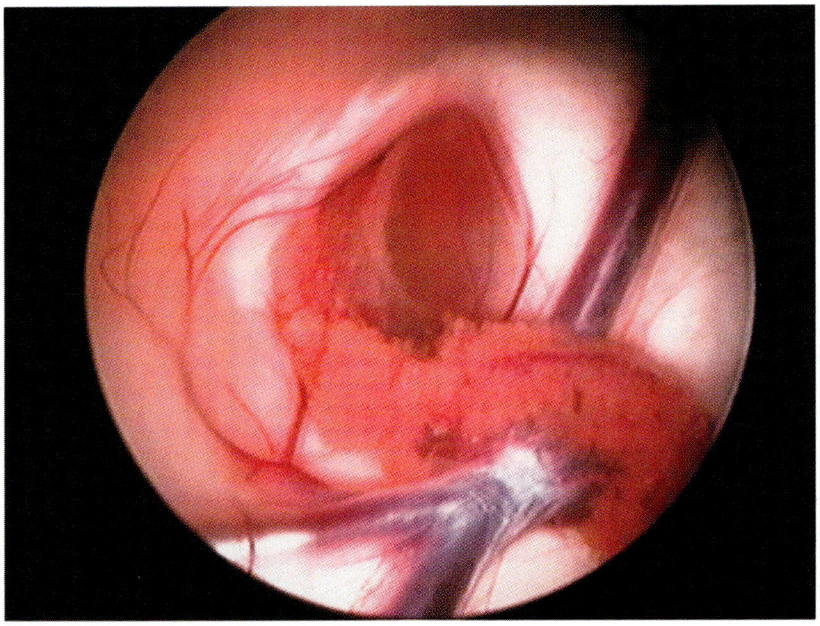

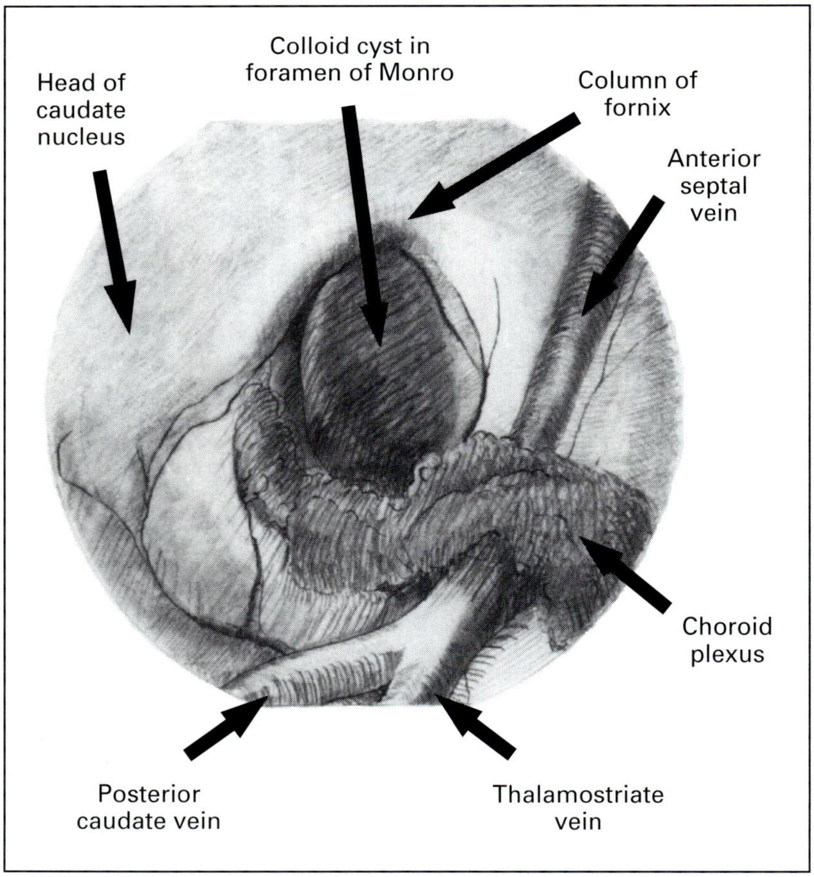

A 26-year-old man admitted to the hospital because he had had headache and vomiting for two months had papilledema but otherwise normal results on neurologic examination. Magnetic resonance imaging of the brain showed noncommunicating hydrocephalus due to occlusion of the anterior third ventricle by a cystic mass.

A small rigid endoscope directed into an asymmetrically enlarged left lateral ventricle through a single coronal burr hole disclosed a colloid cyst that obliterated the left foramen of Monro and blocked the passage of cerebrospinal fluid into the third ventricle. The colloid cyst was removed endoscopically with a fiberoptic neodymium:yttrium–aluminum–garnet laser and microinstruments. The patient's headache and papilledema resolved postoperatively.

Alan R. Cohen, M.D.

Rainbow Babies and Children's Hospital
Cleveland, OH 44106

May 11, 1995

Nail in the Brain

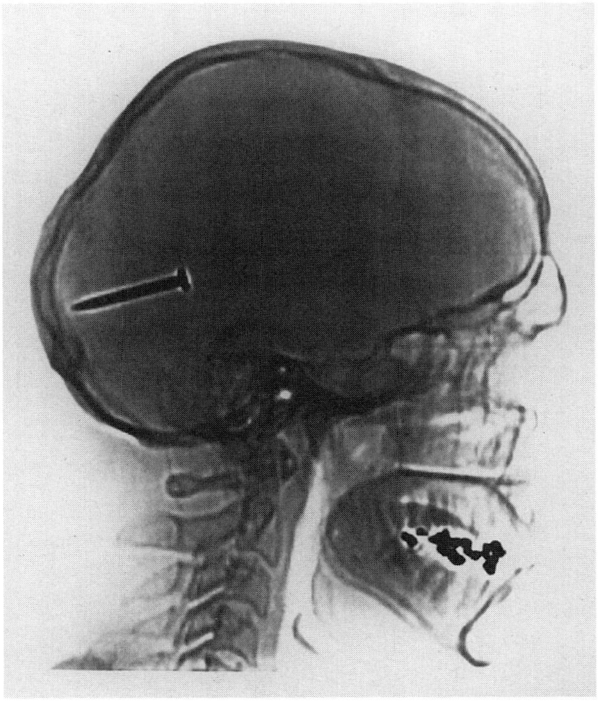

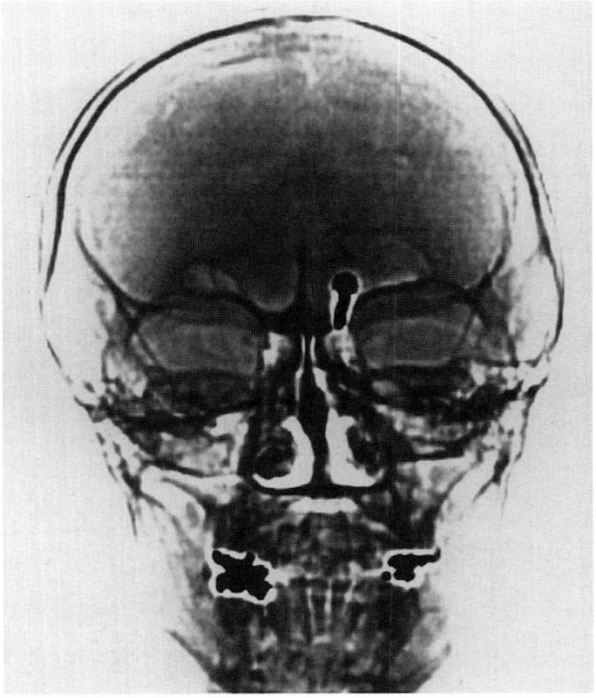

"Scout" films for a computed tomographic scan of the head show a nail in the brain of a stuporous, inebriated man seen in the emergency department. Examination revealed a mild right hemiparesis, which persisted after he became sober and fully articulate. Nine hours after admission, the patient disclosed that during a depressive episode 12 years earlier, he had attempted suicide with a nail gun directed between his eyes. Aside from right-sided facial droop and a slight limp, the patient had been symptom-free since the suicide attempt; he had had neither seizures nor episodes of loss of consciousness.

Michael Schwarzschild, M.D., Ph.D.

Massachusetts General Hospital
Boston, MA 02114

March 4, 1993

Nail in the Aorta

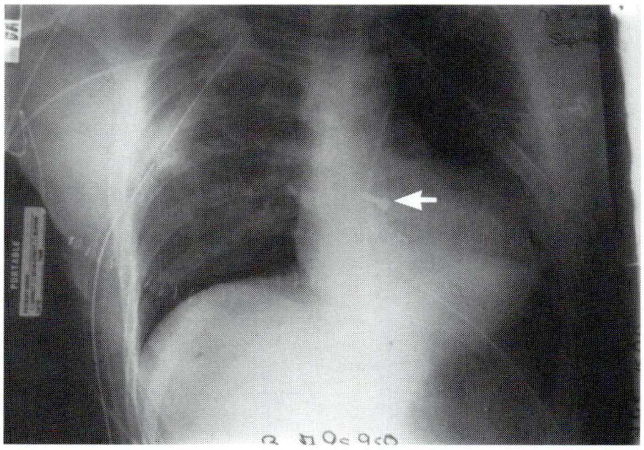

A

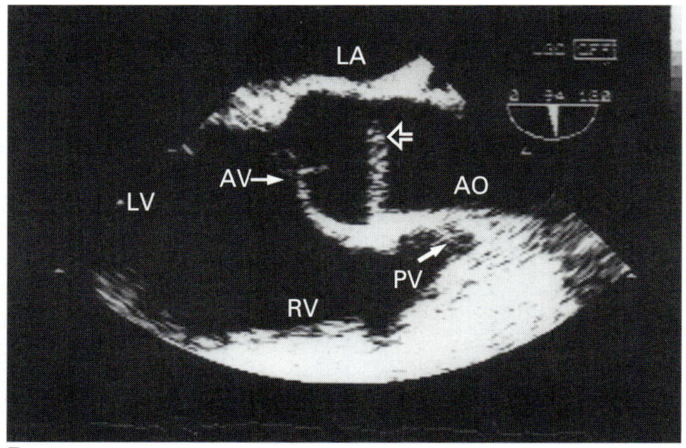

B

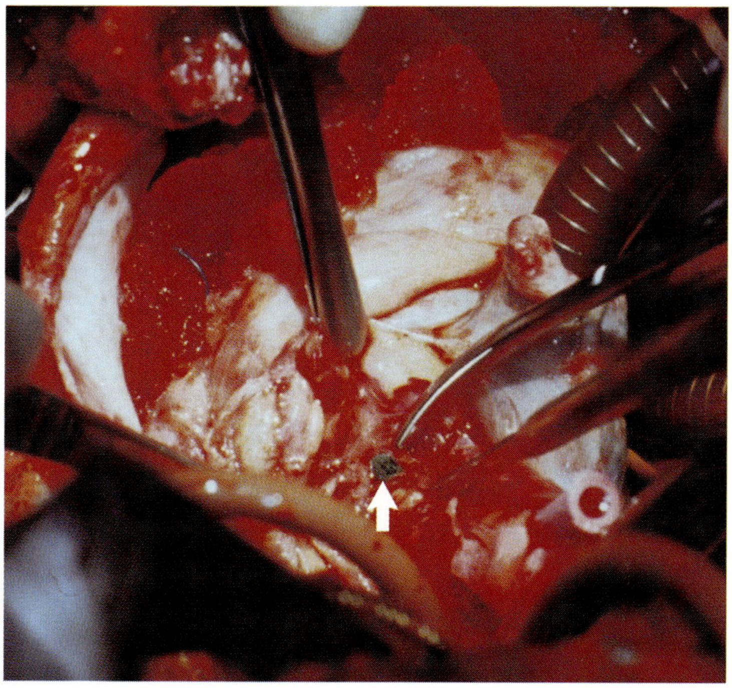

C

A 32-year-old man who had attempted suicide with a nail gun directed at his heart just to the left of the sternum presented to the emergency room with cardiac tamponade. The chest x-ray film (Panel A) revealed a nail (arrow), apparently in the heart. A two-dimensional transesophageal echocardiogram in the transverse plane at the level of the aorta revealed that the nail (open arrow) was 1 cm distal to the aortic leaflets (Panel B). The nail penetrated the right ventricle (RV), just proximal to the pulmonic valve (PV), adhering the right ventricle to the aorta (AO). A horizontal image (not shown) showed that the nail was within 1 mm of the right coronary artery. The color Doppler image (not shown) identified a left-to-right communication from the aorta into the right ventricle. LA denotes left atrium, LV left ventricle, and AV aortic valve.

The patient underwent emergency surgery, and by studying the transesophageal echocardiogram the surgeon was able to pinpoint his incision. Panel C shows the nail (arrow) just before its removal. The nail, with adherent thrombus and pieces of the patient's shirt, was removed without complication, permitting the right ventricular wall to contract normally. The patient was sent home from the hospital one week postoperatively, doing well physically. His mental health was improved.

Joel M. Felner, M.D.

Emory University School of Medicine
Atlanta, GA 30303

January 25, 1996

Abdominal Aortic Aneurysm

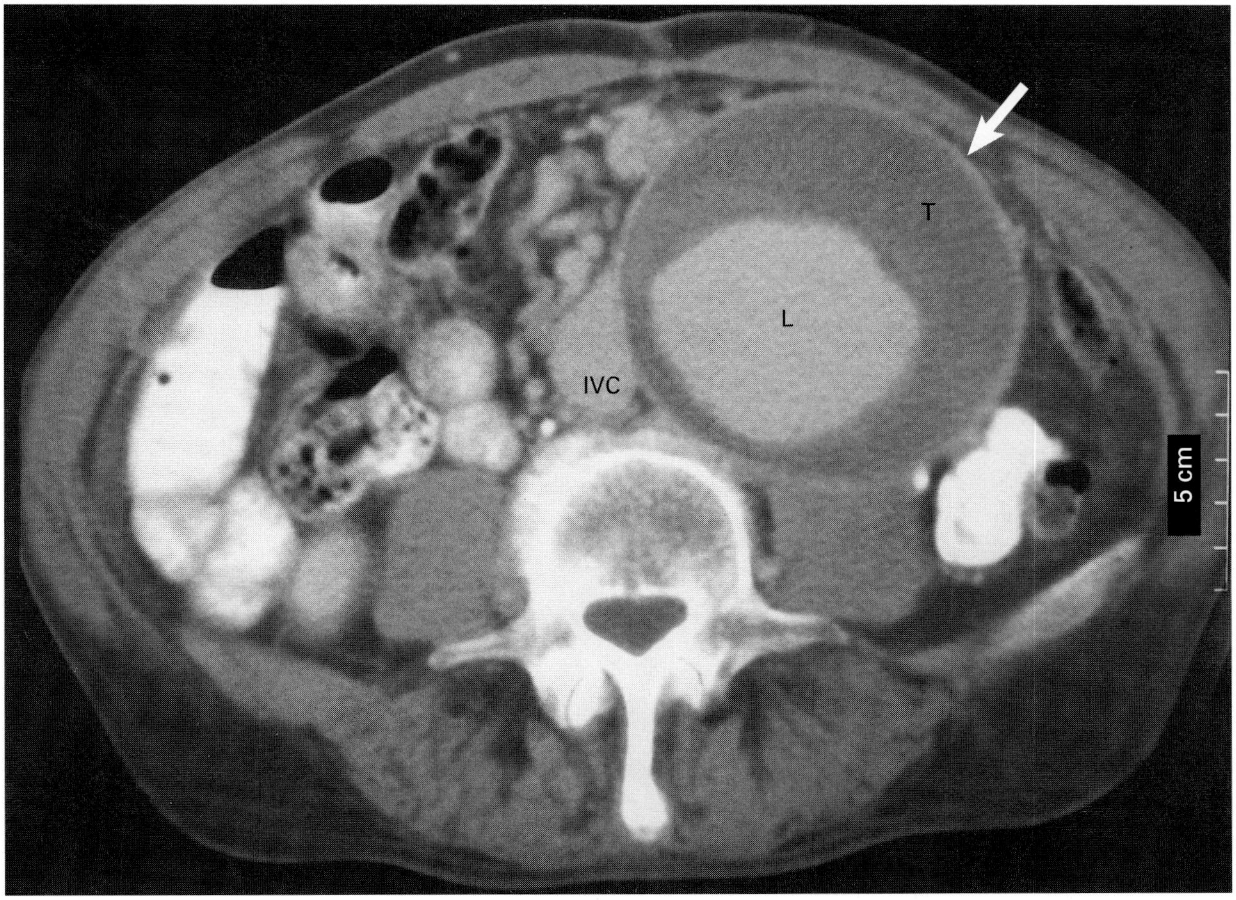

A cross-sectional computed tomographic scan of the abdomen of an 85-year-old man shows an aneurysm (arrow) of the infrarenal aorta measuring 10 cm in diameter. The initial diagnosis was made on physical examination by palpation of a pulsatile abdominal mass and was confirmed by computed tomography. The infrarenal aorta was replaced by a tube graft, and the remaining aneurysmal wall was trimmed and sutured back around the graft as a reinforcement. L denotes lumen, T mural thrombus lining the aneurysm, and IVC inferior vena cava.

Miralem Pasic, M.D., Ph.D.
Marko Turina, M.D.

University Hospital Zurich
CH-8091 Zurich, Switzerland

January 4, 1996

Aortoenteric Fistula

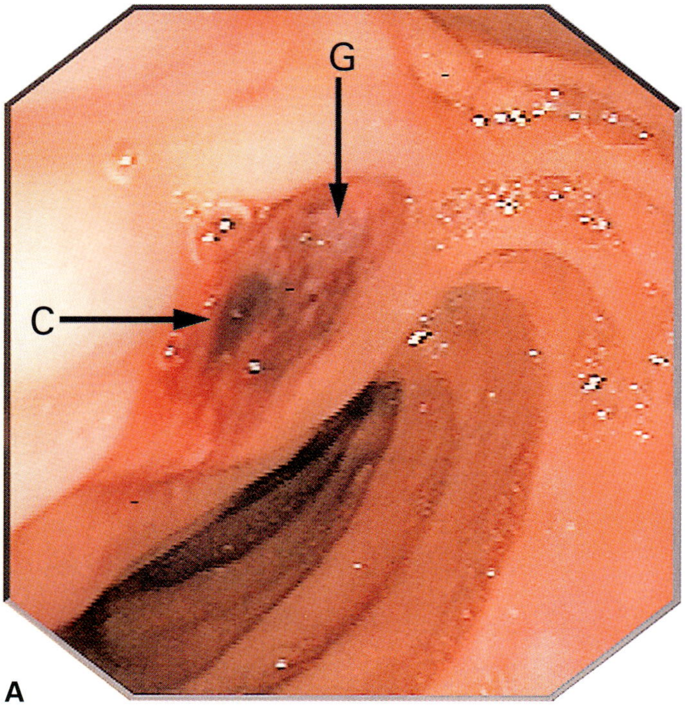

A

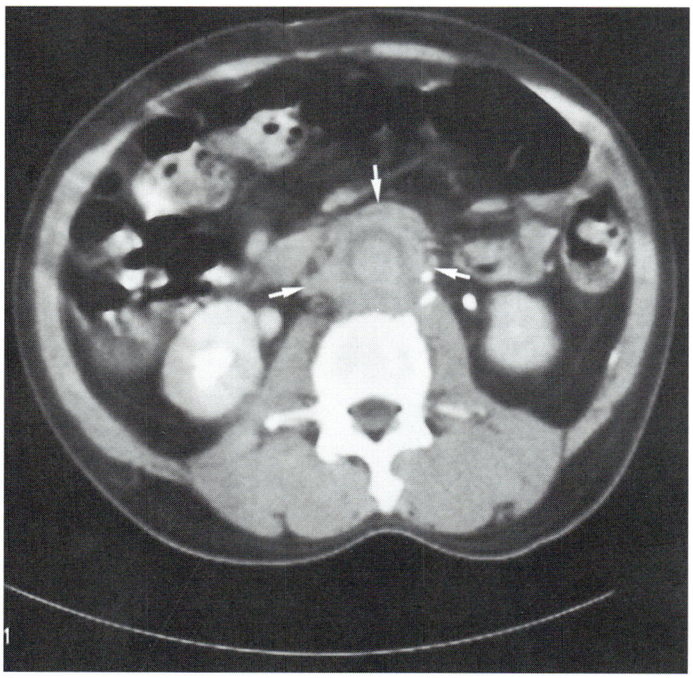

B

A 1.5-cm mucosal defect with the classic appearance of an aortoduodenal fistula was detected by endoscopy in the third portion of the duodenum (Panel A). The patient had a Dacron aortic graft and presented with hematemesis. C indicates the clot overlying the bleeding site, and G the graft with a superimposed collection of infected fluid. Computed tomographic scanning (Panel B) revealed fluid collection in the area of the aorta (arrows). Surgery confirmed the presence of the aortoenteric fistula and an infected graft.

Paul E. Zachary, Jr., M.D.

University of Kansas Medical Center
Kansas City, KS 66160

Donald R. Campbell, M.D.

Veterans Affairs Medical Center
Kansas City, MO 64128

April 22, 1993

Correspondence

Aortoenteric Fistula

August 19, 1993

To the Editor: The photograph of the aortoenteric fistula detected by endoscopy, shown in Images in Clinical Medicine (April 22 issue),[1] is dramatic. The accompanying computed tomographic scan is interesting and confirms the diagnosis, but I am surprised to see it.

This endoscopic finding in a patient known to have an aortic graft would have prompted me to rush the patient to emergency surgery before the aneurysm ruptured. The potential for rupture is so great in these cases that any delay may be fatal.

Herbert Rakatansky, M.D.
Brown University
Providence, RI 02912

1. Zachary PE Jr, Campbell DR. Aortoenteric fistula. N Engl J Med 1993;328:1166.

The authors reply:

To the Editor: The gastroenterologists and surgeons were confident that this lesion, as visualized with a side-viewing duodenoscope, represented an aortoenteric fistula and agreed that the patient should undergo prompt surgical correction before an exsanguinating hemorrhage occurred. Experts[1,2] recommend that patients who are hemodynamically stable undergo a deliberate and orderly, yet expeditious, evaluation to establish this diagnosis. Because the patient's condition was stable, computed tomography was performed, without delay, to define the suspected infectious process in more detail. Detection of a false aneurysm, renal-artery involvement, or suprarenal aneurysmal dilatation (the patient had undergone aortobifemoral grafting seven years earlier) might have influenced the surgical approach. Computed tomography should not be performed in an unstable patient suspected of having an aortoenteric fistula. Studies such as computed tomography and angiography complement upper endoscopy and provide information that can alter the surgical approach to patients with aortoenteric fistulas. The attending surgeon must make the final decision about the benefit to be gained from such studies as compared with the risk entailed by delaying surgery.

Paul E. Zachary, Jr., M.D.
University of Kansas School of Medicine
Kansas City, KS 66160

Donald R. Campbell, M.D.
Veterans Affairs Medical Center
Kansas City, MO 64128

1. Hermreck AS. Prevention and management of surgical complications during repair of abdominal aortic aneurysms. Surg Clin North Am 1989;69:869-94.
2. Ernst CB. Aortic graft enteric fistula. In: Ernst CB, Stanley JC, eds. Current therapy in vascular surgery. 2nd ed. Philadelphia: B.C. Decker, 1991:440-5.

Ruptured Abdominal Aortic Aneurysm

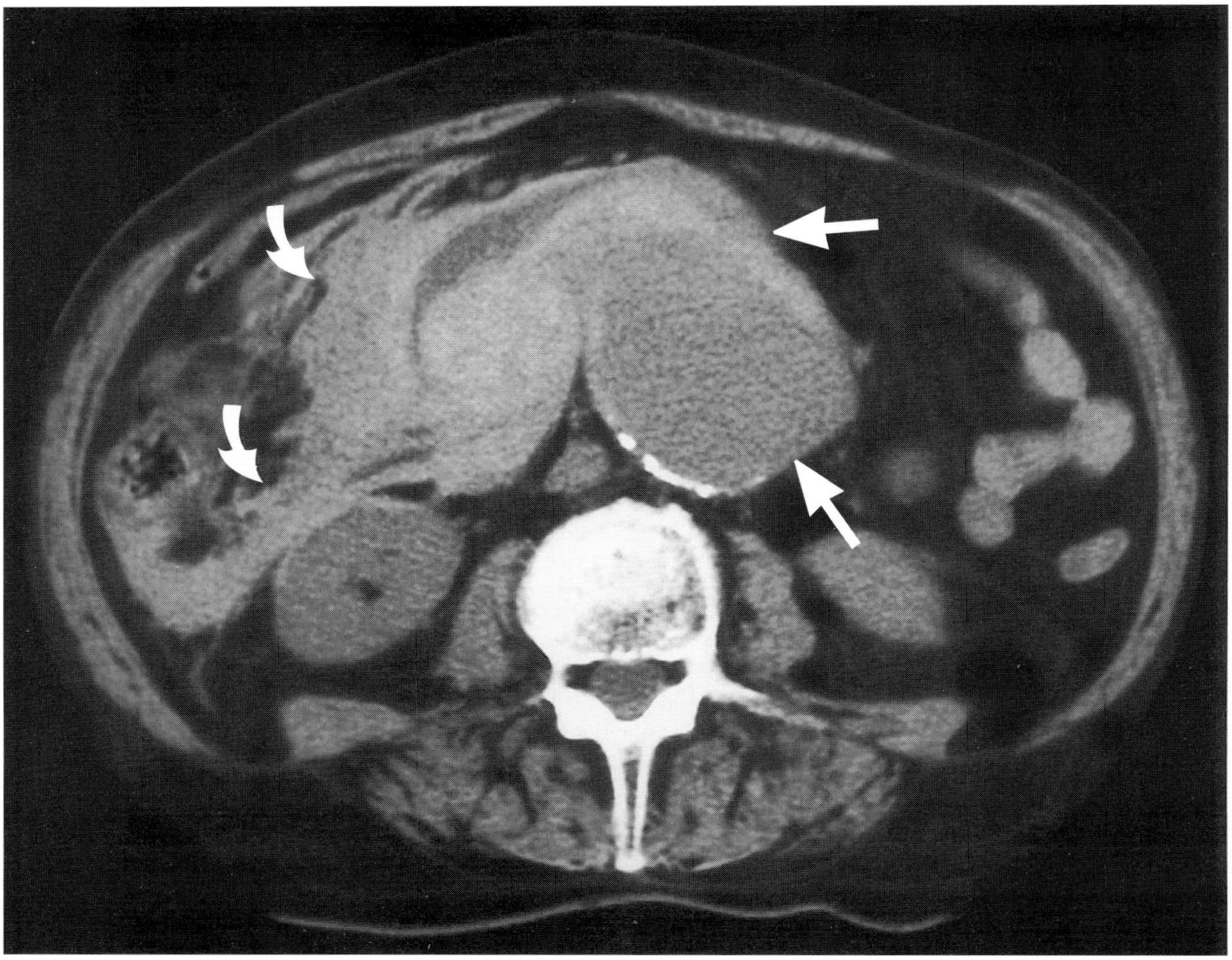

An 85-year-old man was brought to the emergency room after two hours of excruciating abdominal pain, nausea, and vomiting. He was hypotensive on admission. Physical examination revealed a pulsatile mid-abdominal mass. Emergency computed tomography revealed a ruptured abdominal aortic aneurysm (straight arrows). Surgical findings confirmed that the aneurysm had ruptured, with hemorrhage (curved arrows) into the right anterior pararenal space. Cardiac arrest occurred intraoperatively. The patient was resuscitated and taken to the surgical intensive care unit. On arrival, he had a second cardiac arrest and died despite vigorous resuscitative efforts.

Debra A. Gervais, M.D.
Gary J. Whitman, M.D.

Massachusetts General Hospital
Boston, MA 02114

January 4, 1996

Correspondence

Computed Tomography for Ruptured Abdominal Aortic Aneurysm?

May 9, 1996

To the Editor: The last place an 85-year-old patient with hypotension, severe abdominal pain, and a pulsatile abdominal mass should be is in the computed tomographic (CT) scanner (Images in Clinical Medicine, Jan. 4 issue).[1] Instead, this patient should have been taken immediately to the operating room, bypassing the radiology department altogether. This is a classic example of a situation in which physicians must rely on the signs and symptoms found at the bedside and act on their intuition, rather than falling back on unnecessary confirmatory tests.

Steven J. Eskind, M.D.
Surgical Specialists of Nashville
Nashville, TN 37205

1. Gervais DA, Whitman GJ. Ruptured abdominal aortic aneurysm. N Engl J Med 1996;334:27.

To the Editor: What in the world could have motivated Drs. Gervais and Whitman to obtain an emergency abdominal CT scan in a patient with a clinically obvious ruptured abdominal aortic aneurysm? This image provided an opportunity to teach a valuable lesson, but unfortunately the wrong lesson has been taught. The *Journal* should have used the submission of the image to condemn the practice and recommend clinical diagnosis and immediate transfer of the patient to an operating room where personnel have been alerted to the emergency. One is left to wonder what responses this case would have prompted if it had appeared as a Clinical Problem-Solving article.

George Andros, M.D.
2701 W. Alameda Ave.
Burbank, CA 91505

The authors reply:

To the Editor: We agree with Dr. Eskind and Dr. Andros that hemodynamically unstable patients with clinically obvious ruptured abdominal aortic aneurysms should be taken directly to the operating room, without diagnostic studies. The patient in this case was not hemodynamically unstable at the time of the CT scan, but had experienced transient hypotension, accompanied in part by bradycardia, which suggested a possible vagal cause. Because he had a known abdominal aortic aneurysm and a history of peptic ulcer disease, his presentation with epigastric pain, nausea, and vomiting led his physicians to consider a gastrointestinal cause in the differential diagnosis. An emergency CT scan was requested and given top priority by both the surgeons and the radiologist in the CT suite, as is consistent with recent suggestions for the close monitoring of patients with symptomatic abdominal aortic aneurysms in the CT suite.[1]

Among hemodynamically stable patients with symptomatic abdominal aortic aneurysm, Kvilekval et al. have found no difference in mortality between those who undergo CT and those who do not.[2] CT is useful, however, in evaluating

Correspondence Continued

the extent of the aneurysm, anatomical variants (especially venous and renal), frank as compared with "contained" rupture, and potential inflammatory components.[3] Identifying symptomatic nonruptured abdominal aortic aneurysm is important, because the perioperative morbidity from cardiovascular events is lower if repair is deferred until the cardiac issues are addressed.[2] CT may also identify clinical conditions that mimic symptomatic abdominal aortic aneurysm, especially in a patient such as ours, in whom there is an alternative diagnostic consideration.[4]

All hemodynamically unstable patients with clinically obvious ruptured abdominal aortic aneurysms should be taken directly to the operating room. Hemodynamically stable patients with this condition or in whom the diagnosis may be uncertain may benefit from CT, which should be done expeditiously, in consultation with the surgical service. Because the condition of such patients can become unstable at any time, radiologists and surgeons must be prepared to respond rapidly.

Debra A. Gervais, M.D.
Gary J. Whitman, M.D.
Massachusetts General Hospital
Boston, MA 02114

1. Cohan RH, Siegel CL. CT of "stable" patients with suspected abdominal aortic aneurysm with leak or contained rupture. AJR Am J Roentgenol 1995;164:1302-3.
2. Kvilekval KH, Best IM, Mason RA, Newton GB, Giron F. The value of computed tomography in the management of symptomatic abdominal aortic aneurysms. J Vasc Surg 1990; 12:28-33.
3. Siegel CL, Cohan RH. CT of abdominal aortic aneurysms. AJR Am J Roentgenol 1994; 163:17-29.
4. Kadir S, Athanasoulis CA, Brewster DC, Moncure AC. Tender pulsatile abdominal mass: abdominal aortic aneurysm or not? Arch Surg 1980;115:631-3.

Transfemoral Repair of Abdominal Aortic Aneurysm

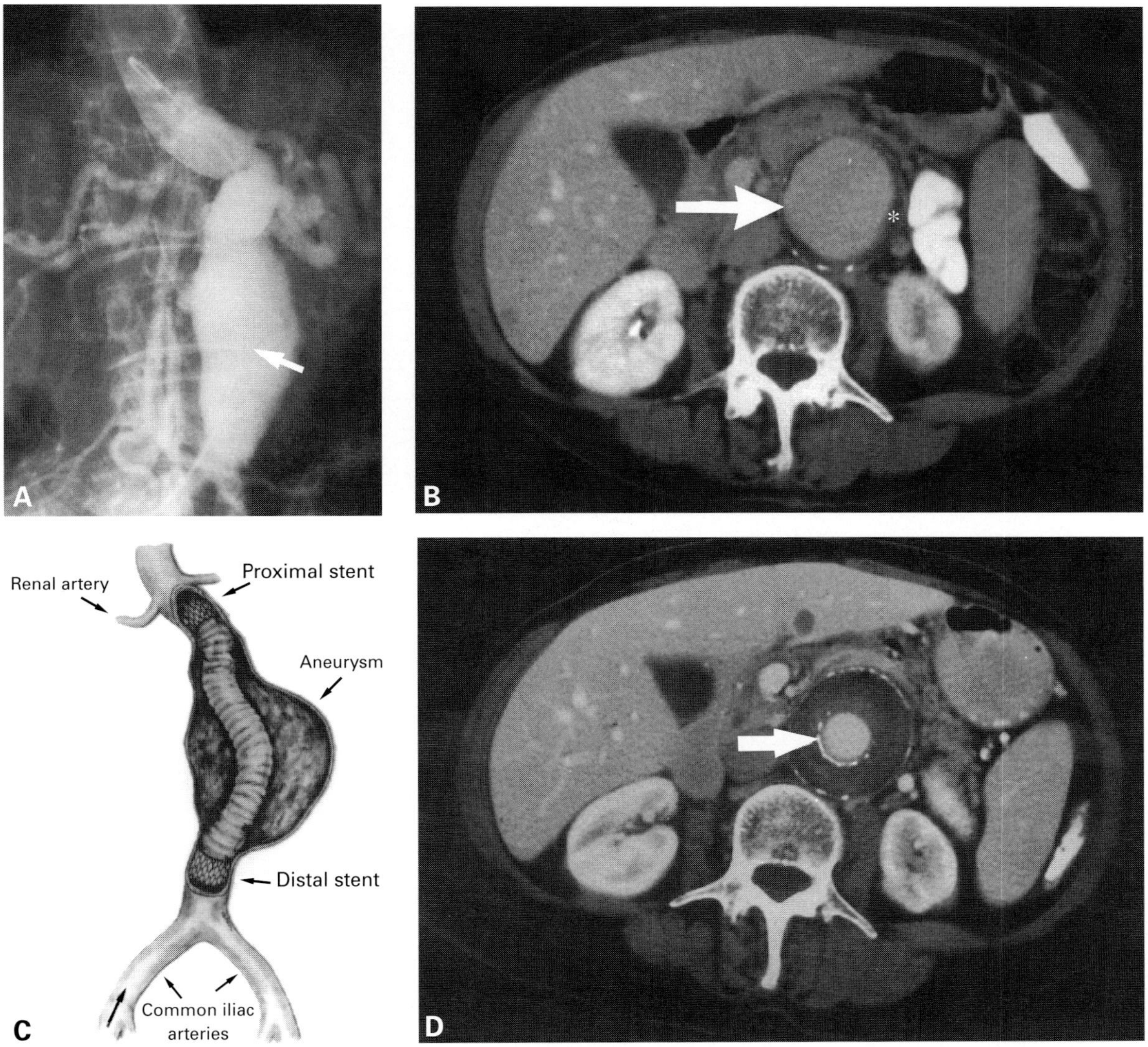

A Dacron prosthetic graft was sutured to a balloon-expandable metallic stent and inserted under local anesthesia through a right femoral-artery cutdown in a 70-year-old woman with an enlarging, tender 5.6-cm abdominal aortic aneurysm. Surgical repair was deemed too risky because the patient required oxygen for chronic pulmonary disease and had coronary artery disease. Aortography (Panel A) revealed the aneurysm (arrow) and a tortuous aorta, and computed tomography (CT) (Panel B) identified the aneurysm (arrow) and minimal mural thrombus (asterisk). The aortic reconstruction is illustrated in Panel C. The stent–graft device was packaged in a Teflon catheter and inserted retrogradely over a wire from the right femoral artery into the aorta along the course indicated by the large arrow. Balloon-expandable stents attached the Dacron graft to the neck of the aneurysm proximally and distally. The aneurysmal sac around the stent–graft thrombosed. A follow-up CT scan (Panel D) after placement of the stent–graft device showed a decrease in the size of the aneurysm, with thrombus surrounding the patent stent–graft (arrow). The patient has had no complications in the 14 months since the procedure, and follow-up CT scans show persistent exclusion of the aneurysm and arterial flow limited to the lumen of the graft.

Michael L. Marin, M.D.
Frank J. Veith, M.D.

Montefiore Medical Center
New York, NY 10467

December 29, 1994

Cholesterol and Lipid Deposits

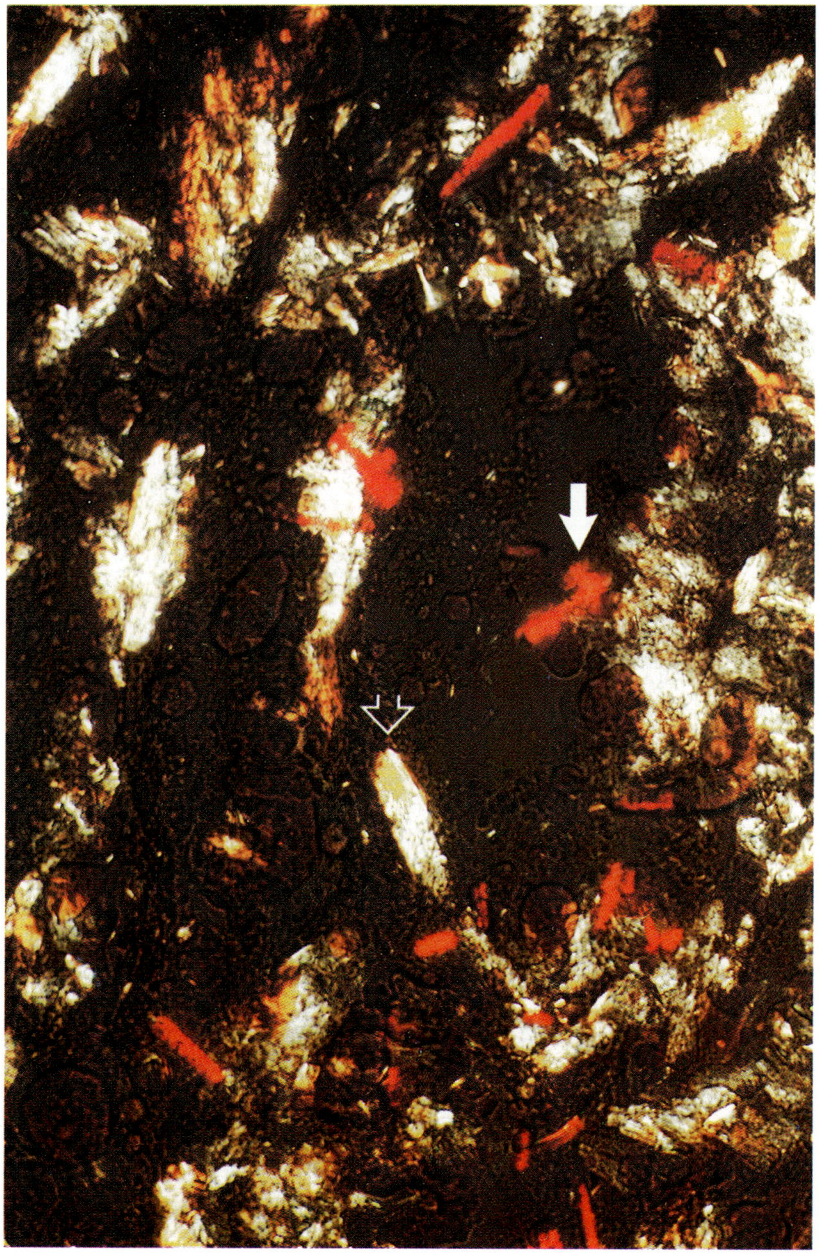

A specimen from the wall of the ascending aorta was excised from a 55-year-old patient at the time of aortocoronary bypass grafting. In a Sudan-stained cryosection viewed under polarized light, cholesterol (open arrow) and neutral lipid deposits (solid arrow) are evident in this atherosclerotic lesion (×710).

Markus M. Lerch, M.D.
Guido Adler, M.D.

Ulm University
7900 Ulm, Germany

February 4, 1993

Gas in the Portal Venous System

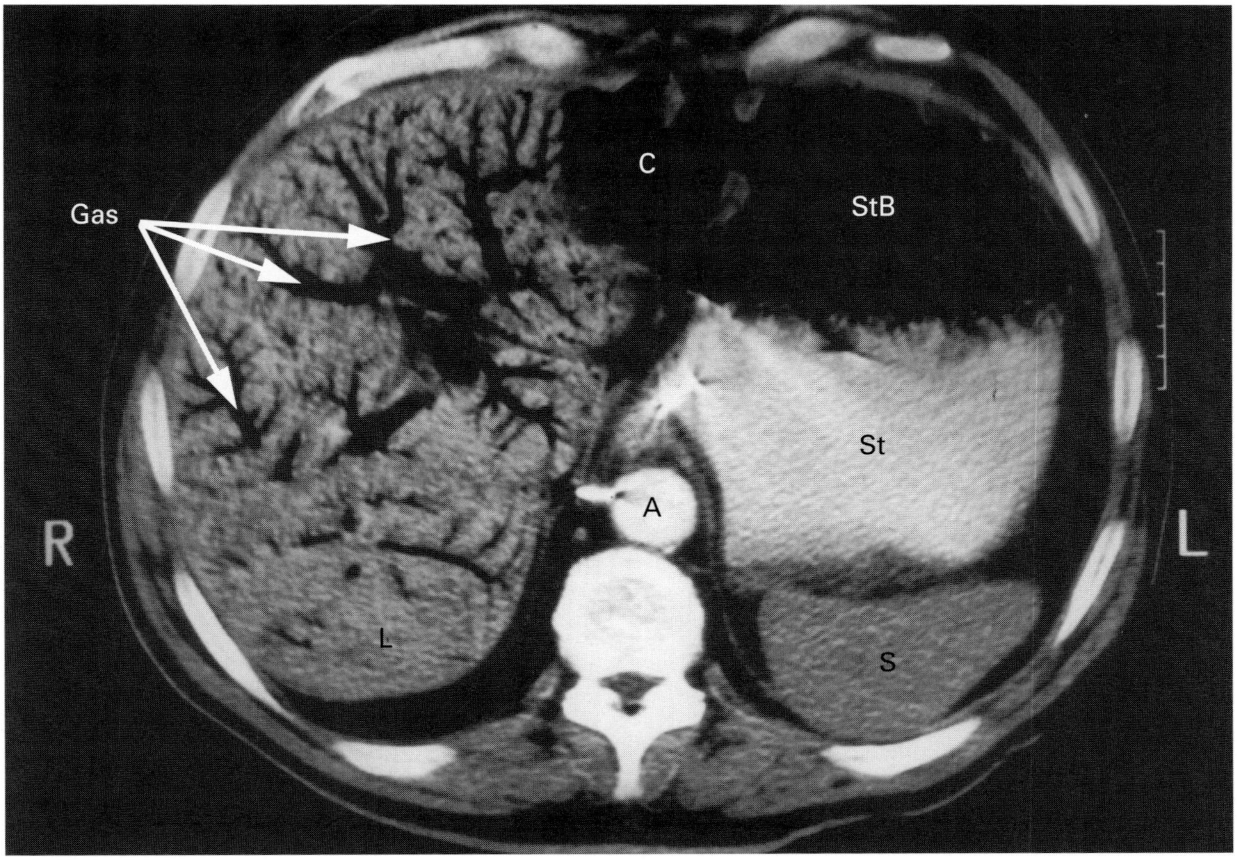

A computed tomographic scan of a 73-year-old man with acute epigastric pain and abdominal distention shows gas in the portal venous system (arrows). A plain film of the abdomen did not reveal the gas within the liver. The patient was taken to the operating room, where he was found to have mesenteric ischemia from stenosis of the celiac axis, superior mesenteric artery, and inferior mesenteric artery and a massive infarction of the small bowel. The patient survived a small-bowel resection. C denotes colon; StB, gas in the stomach lumen; St, stomach partially filled with contrast agent; S, spleen; A, aorta; and L, liver.

Leon W. Kundrotas, M.D., Lt. Col., M.C., U.S.A.F.
A. Brian Robinson, M.D., Maj., M.C., U.S.A.F.

Wilford Hall Medical Center
Lackland AFB, TX 78236-5300

September 19, 1996

Endovascular Stents for Iliac Arterial Disease

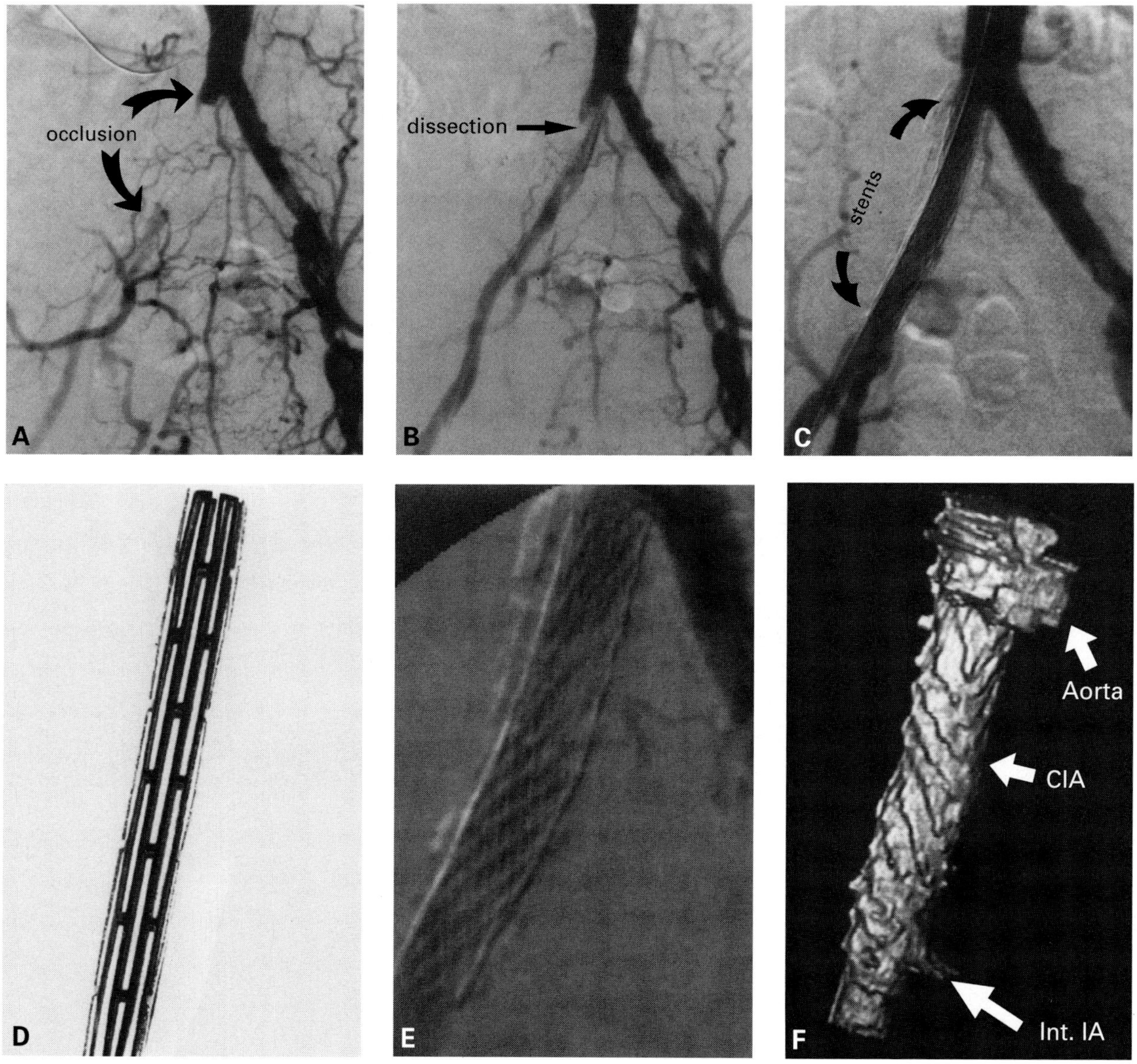

The angiogram shown in Panel A was recorded in a 57-year-old man with no right femoral pulse; arrows indicate a 5-cm total occlusion of the right common iliac artery. The occlusion was crossed with a hydrophilic guidewire. An angiogram recorded after angioplasty (Panel B) shows a patent common iliac artery with extensive dissection. A final angiogram (Panel C) was recorded after the tandem insertion of two endovascular stents and shows that the artery is widely patent.

The non-expanded iliac stent (Johnson and Johnson, Piscataway, N.J.) is shown in Panel D, and the radiographic appearance of the balloon-expanded stents is shown in Panel E. A three-dimensional view of the stented right common iliac artery was reconstructed (Panel F) from two-dimensional images obtained by intravascular ultrasonography; the aorta, common iliac artery (CIA), and internal iliac artery (Int. IA) are shown.

Kenneth Rosenfield, M.D.
Jeffrey M. Isner, M.D.

St. Elizabeth's Hospital
Boston, MA 02135

August 26, 1993

Hypertension and Renal Insufficiency due to Renovascular Disease

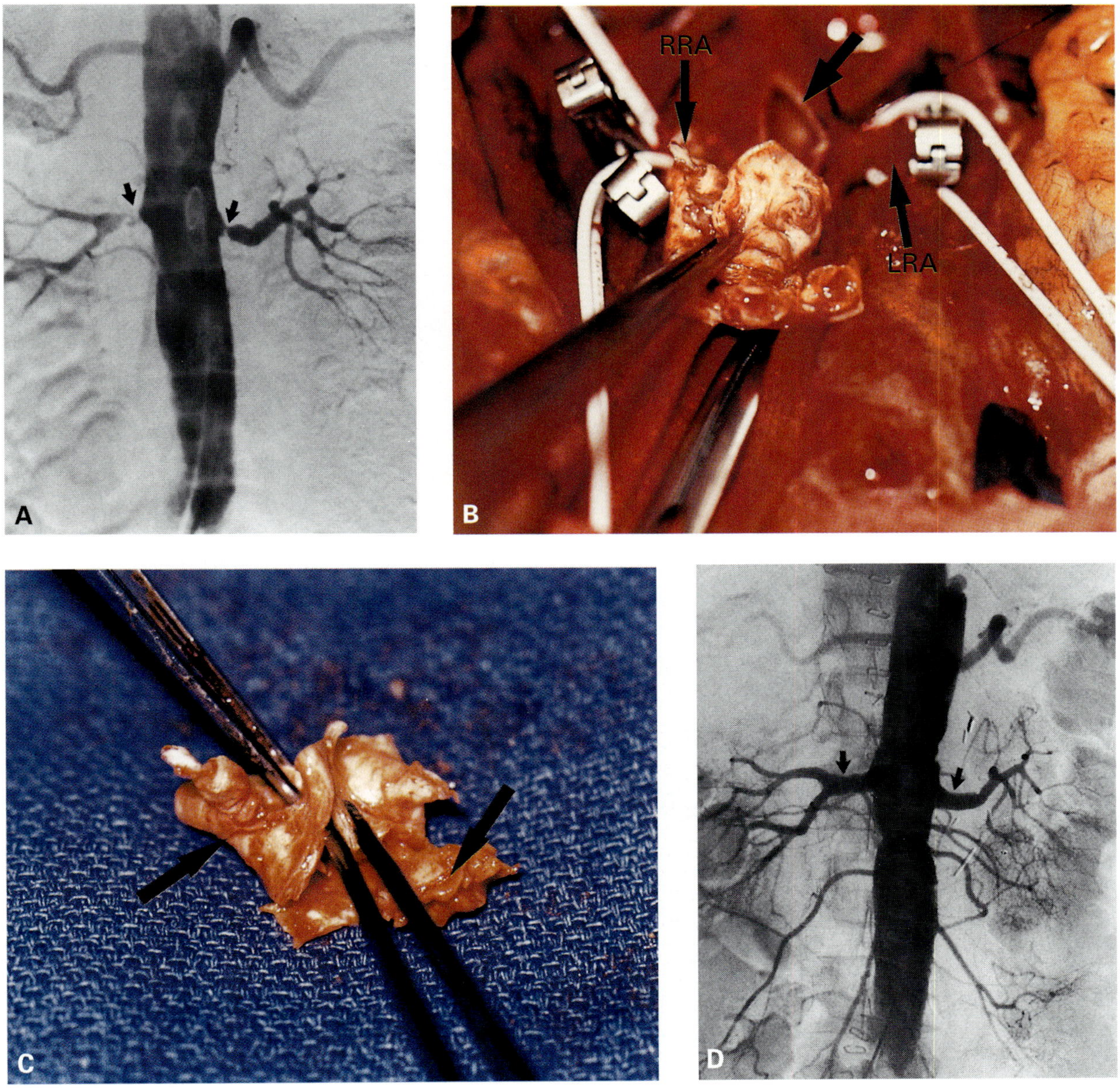

The images illustrate renovascular hypertension and renal insufficiency in a 57-year-old woman. Arteriography (Panel A) reveals severe bilateral renal-artery stenoses (arrows). A photograph taken during transaortic bilateral renal-artery endarterectomy (Panel B) shows the specimen being removed; the aortotomy is evident (large arrow) in the background. A close-up of the specimen (Panel C) shows the tongues of atheroma (arrows) that extended into and obstructed the renal arteries. A postoperative arteriogram (Panel D) demonstrates widely patent renal arteries (arrows). After surgery the patient no longer required antihypertensive medications, and her serum creatinine level decreased from 2.1 to 1.2 mg per deciliter (186 to 106 μmol per liter). LRA denotes left renal artery, and RRA right renal artery.

Richard P. Cambria, M.D.

Massachusetts General Hospital
Boston, MA 02114

November 19, 1992

Pott's Disease with Paraparesis

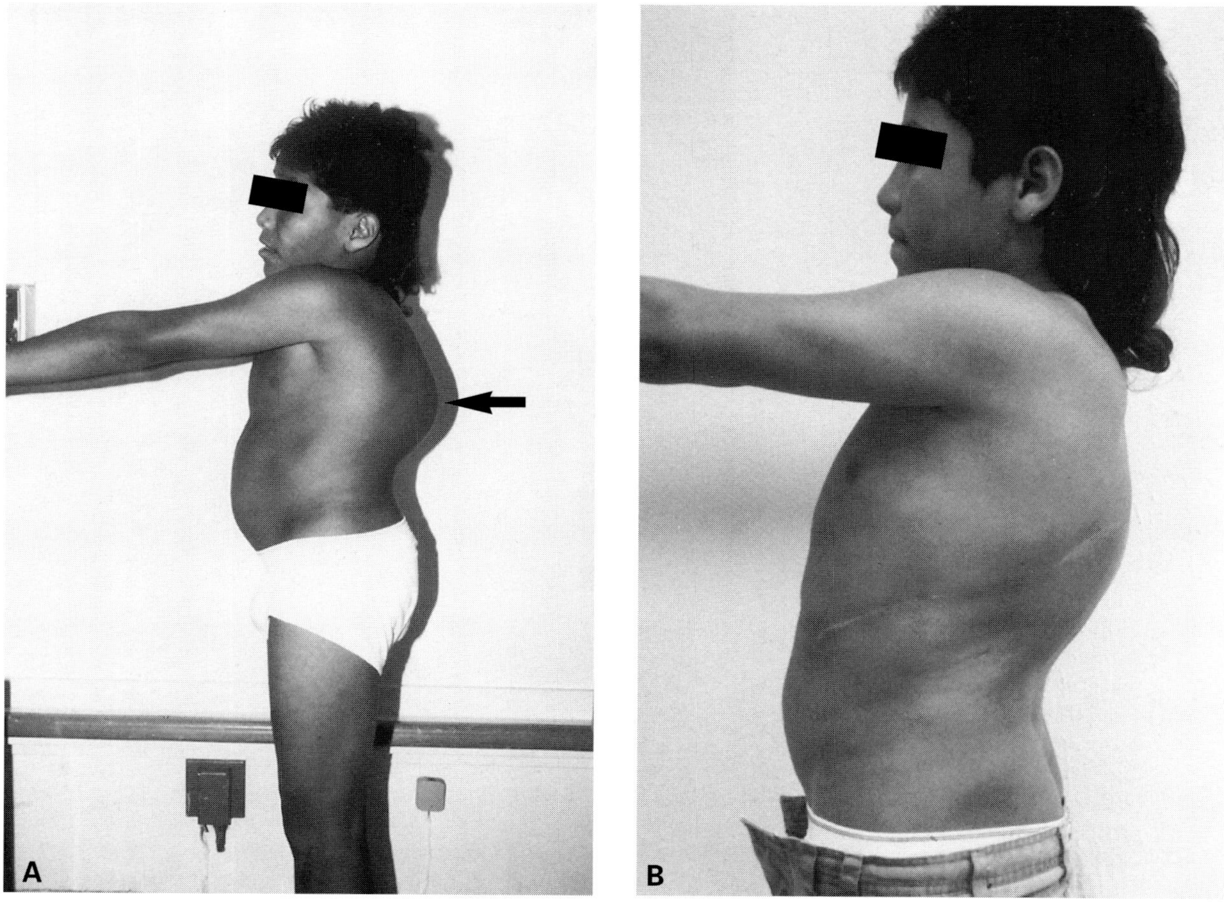

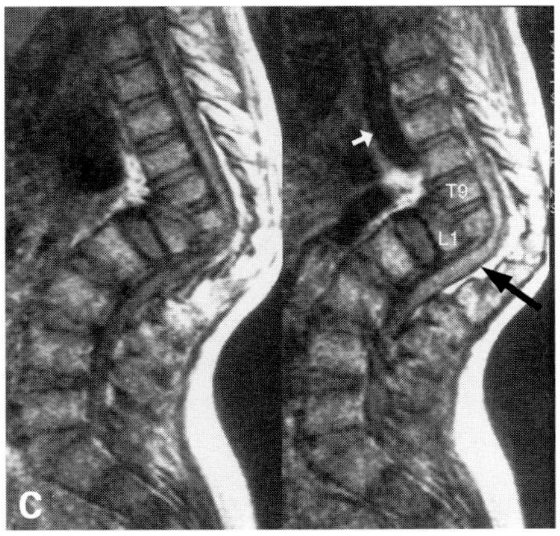

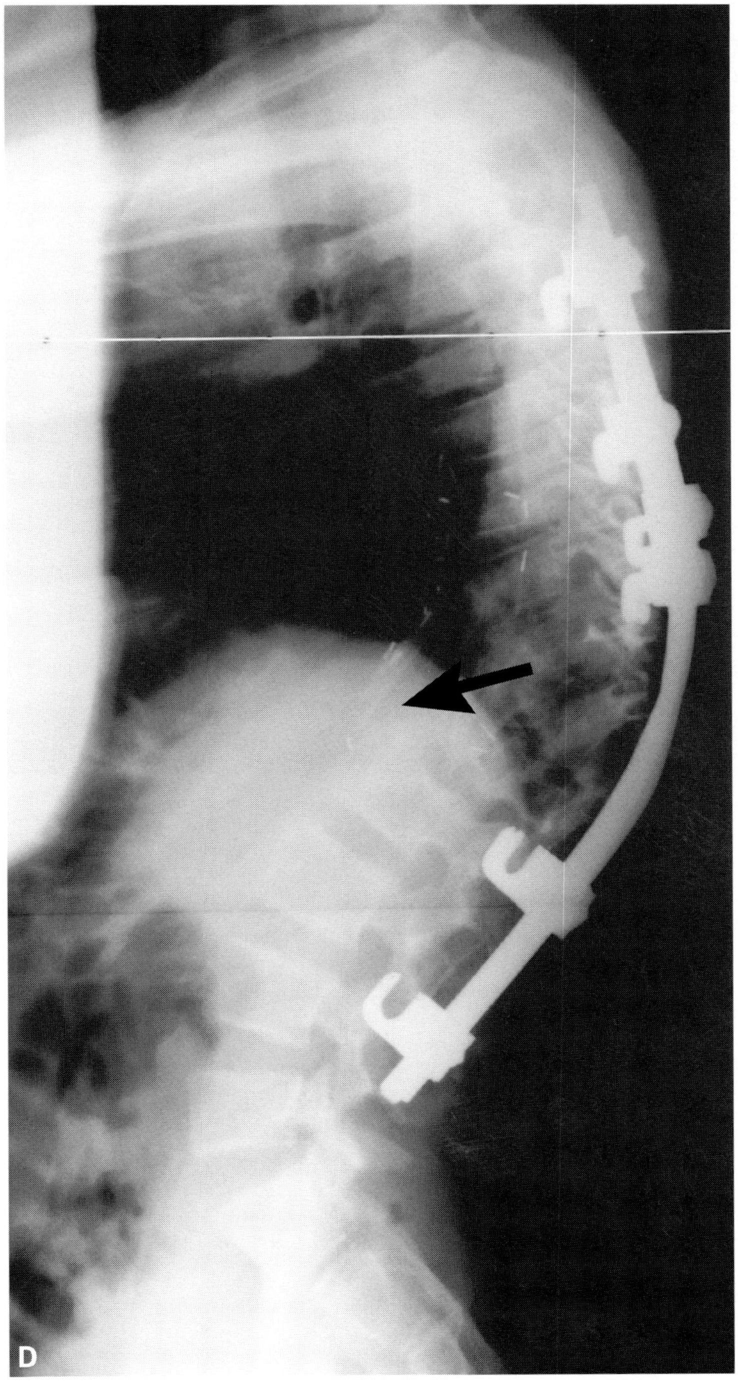

A 13-year-old boy presented with increasing kyphotic deformity, back pain, and progressive paraparesis seven years after a one-year course of medical therapy for tuberculosis. He reported shock-like sensations in his legs whenever he bent forward and fatigue in his thighs and calves, which limited his activities. Physical findings included a rigid gibbus (Panel A, arrow), inability to tiptoe, hyperreflexia of the ankles with mild clonus, and normal proprioception and sensation to light touch. A magnetic resonance imaging scan (Panel C) showed that the bodies of T9 through L1 had collapsed into one mass, compressing the spinal cord to about half its usual diameter (large arrow) and kinking his aorta (small arrow). He underwent a single operative procedure including anterior decompression and vertebrectomy with strut grafting with autologous iliac bone and rib (Panel D, arrow) followed by posterior spinal instrumentation and fusion. Histologic examination and culture showed no active tuberculous disease, and no further medical treatment was given. As of the most recent follow-up three years later (Panel B), he had made a complete neurologic recovery and was participating in all noncontact sports at his high school.

Brian A. Shaw, M.D.

Valley Children's Hospital
Fresno, CA 93703

April 11, 1996

Cholesteatoma

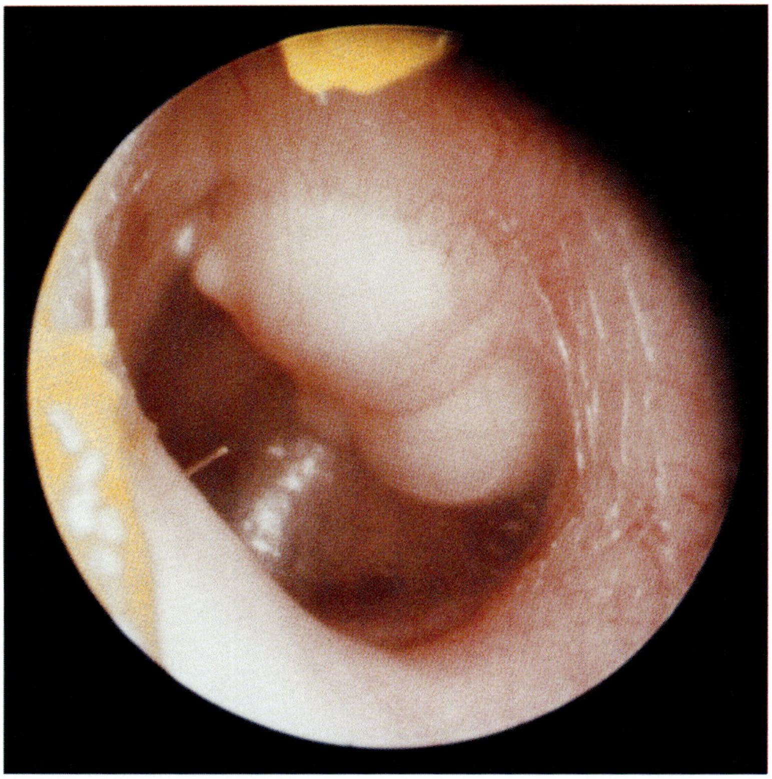

A cholesteatoma medial to an intact translucent tympanic membrane is shown in the left ear of a five-year-old girl. This abnormality was found by an audiologist during screening at school. The tympanic membrane was illuminated with a tungsten lamp and photographed through a Hopkins rod mounted on a 35-mm camera with Fuji 1600 film. The color was corrected to a reference standard during processing.

N. Wendell Todd, M.D.

Emory University
Atlanta, GA 30322

November 17, 1994

Paraganglioma of the Middle Ear

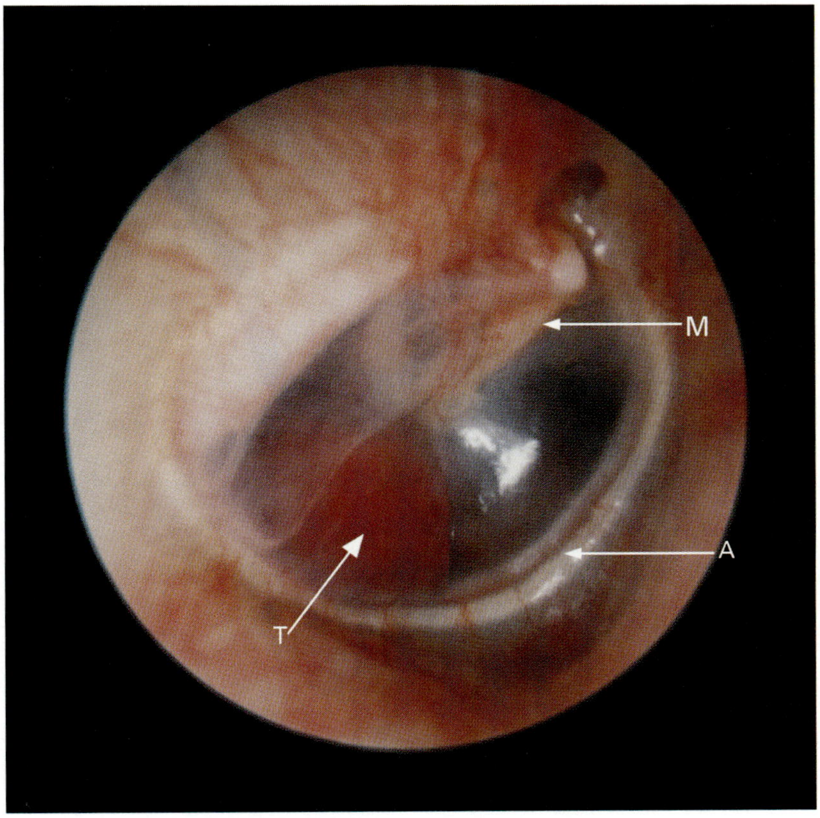

A 40-year-old woman presented with pulsatile tinnitus in her right ear. In this photograph, a red glomus tumor (T), or paraganglioma, is apparent in the right tympanic membrane. The malleus (M) and annulus tympanicus (A) are labeled. The tumor was removed through the external auditory canal, and the patient has been free of symptoms and of the tumor for more than five years.

Edward L. Applebaum, M.D.
University of Illinois at Chicago
Chicago, IL 60612

December 21, 1995

Three-Dimensional CT Diagnosis of Maxillofacial Trauma

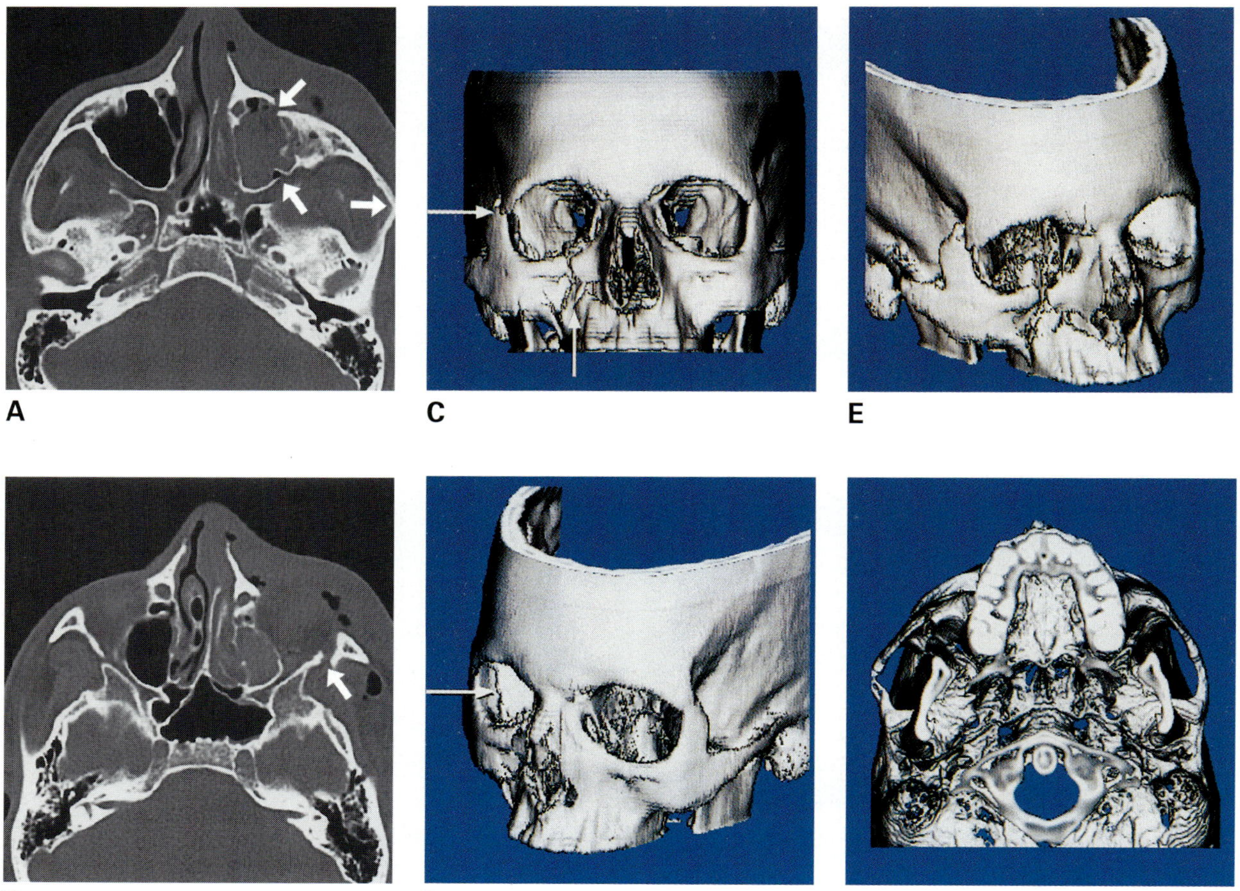

A C E

B D F

Spiral computed tomographic (CT) slices (Panels A and B) from which three-dimensional images were reconstructed (Panels C, D, E, and F) were obtained in a 16-year-old boy with facial fractures sustained in a head-on collision. The boy was not wearing a seat belt, and his car was traveling at 50 mph (80 km per hour). He had a slightly limited upward gaze on the right side, a small subconjunctival hemorrhage, and infraorbital pain. There were no other findings on physical examination.

A zygomaticomaxillary complex ("tripod") fracture is present. The zygomatic arch is fractured, and the zygomaticomaxillary complex is displaced posteromedially. There are comminuted fractures of the anterior and posterolateral walls of the maxillary sinus, as well as fractures of the medial, lateral, and inferior orbital walls.

Three-dimensional images reconstructed from the spiral CT slices are shown in four views. The frontal view (Panel C) shows the fractured frontal and maxillary processes of the zygomatic bone and the comminuted fracture of the anterior maxillary-sinus wall. The left oblique view (Panel D) shows the course of the fracture along the lateral wall of the right orbit. The right oblique view (Panel E) shows the zygomatic displacement, as well as the fracture of the orbital floor. The basal view (Panel F) shows the posterolateral displacement of the right zygomatic arch and the intact left arch for comparison.

The patient was admitted for observation and discharged the next day. He returned to the hospital eight days after the injury for surgical repair involving an open reduction and internal fixation. The postoperative course was uncomplicated, and he was discharged two days later.

Lee A. Fox, B.S.

Mallinckrodt Institute of Radiology
St. Louis, MO 63110

July 8, 1993

Correspondence

Three-Dimensional CT Diagnosis of Maxillofacial Trauma

January 6, 1994

To the Editor: The "Three-Dimensional CT Diagnosis of Maxillofacial Trauma" (Images in Clinical Medicine, July 8 issue)[1] contains remarkable pictures. At first I thought they were a Steven Spielberg creation. They surely represent the technological wizardry of American medicine. Unfortunately, this image does not tell the entire story.

It is clear that technological advances have fueled increases in health care costs. Although it is unlikely that we will ever shy away from new forms of technology, their inappropriate use arouses greater concern than do their costs.

These reconstructed computed tomographic (CT) images are appealing. I could not help but be drawn to them. If I were a medical student, they would certainly make me think about pursuing a career in diagnostic radiology. However, there is no mention either of their cost or of whether they are any more helpful in diagnosis than a plain radiograph, a simple CT scan, or even physical diagnosis. Even in medicine, what we learn can be influenced by the presentation of incomplete information.

Howard Bauchner, M.D.
Boston University School of Medicine
Boston, MA 02118

1. Fox LA. Three-dimensional CT diagnosis of maxillofacial trauma. N Engl J Med 1993; 329:102.

To the Editor: The CT scans entitled "Three-Dimensional CT Diagnosis of Maxillofacial Trauma" actually reveal a more extensive injury than is described. The patient has not only a fractured zygoma, but also a minimally displaced heminasoethmoidal orbital fracture, with fracture lines extending across the piriform buttress and the lower maxilla on the right and through the medial portion of the orbit. These fractures are barely visible on the axial images shown in Panels A and B and actually are seen most clearly in Panels C and E.

Paul N. Manson, M.D.
Maryland Institute for Emergency Medical Services Systems
Baltimore, MD 21201

The authors reply:

To the Editor: CT scans are the standard of care for skull fractures, since physical examination and plain radiography have been shown to be inadequate for the study of many correctable abnormalities.[1] The relative diagnostic performance of three-dimensional CT-scan reconstructions in the evaluation of complex facial fractures is less well established. The scans reproduced in the *Journal* were created on a Sun Workstation with Analyze software.[2] Similar software was available with the CT scanner located in the emergency room where the patient was examined. The cost of the software used in the three-dimensional reconstruction was approximately $20,000 (list price). This scanner has performed about 20,000 scans in the past five years. Perhaps 3 to 5 percent of examinations involve subsequent processing, and one sheet of film (costing about $5) is used for each three-dimensional study. Processing of data on the CT console has become a routine procedure. The marginal

Correspondence Continued

cost (an extra 5 to 10 percent, we estimate) of adding a three-dimensional reconstruction is small in terms of the total cost of the examination.

The benefit to patients and the cost effectiveness of a three-dimensional display are difficult to isolate and measure. CT scanners are expensive capital items with high costs, both fixed and variable.[3] Improvements that make their results more useful or convenient may provide benefits that can justify their use in selected institutions. Three-dimensional CT reconstructions are a prime example. The resulting images have been shown to provide improved diagnostic performance as compared with conventional imaging methods in certain applications.[4] Anatomical information is displayed in a form that is familiar and consistent with the clinician's everyday experience.

Dr. Manson is correct. The caption to the image concentrated on the most obvious component of the fractures and used the case to illustrate the classic "tripod" fracture.

Lee A. Fox, B.S.
Michael W. Vannier, M.D.
Ronald G. Evens, M.D.
Washington University School of Medicine
St. Louis, MO 63110

1. Kuhns LR, Thornbury JR, Fryback DG. Decision making in imaging. Chicago: Year Book, 1989:673-7.
2. Robb RA, Barillot C. Interactive display and analysis of 3-D medical images. IEEE Trans Med Imag 1989;8:217-26.
3. Evens RG. The economics of computed tomography: comparison with other health care costs. Radiology 1980;136:509-10.
4. Gillespie JE, Gholkar A, Isherwood I. Three-dimensional computed tomographic reformations: assessment of clinical efficacy. In: Udupa JK, Herman GT, eds. 3D imaging in medicine. Boca Raton, Fla.: CRC Press, 1991:104-43.

Knotted Umbilical Cord

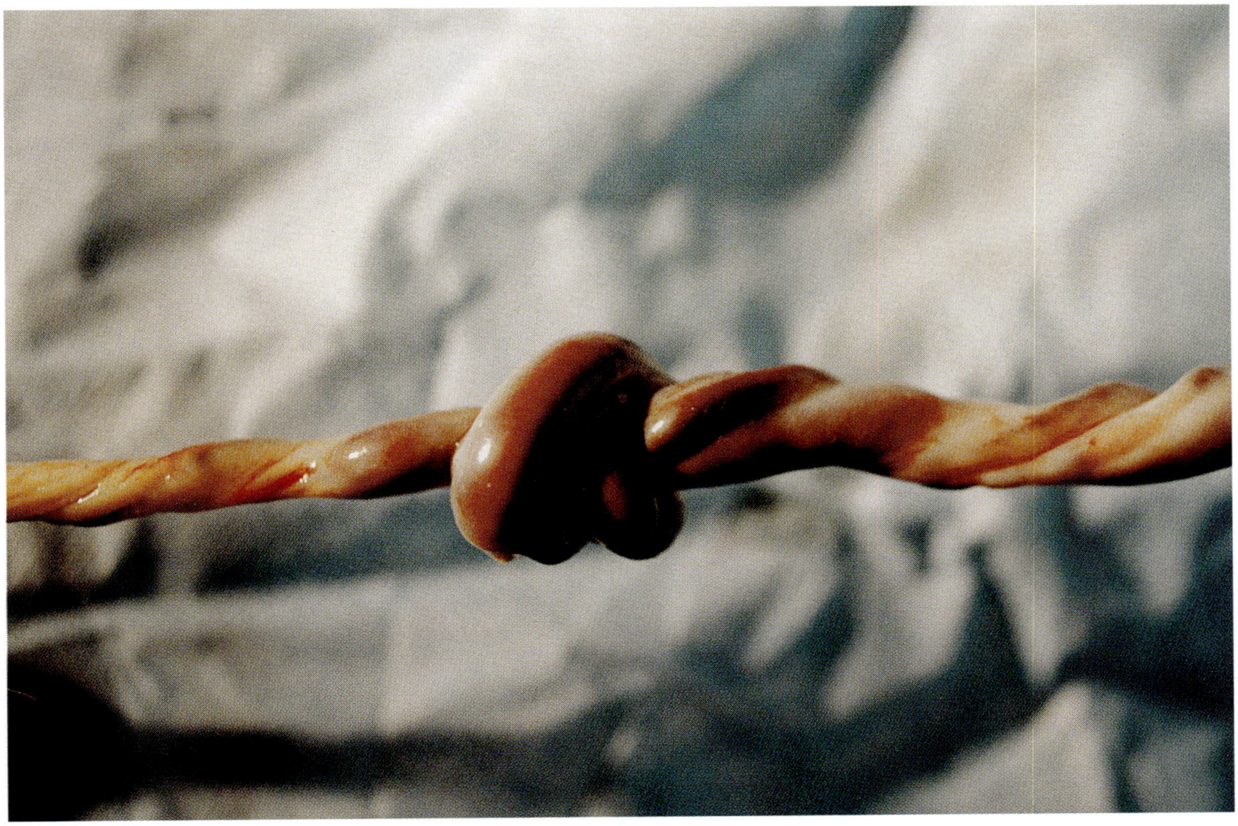

An umbilical cord with a true knot was discovered immediately after delivery of a baby girl to a 33-year-old woman. The mother had had two previous pregnancies and had delivered at full term with no complications. This pregnancy was complicated by gestational diabetes, and labor was induced with intravenous oxytocin at 39 weeks. The knot was not noticed during either of two ultrasound examinations performed during gestation. The baby also presented with the umbilical cord wrapped around her neck. Congestion of the umbilical vessels can be seen within the knot and on the maternal (right) side. The child's Apgar scores were 8 at one minute and 9 at five minutes. Both mother and daughter were discharged from the hospital within 24 hours with no complications. The mother's blood glucose concentration returned to normal within three days after delivery.

Russ B. Altman, M.D., Ph.D.
Jeanne E. Merino, J.D.

Stanford University School of Medicine
Stanford, CA 94305

February 29, 1996

Neurology

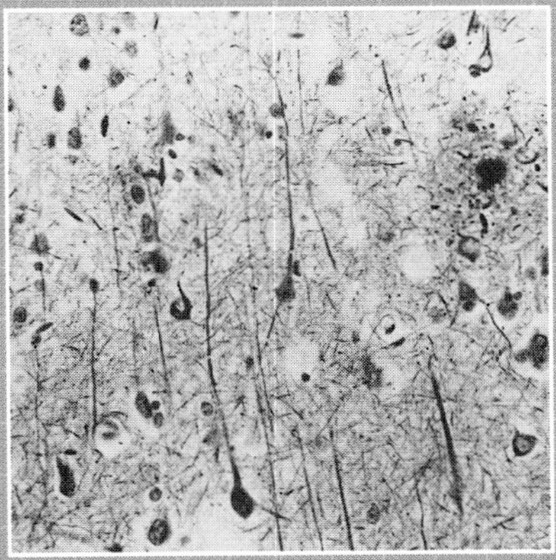

Periodic Breathing in an Infant with Hydrocephalus

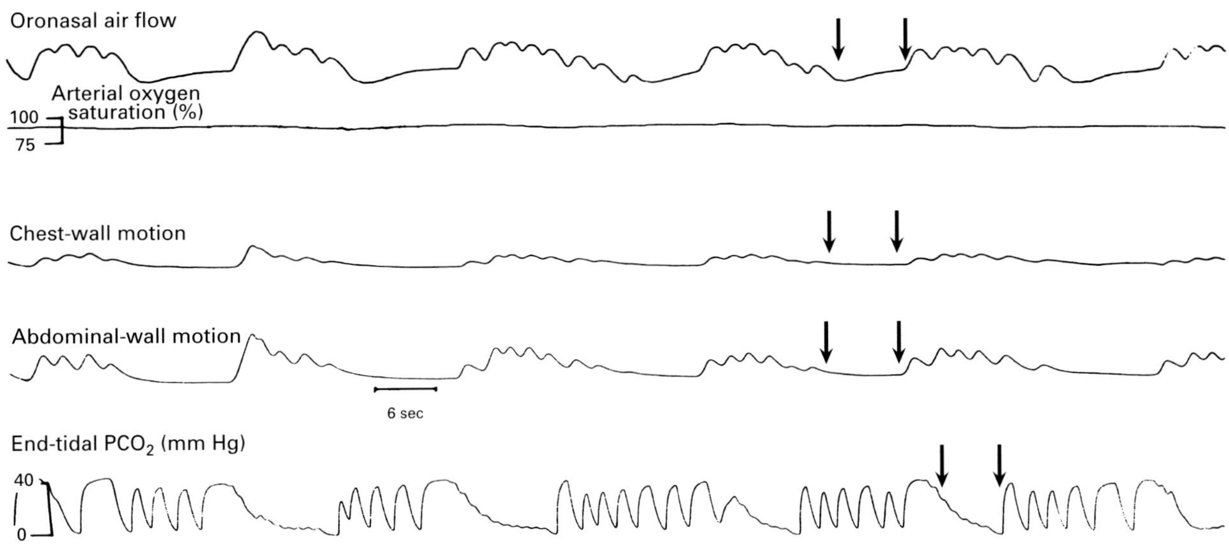

A portion of a polysomnogram recorded in a neonate with congenital hydrocephalus and resultant periodic breathing shows frequent, short periods of central apnea, as demonstrated by the cessation of oronasal air flow and the absence of a wave form on the tracing for end-tidal partial pressure of carbon dioxide (PCO_2), in association with the absence of chest- and abdominal-wall motion (arrows). Inspiration is represented by an upward deflection in the air-flow and chest- and abdominal-wall signals. There is a six-second delay in the recording of end-tidal PCO_2. Oronasal air flow was measured with a thermistor.

During the night while sleeping, the infant had periodic breathing 50 percent of the time. Although no arterial oxygen desaturation is evident on this portion of the tracing, desaturation to 75 percent occurred during active sleep. The infant received a ventriculoperitoneal shunt as well as a blood transfusion for the treatment of coexisting anemia. Subsequent polysomnography while the infant was receiving 0.25 liter of supplemental oxygen per minute demonstrated periodic breathing 3 percent of the total sleep time, with no desaturation. The infant was sent home with an apnea monitor while still receiving supplemental oxygen. Polysomnography repeated at six months of age with the infant breathing room air demonstrated periodic breathing 12 percent of the total sleep time, with an arterial-oxygen-saturation nadir of 93 percent.

Carole L. Marcus, M.D.

Johns Hopkins Children's Center
Baltimore, MD 21287

June 13, 1996

Cerebral Arteriovenous Malformation

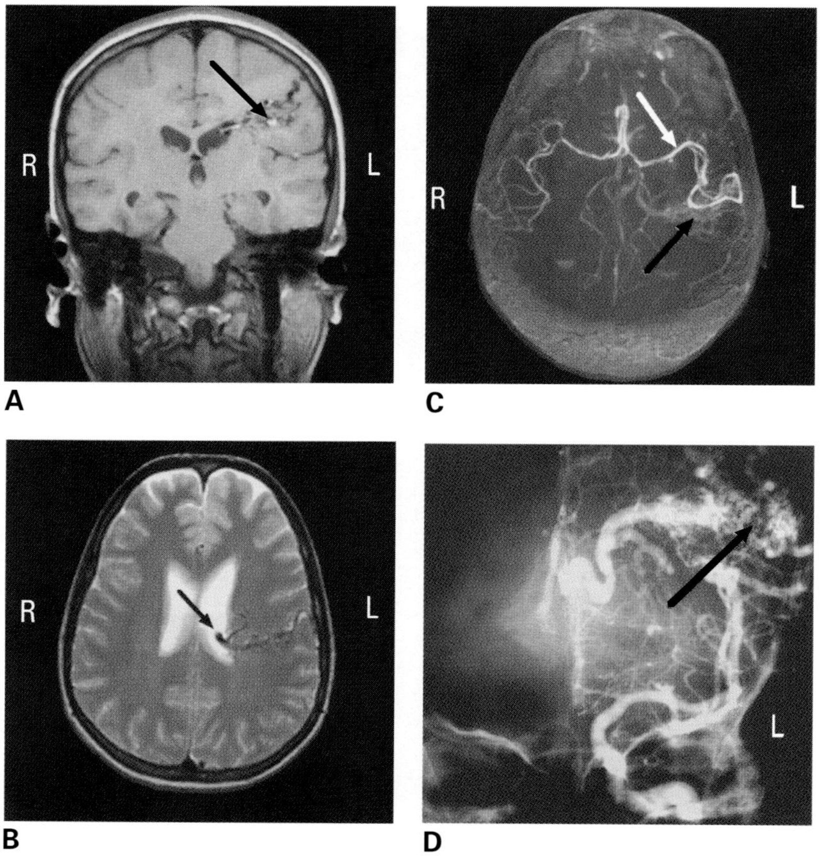

Magnetic resonance imaging and angiography of the brain revealed a left parietal arteriovenous malformation measuring 2.5 cm in diameter in a 32-year-old woman who presented with severe headache. Panel A, a coronal T_1-weighted magnetic resonance image, and Panel B, an axial T_2-weighted magnetic resonance image, demonstrate a tangle of abnormal vascular channels. Rapid blood flow causes a lack of signal intensity within the larger vessels of the arteriovenous malformation. Interspersed areas of higher signal intensity within the nidus of the arteriovenous malformation may represent regions of slow blood flow or hemorrhage (arrow, Panel A). An enlarged subependymal draining vein extends into the left lateral ventricle (arrow, Panel B), and an enlarged cortical draining vein is visible. As seen on the magnetic resonance angiogram (Panel C), the arteriovenous malformation (black arrow) is fed predominantly by the left middle cerebral artery (white arrow). There is also an aneurysm (2 to 3 mm) of the left middle cerebral artery proximal to its bifurcation. Cerebral angiography confirms the presence of the arteriovenous malformation (arrow, Panel D). The patient received stereotactic radiation therapy and is currently asymptomatic. R denotes right, and L left.

Kathleen Lee, M.D.
B. Leonard Holman, M.D.

Brigham and Women's Hospital
Boston, MA 02115

April 6, 1995

Cerebral Infarction

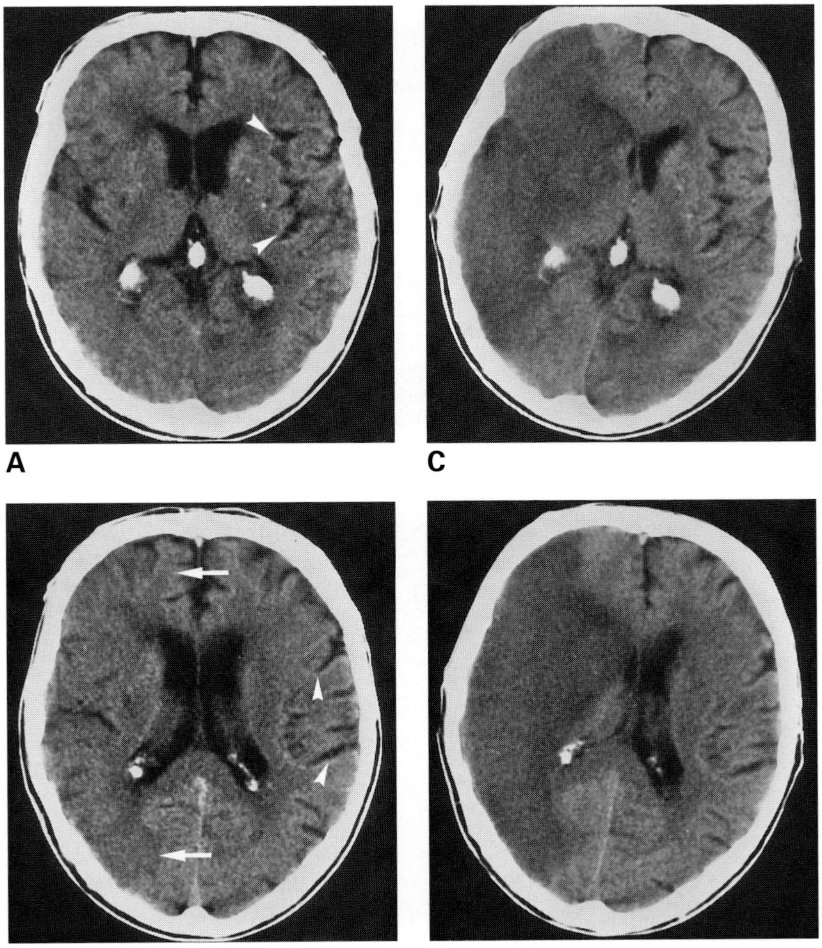

A C B D

Computed tomographic scans were obtained in a 77-year-old man with sudden onset of dense left-sided hemiparesis. Noncontrast scans performed 2½ hours after the onset of symptoms (Panels A and B) show early changes in the distribution of the right middle cerebral artery characteristic of an infarct. In Panel A, the normal gray–white differentiation is seen at the insular cortex on the left (arrowheads) but is absent on the right, a finding referred to as the insular ribbon sign. In addition, the right sylvian fissure is effaced relative to the left fissure. The scan in Panel B was taken slightly cephalad to the scan in Panel A. In Panel B, the left-sided sulci are better seen and the cortical gyri have preserved gray–white differentiation (arrowheads). In addition, there is slightly diminished density in the distribution of the right middle cerebral artery, best seen in the frontal and occipital regions (arrows). Follow-up scans at comparable levels obtained two days later because of a progressive decline in the level of consciousness show severe hypodensity in the distribution of the right middle cerebral artery, with a mass effect on the ventricular system and a shift in the midline from right to left (Panels C and D).

Lawrence E. Ginsberg, M.D.
Daniel W. Williams III, M.D.

Bowman Gray School of Medicine
Winston-Salem, NC 27157

June 2, 1994

Traumatic Carotid-Artery Dissection

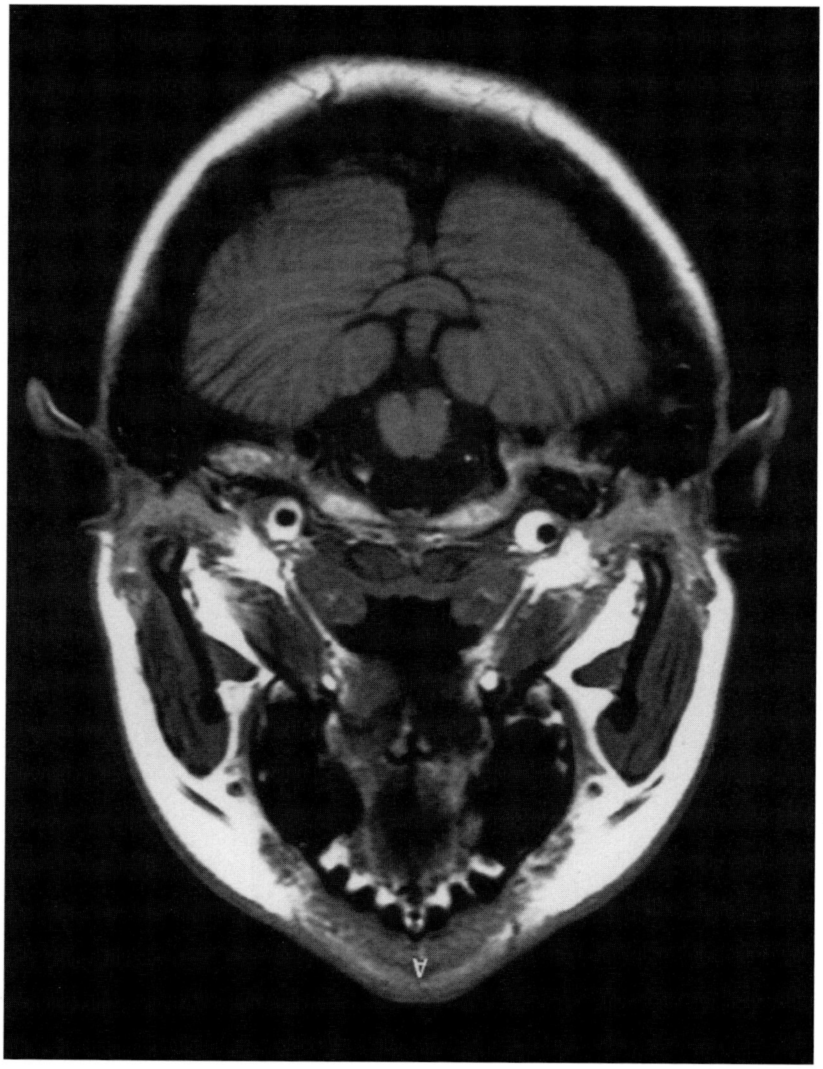

A 35-year-old woman fell off her bicycle, striking her chin on the pavement. She initially reported bilateral neck pain and headache and later had photophobia and weakness and paresthesia in the right arm. Examination revealed anisocoria but no other neurologic findings.

Magnetic resonance imaging confirmed the presence of bilateral dissections, beginning with tears in the extracranial internal carotid arteries anterior to the upper cervical vertebrae and extending distally into the intracranial siphon. (The inverted A denotes anterior orientation.) These lesions are uncommon, accounting for less than 5 percent of all carotid injuries, but they are diagnosed more frequently with improved cerebrovascular imaging. The "eyes of dissection" are composed of the dark flow-void "pupils" surrounded by the high-intensity signal of intramural hematoma. A small pseudoaneurysm was present on the left side. The patient was given anticoagulant therapy and had no further focal neurologic symptoms. After 10 months and radiographic confirmation of healing, the anticoagulation was discontinued and the patient was well.

Jon S. Matsumura, M.D.
William H. Pearce, M.D.

251 E. Chicago Ave., Suite 626
Chicago, IL 60611

October 31, 1996

Correspondence

The Scary MRI

April 17, 1997

To the Editor: I must congratulate you on the wonderful reproduction of the magnetic resonance imaging (MRI) scan of traumatic carotid-artery dissection (Image in Clinical Medicine, Oct. 31 issue).[1] Perhaps you could market it as a mask for radiologists who party on Halloween.

Mark C. Levine, M.D.
1662 E. Main St.
El Cajon, CA 92021

1. Matsumura JS, Pearce WH. Traumatic carotid-artery dissection. N Engl J Med 1996; 335:1368.

To the Editor: Medicine aside, could you possibly have chosen a better item for the *Journal* dated October 31, 1996 — the day of Halloween? What great selection and timing, or was it just serendipity?

Lester I. Leonard, M.D.
2750 Ocean Shore Blvd.
Ormond Beach, FL 32176

Dr. Kassirer replies: Not serendipity this time,[1] Dr. Leonard.

Jerome P. Kassirer, M.D.

1. Kassirer JP. Smallpox. N Engl J Med 1996;335:902.

Progressive Multifocal Leukoencephalopathy

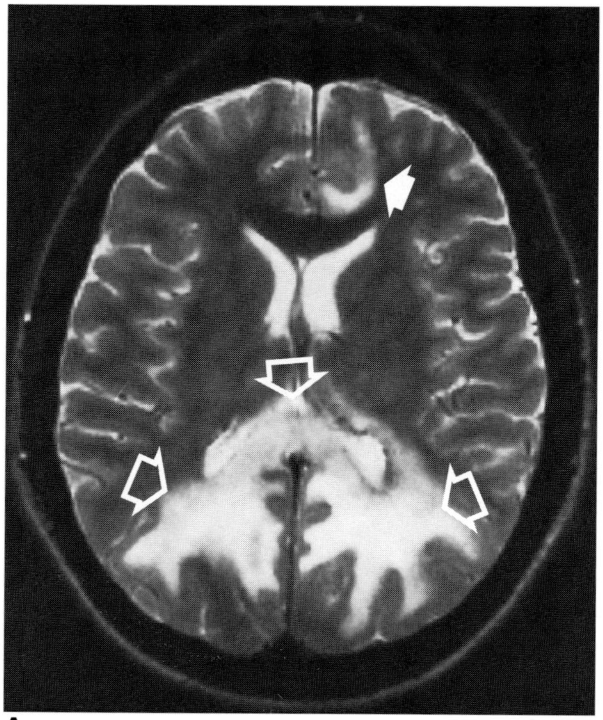

A

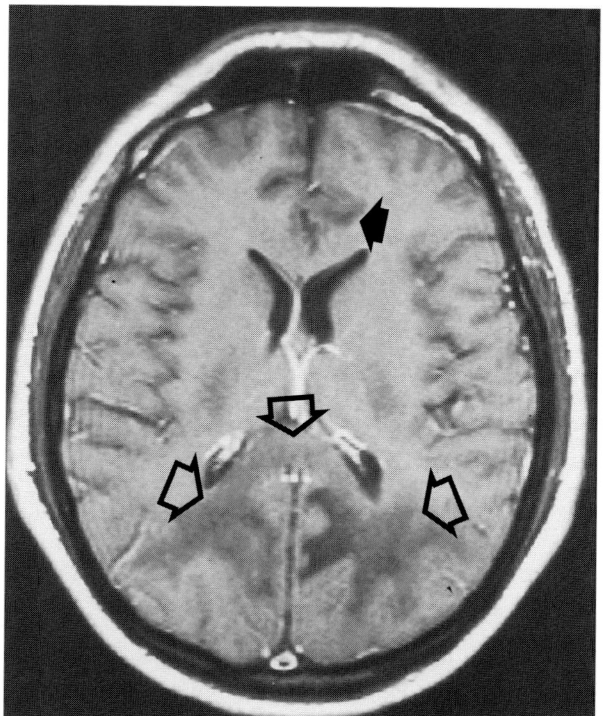

B

Magnetic resonance images of the brain were obtained in a 40-year-old man with the acquired immunodeficiency syndrome who had a six-week history of decreased memory and visual impairment. The changes associated with progressive multifocal leukoencephalopathy are best seen on the T_2-weighted image (Panel A) as high-intensity abnormalities isolated in the white matter (arrows). A large, bilateral parieto-occipital lesion crosses the splenium of the corpus callosum (open arrows); a smaller frontal-lobe lesion is also present (solid arrow). On the T_1-weighted image (Panel B), the lesions appear as low-intensity abnormalities that are not enhanced with gadolinium, which helps differentiate progressive multifocal leukoencephalopathy from primary lymphoma of the central nervous system. Progressive neurologic deterioration occurred, and the patient died 14 weeks after the onset of symptoms.

Peter J. Weiss, M.D.
J. Kevin DeMarco, M.D.

Naval Medical Center
San Diego, CA 92134

April 28, 1994

Tripolar Mitotic Figure

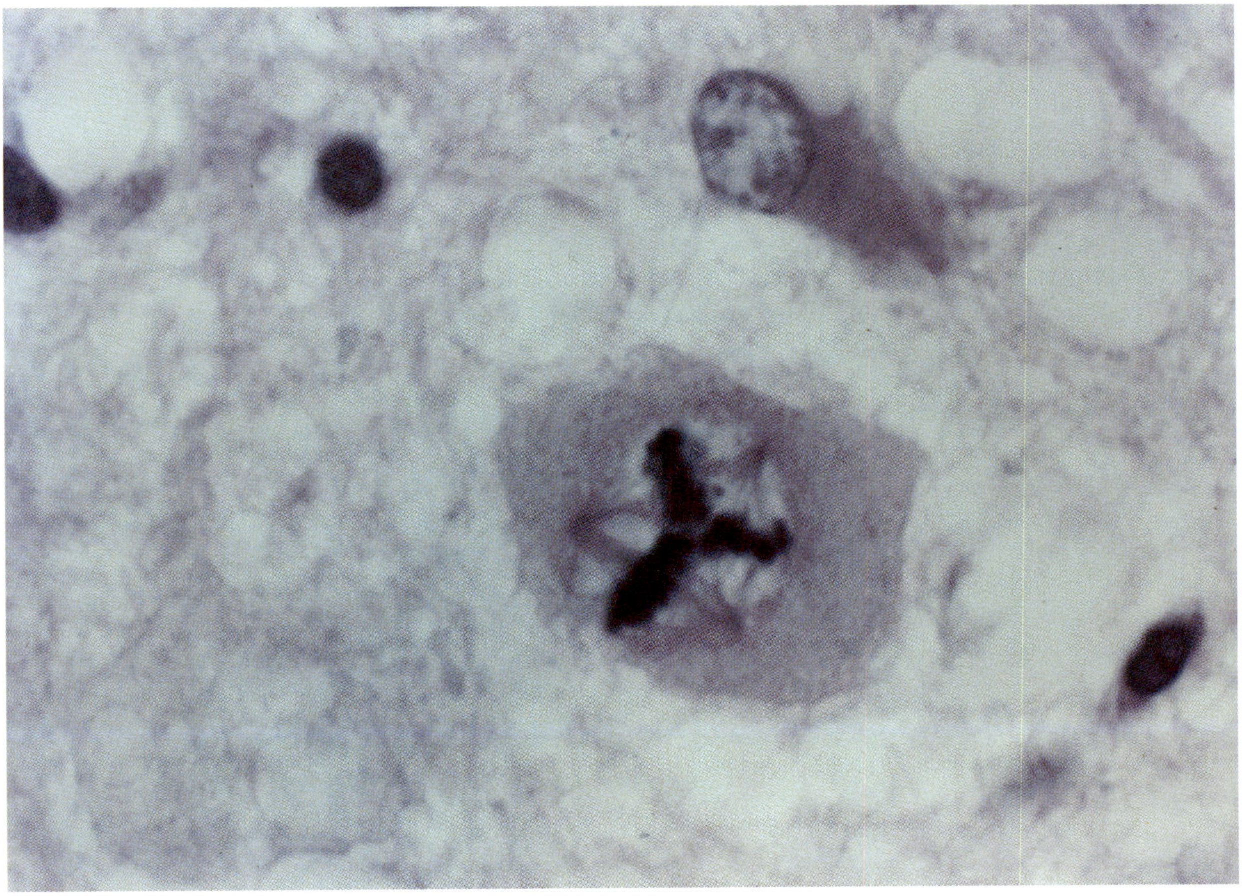

Dysfunctional tripolar mitotic figures usually indicate neoplasia. The cell shown here, however, represents an abnormal but nonneoplastic astrocyte, presumably infected with papovavirus, in a patient with progressive multifocal leukoencephalopathy. (Hematoxylin and eosin, ×1500.)

Robert E. Mrak, M.D., Ph.D.

Veterans Affairs Medical Center
Little Rock, AR 72205

March 16, 1995

Wallerian Degeneration of the Pyramidal Tract

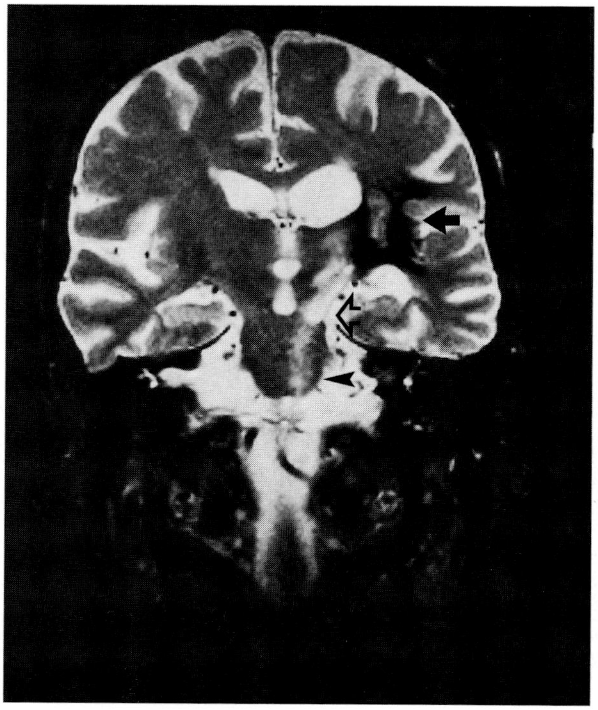

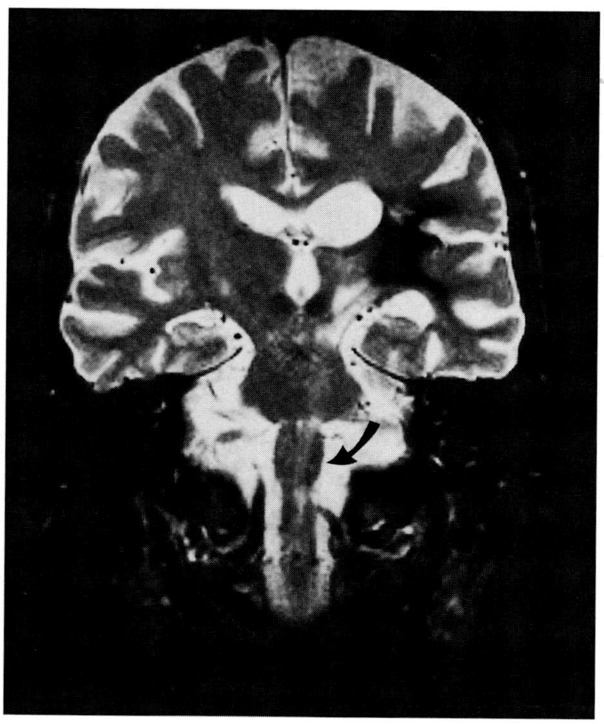

Coronal views of the brain of a 41-year-old man with the acquired immunodeficiency syndrome and right-sided spastic hemiplegia, aphasia, and hemianopia were obtained by magnetic resonance imaging (MRI) eight months after the patient had an intracerebral hemorrhage. The consecutive T_2-weighted coronal MRI slices show the old hematoma as an irregular lesion, which is hypointense because of hemosiderin deposition; dilatation of the left lateral ventricle is also evident. In addition, a long band of increased signal intensity traces the anatomical course of the pyramidal tract from the lesion in the internal capsule (upper panel, solid arrow) down to the left cerebral peduncle (open arrow), reaching the pons (arrowhead) and the medulla oblongata (lower panel, curved arrow). This finding is compatible with wallerian degeneration of the pyramidal tract. Wallerian degeneration is the descending destruction of axons and myelin sheaths resulting from neuronal damage, such as that due to ischemic infarction or hemorrhage. The degeneration leads to an increase in extracellular water, producing increased signal intensity on T_2-weighted MRI scans.

Johan A. Dol, M.D.
Elisabeth S. Louwerse, M.D.

Academic Medical Center
1105 AZ Amsterdam, the Netherlands

July 14, 1994

Alzheimer's Disease

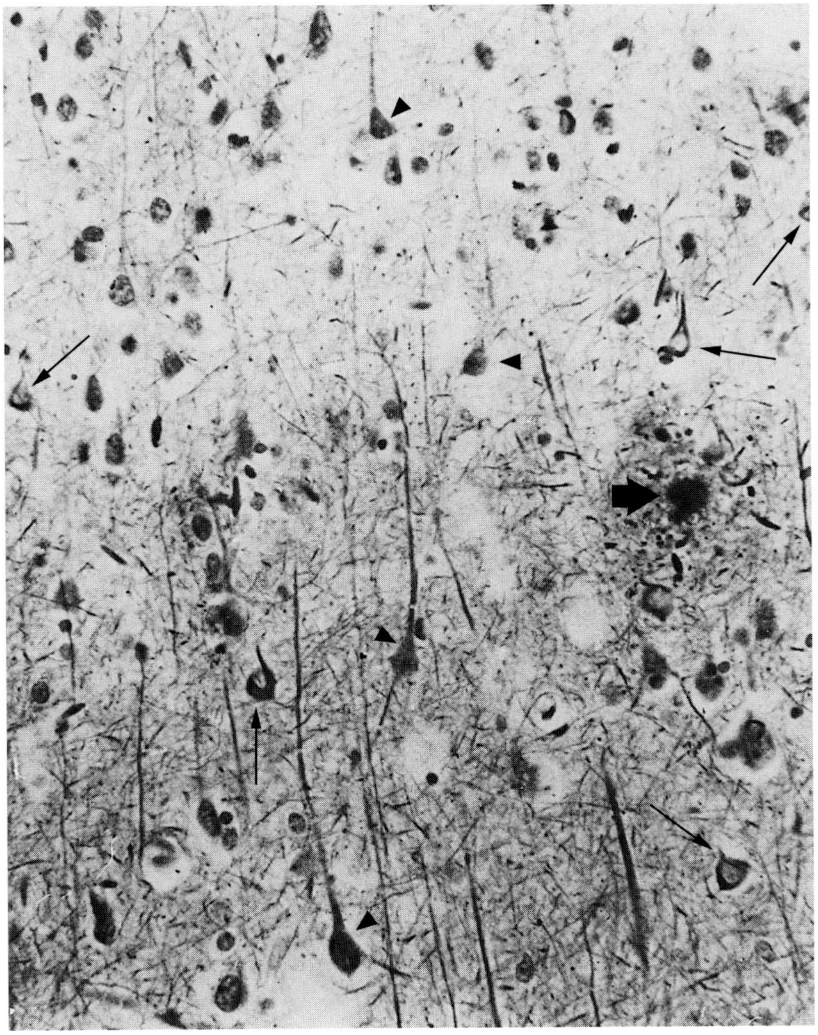

A section of cerebral cortex (frontal region) from a patient with Alzheimer's disease is shown, stained with the Cajal silver method for axons and neurofibrils. On the right is a neuritic plaque (broad arrow) with a darkly stained core of amyloid. Surrounding the core are irregular fragments of stained material composed of pathologically altered, distorted axons and dendrites, collectively referred to as neurites. Scattered medium-sized neurons (thin arrows) have the dense fibrillary deposits first described by Alzheimer and now generally referred to as neurofibrillary tangles. The appearance of other neurons is normal (a few of these are indicated by arrowheads). The weblike meshwork in the background is formed by interlacing normal axons and dendrites (×210).

E.P. Richardson, M.D.
Charles S. Kubik, M.D.

Massachusetts General Hospital
Boston, MA 02114

October 29, 1992

Syphilitic Gummas in a Patient with Human Immunodeficiency Virus Infection

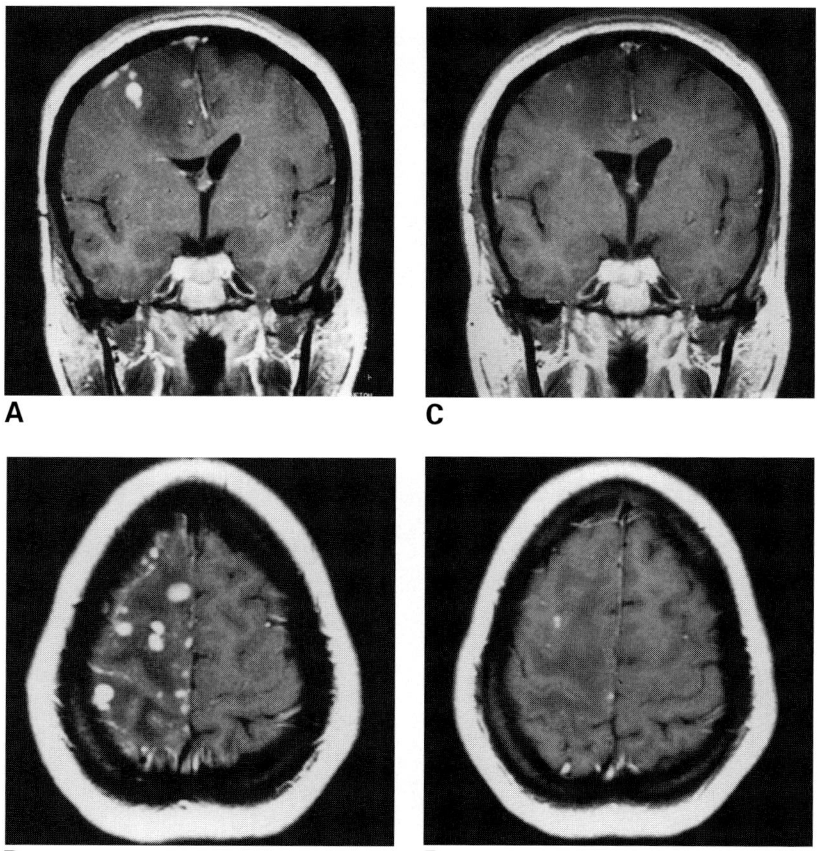

A 26-year-old woman who was positive for the human immunodeficiency virus presented with focal motor seizures, a CD4 cell count of 238 per cubic millimeter, a rapid plasma reagin titer of 1:32, and a positive test for serum treponemal IgG antibody. One year earlier, she had received a single dose of intramuscular penicillin (dose and rapid plasma reagin titer not known). On admission, gadolinium-enhanced T_1-weighted magnetic resonance imaging showed multiple syphilitic cerebral gummas (Panels A and B). Studies of cerebrospinal fluid revealed a white-cell count of 20 per cubic millimeter (92 percent lymphocytes and 8 percent monocytes), protein concentration of 27 mg per deciliter, glucose concentration of 53 mg per deciliter (2.9 mmol per liter), and a nonreactive Venereal Disease Research Laboratory test. The patient was treated with 12 million U of penicillin G per day intravenously for seven days, followed by 24 million U per day for an additional seven days. After nine days of treatment, imaging demonstrated a dramatic improvement (Panels C and D). Corticosteroids were not administered. The patient voluntarily stopped taking phenytoin one month after discharge. Seven months later, she continues to be seizure-free, with a CD4 cell count of 78 per cubic millimeter and a rapid plasma reagin titer of 1:8. Other possible causes of this radiographic appearance, such as toxoplasmosis, bacterial or fungal cerebral abscess, sarcoidosis, neuroborreliosis, tuberculosis, and lymphoma, were ruled out by tests and by the patient's clinical response to penicillin.

Lisa C. Roeske, M.D.
Philip R. Kennedy, M.D., Ph.D.

Emory University School
of Medicine
Atlanta, GA 30322

October 10, 1996

Correspondence

Cerebral Syphilitic Gumma

April 3, 1997

To the Editor: The Image in Clinical Medicine involving syphilitic gummas in a patient with human immunodeficiency virus (HIV) infection who presented with focal seizures (Oct. 10 issue)[1] caused us much concern. Our concern was heightened by the letter from Suarez et al. about a syphilitic gumma in an HIV-negative patient with focal seizures.[2] Both patients had important focal neurologic findings coupled with severely abnormal magnetic resonance imaging (MRI) findings (in the case of the HIV-positive patient, there was a clear mass effect from the lesions and subfalcine herniation). Both patients underwent a lumbar puncture on the basis of which, according to the authors, the diagnosis of neurosyphilitic gummas was made.

However, the cerebrospinal fluid findings described in the HIV-positive patient do not establish the diagnosis of neurosyphilis. The patient had a negative serologic test for syphilis and the lymphocytic pleocytosis could have been consistent with HIV meningitis. In the case of the HIV-negative patient, the cerebrospinal fluid Venereal Disease Research Laboratory (VDRL) titer did not show a fourfold increase. In both patients, the diagnosis was established by empirical antibiotic therapy, with subsequent improvement in the imaging findings. The cerebrospinal fluid findings did not appear to be as important in establishing the diagnosis. With the potential risk of untoward tragic effects, the need for lumbar puncture can be seriously questioned in both cases.

Lumbar puncture is contraindicated in the presence of mass lesions, because the risk of transtentorial herniation and death is quite high. The risk appears to be even greater in HIV-positive patients than in HIV-negative patients. Fortunately, these two patients had no serious complications. When neurosyphilitic gummas are suspected, the patients should be presumptively treated and followed with serial radiologic studies.

Pamela Quinn, M.D., and Leon Weisberg, M.D.
Tulane University Medical Center, New Orleans, LA 70112

1. Roeske LC, Kennedy PR. Syphilitic gummas in a patient with human immunodeficiency virus infection. N Engl J Med 1996;335:1123.
2. Suarez JI, Mlakar D, Snodgrass SM. Cerebral syphilitic gumma in an HIV-negative patient presenting as prolonged focal motor status epilepticus. N Engl J Med 1996;335:1159-60.

The authors reply:

To the Editor: We appreciate the concern of Drs. Quinn and Weisberg and agree that in the presence of a mass lesion, the risks associated with lumbar puncture must be carefully considered. At the time of the lumbar puncture, our patient had no signs of increased intracranial pressure and was awake and alert. The basilar cisterns were widely patent on both the initial computed tomographic (CT) scan and subsequent MRI.

We disagree with Drs. Quinn and Weisberg about the need for lumbar puncture. In our patient, who had a history of drug abuse, mouth sores, and recent incarceration and whose HIV status was unknown, it was necessary to exclude bacterial abscess, tuberculosis, toxoplasmosis, and cryptococcal meningitis as potential causes. Although the MRI findings of peripherally enhancing nodules with leptomeningeal and dural components are characteristic of syphilitic gummas,[1,2] the diagnosis cannot be established on the basis of the radiographic appearance alone. Furthermore, although the latency period before the development of tertiary neurosyphilis may be shortened in an HIV-positive patient,[3] syphilitic gummas are rare enough to warrant the consideration of other causes.

The diagnosis of syphilitic gummas was not based on the results of the lumbar

Correspondence Continued

puncture alone. It was based on the combination of several factors: the prior treatment of asymptomatic syphilis, the clinical presentation of focal seizures,[1] the positive serologic status, the characteristic MRI findings, and the clinical response to penicillin. The cerebrospinal fluid findings were nonspecific but compatible with neurosyphilis, and they helped rule out other treatable infectious processes. The patient's positive syphilitic serologic status was stated in the legend (the rapid plasma reagin titer was 1:32, and the fluorescent treponemal-antibody-absorption test of serum was positive).

Lisa C. Roeske, M.D., and Philip R. Kennedy, M.D., Ph.D.
Emory University School of Medicine, Atlanta, GA 30322

1. Berger JR, Waskin H, Pall L, Hensley G, Ihmedian I, Post MJ. Syphilitic cerebral gumma with HIV infection. Neurology 1992;42:1282-7.
2. Brightbill TC, Ihmeidan IH, Post MJ, Berger JR, Katz DA. Neurosyphilis in HIV-positive and HIV-negative patients: neuroimaging findings. AJNR Am J Neuroradiol 1995;16:703-11.
3. Johns DR, Tierney M, Felsenstein D. Alteration in the natural history of neurosyphilis by concurrent infection with the human immunodeficiency virus. N Engl J Med 1987;316:1569-72.

To the Editor: Regarding the concern expressed by Drs. Quinn and Weisberg about the diagnosis of neurosyphilis and the safety of lumbar puncture in our HIV-negative patient with syphilitic gumma,[1] the recommended criteria for the diagnosis of active neurosyphilis in an HIV-negative patient include a reactive cerebrospinal fluid VDRL test, a reactive serum fluorescent treponemal-antibody-absorption test, and pleocytosis of more than 5 to 10 leukocytes per cubic millimeter.[2] In the presence of a nontraumatic lumbar puncture and a truly reactive cerebrospinal fluid VDRL test, we believe that our patient most certainly had neurosyphilis and thus that the treatment was not instituted empirically.

The report of the quality-standards subcommittee of the American Academy of Neurology on practice guidelines for lumbar puncture contraindicates the use of that procedure in the presence of suspected elevated intracranial pressure and recommends obtaining a head CT scan to screen patients at risk for herniation.[3] Although we strongly agree with those recommendations, there are several points to consider. First, in the era before CT scanning, nonrandomized studies showed that the incidence of actual complications of careful diagnostic lumbar puncture in the presence of papilledema was 1.2 percent.[4] Second, with the advent of CT scanning, several anatomical criteria have been proposed as risk factors for herniation, including lateral shifting of midline structures, sulcal effacement, loss of the suprachiasmatic and basilar cisterns, obliteration of the fourth ventricle, and obliteration of the superior cerebellar and quadrigeminal-plate cisterns with sparing of the ambient cisterns.[5] Since our patient did not meet those clinical or radiologic criteria, we believed that he was at low risk for cerebral herniation. The analysis of cerebrospinal fluid helped rule out other neurologic conditions, such as inflammatory or neoplastic vasculitis, and other infectious processes that require different treatment methods.

Jose I. Suarez, M.D., Diane Mlakar, R.N., and Susan M. Snodgrass, M.D.
University Hospitals of Cleveland, Cleveland, OH 44106

1. Suarez JI, Mlakar D, Snodgrass SM. Cerebral syphilitic gumma in an HIV-negative patient presenting as prolonged focal motor status epilepticus. N Engl J Med 1996;335:1159-60.
2. Jordan KG. Modern neurosyphilis — a critical analysis. West J Med 1988;145:47-57.
3. Practice parameters: lumbar puncture (summary statement): report of the Quality Standards Subcommittee of the American Academy of Neurology. Neurology 1993;43:625-7.
4. Korein J, Cravioto H, Leicach M. Reevaluation of lumbar puncture: a study of 129 patients with papilledema or intracranial hypertension. Neurology 1959;9:290-7.
5. Gower DJ, Baker AL, Bell WO, Ball MR. Contraindications to lumbar puncture as defined by computed cranial tomography. J Neurol Neurosurg Psychiatry 1987;50:1071-4.

Acute Bacterial Meningitis

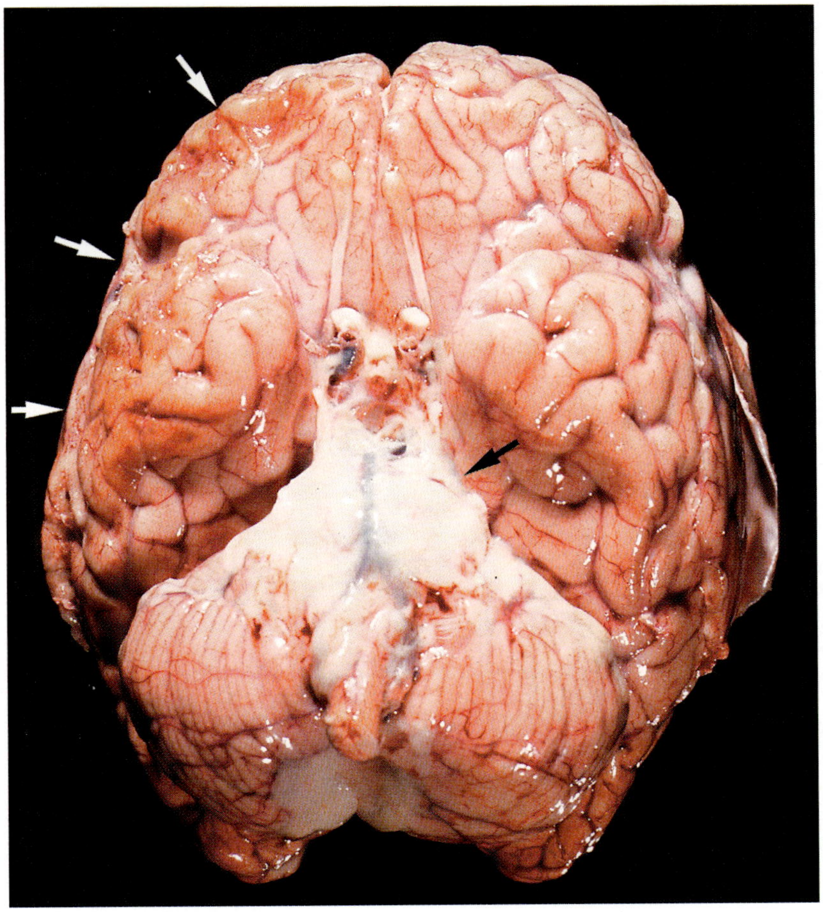

A basal view of the brain of a 76-year-old man who died of acute *Streptococcus pneumoniae* meningitis is shown. A thick, purulent exudate (black arrow) obscures the ventral aspect of the brain stem, encasing the basilar artery and cranial nerves. The exudate tracks over the ventral cerebellar hemispheres and fills the basal cisterns, including the cisterna magna. A large depressed and pigmented scar is visible on the left (white arrows), in the right frontal and temporal lobes, presumably the result of an old contusion and focal tissue loss.

Jeffrey A. Golden, M.D.
David N. Louis, M.D.

Massachusetts General Hospital
Boston, MA 02114

August 11, 1994

Multiple Brain Abscesses

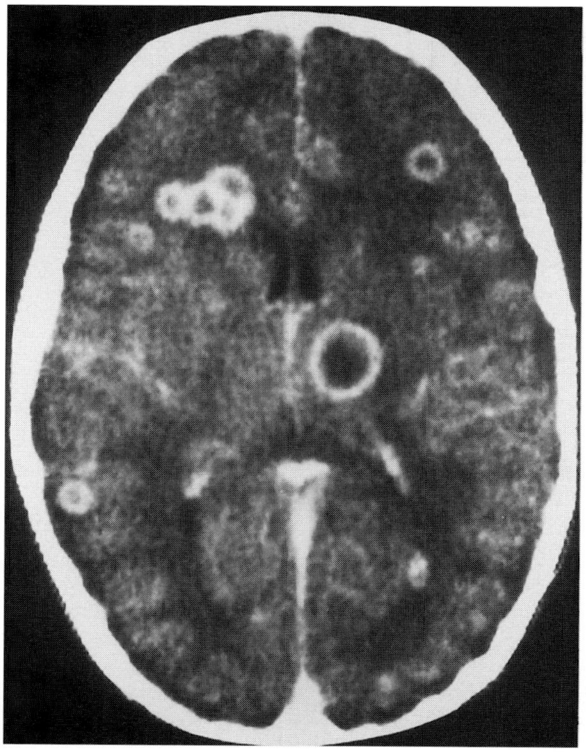

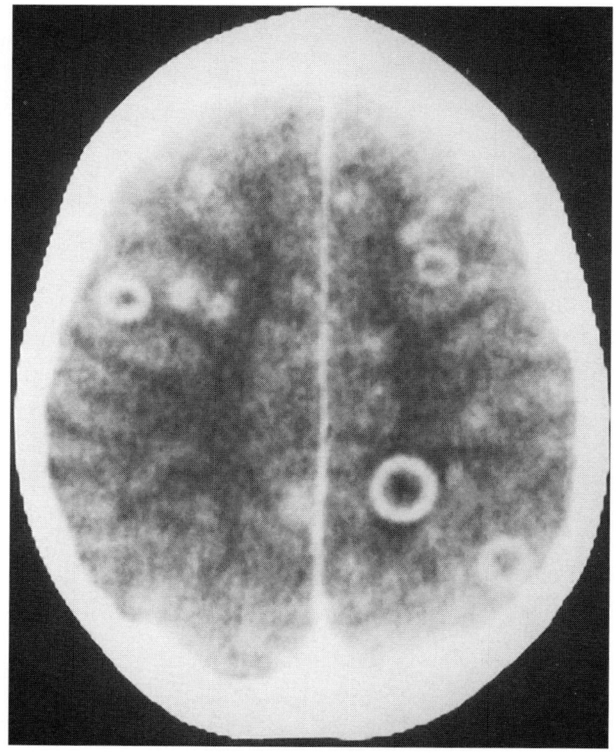

Both images are computed tomographic scans (with contrast) of the head of an eight-year-old boy with a 10-day history of headaches, vomiting, fever, altered mental status, and frontal-lobe signs. More than 30 ring-enhancing lesions are present. The precontrast study showed only one low-density lesion in the left thalamus. The abscesses resolved completely after antibiotic therapy, although the left thalamic lesion grew larger during the first 10 days. Initially, treatment consisted of nafcillin and chloramphenicol; nafcillin was replaced by penicillin G after one week. Extensive studies failed to uncover the source or type of infection.

Masanori Igarashi, M.D.

University of Tennessee
Memphis, TN 38105

October 7, 1993

Intraventricular Rupture of a Cerebral Abscess

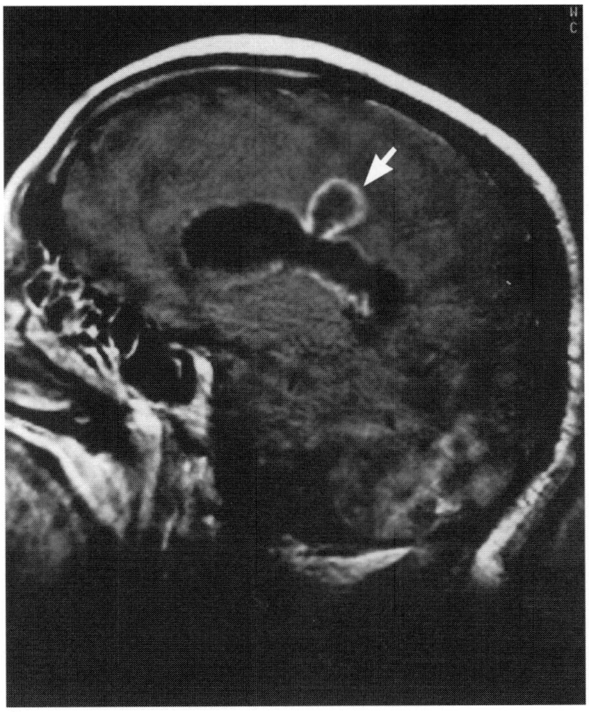

A

Cerebral imaging studies were performed in a 53-year-old man with a one-week history of headache, ataxia, and disorientation that culminated in right hemiparesis and coma. He had a remote history of dental abscesses. Magnetic resonance imaging with gadolinium enhancement (Panel A) shows a left frontal lesion (arrow) in communication with the left lateral ventricle. Purulent material containing *Streptococcus anginosus* was obtained by ventriculostomy, and both intrathecal and intravenous antibiotics were given. A contrast-enhanced computed tomographic scan obtained after four weeks of treatment (Panel B) shows loculation of the left lateral ventricle (arrowheads) and transependymal edema (arrows). The patient later required bifrontal ventriculoperitoneal shunts but recovered with only mild cognitive deficits.

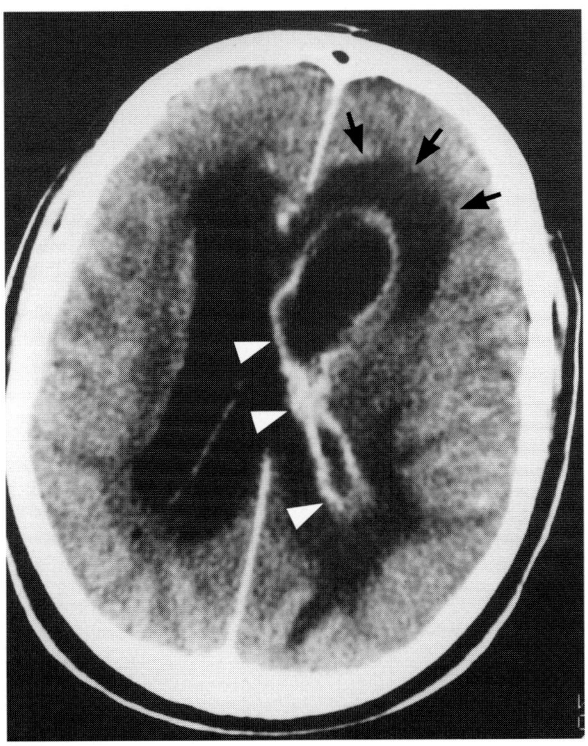

B

David M. McKalip, M.D.
Steven K. Gudeman, M.D.

University of North Carolina at Chapel Hill
Chapel Hill, NC 27599

August 29, 1996

Miliary Tuberculosis Involving the Central Nervous System

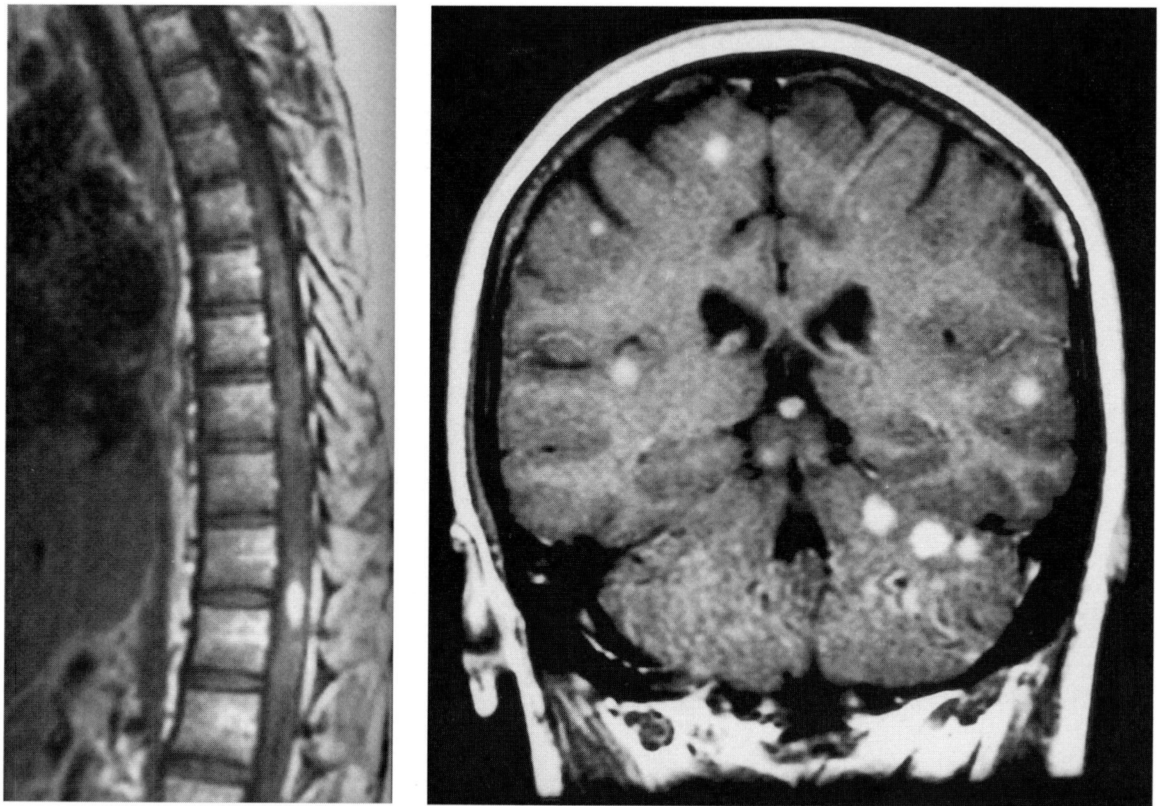

A B

A 28-year-old woman with a 10-year history of systemic lupus erythematosus presented with fever, back pain, and bilateral paresthesias and weakness of the legs of 10 days' duration. She had been taking prednisone for the preceding nine months for the management of flares. On examination her neck was supple. She had decreased power and sensation in her legs, with diminished knee and ankle reflexes, an extensor right-plantar response, and an equivocal left-plantar response. T_1-weighted magnetic resonance imaging after the administration of contrast medium revealed an enhancing lesion within the spinal cord at the T11 level (Panel A) and multiple enhancing lesions at the junction of the cerebrum and cerebellum (Panel B). Lumbar puncture revealed a glucose concentration below 20 mg per deciliter (1.1 mmol per liter), a protein concentration of 92 mg per deciliter, a red-cell count of 13 per high-power field, and a white-cell count of 227 per high-power field (differential count, 88 percent segmented neutrophils and 12 percent lymphocytes). Culture of cerebrospinal fluid was positive for a strain of *Myobacterium tuberculosis* that was not resistant to multiple drugs. Bacterial, fungal, and viral cultures of blood and antigen tests for these agents were negative. An x-ray film and computed tomographic scan of the chest showed multiple miliary nodules. Bronchoscopic biopsy revealed caseating granulomata containing acid-fast bacilli. Culture of this tissue was also positive for *M. tuberculosis.*

The patient was treated with ethambutol, rifampin, isoniazid, and pyrazinamide, and tapering doses of prednisone. Repeated magnetic resonance imaging one month later revealed a reduction in the size, level of enhancement, and conspicuousness of the brain and spinal cord lesions. On subsequent clinic visits, the patient's condition improved, but the weakness of the legs persisted.

Kieran Murphy, M.B., B.Ch.
James A. Brunberg, M.D.

University of Michigan
Ann Arbor, MI 48109-0030

March 21, 1996

Brain Herniation in Toxoplasmosis

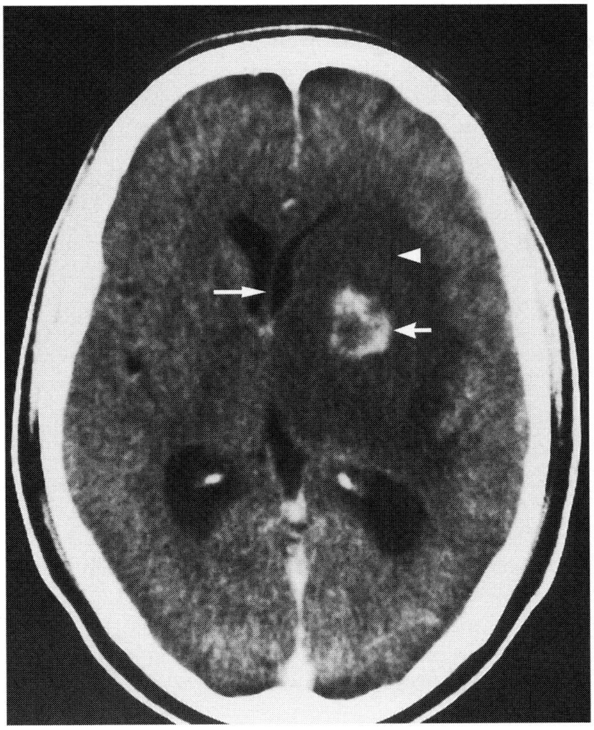

A

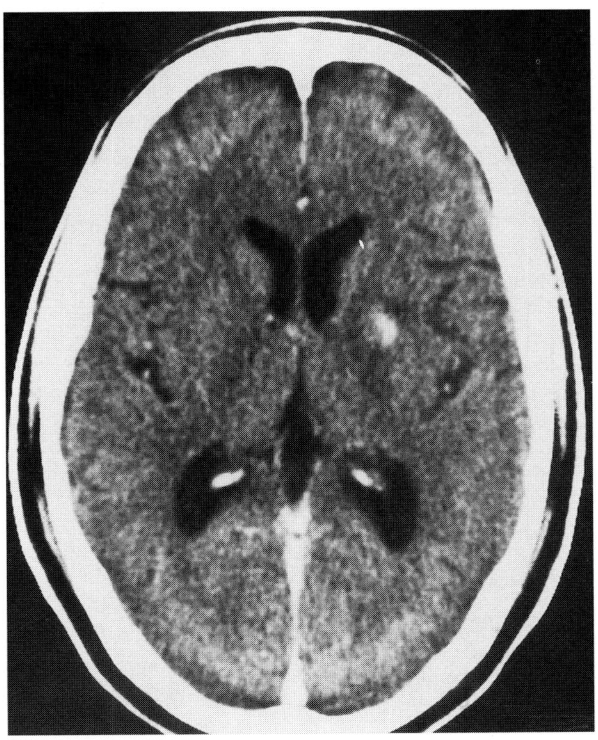

B

A computed tomographic scan of the head (Panel A) shows subfalcial brain herniation in an outpatient who was seropositive for the human immunodeficiency virus and who had subtle changes in cognitive function but an otherwise normal neurologic examination. A ring-enhancing mass with irregular borders measuring 1.8 by 1.4 cm is present in the left basal ganglia (short arrow), associated with marked edema (arrowhead). The mass effect has caused compression of the left lateral ventricle, with a 0.8-cm ventricular shift toward the right (long arrow) and displacement of the falx cerebri to the right of midline (in a manner consistent with subfalcial herniation). The patient was seropositive for toxoplasma antibodies and was treated with pyrimethamine, leucovorin, and clindamycin. Panel B shows the near-complete reversal of Four months after treatment ended, the patient had no overt cognitive disturbances.

Nina Singh, M.D.
Kevin Stempel, M.D.

Veterans Affairs Medical Center
Pittsburgh, PA 15240

September 15, 1994

Osmotic Myelinolysis

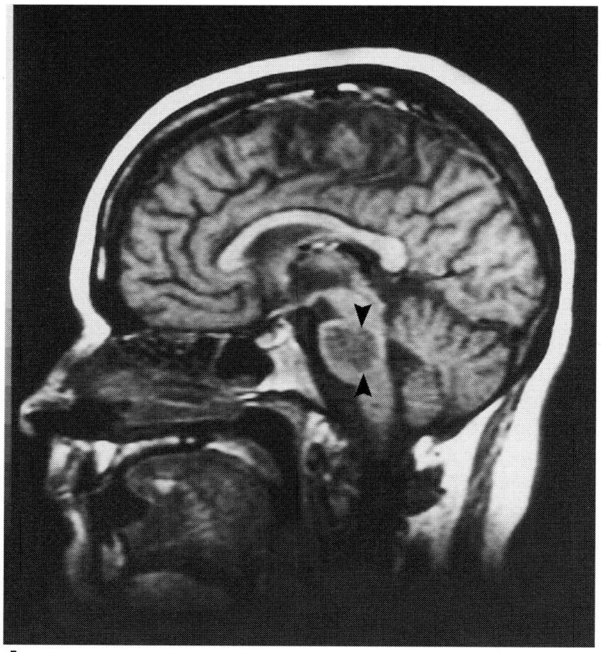

A

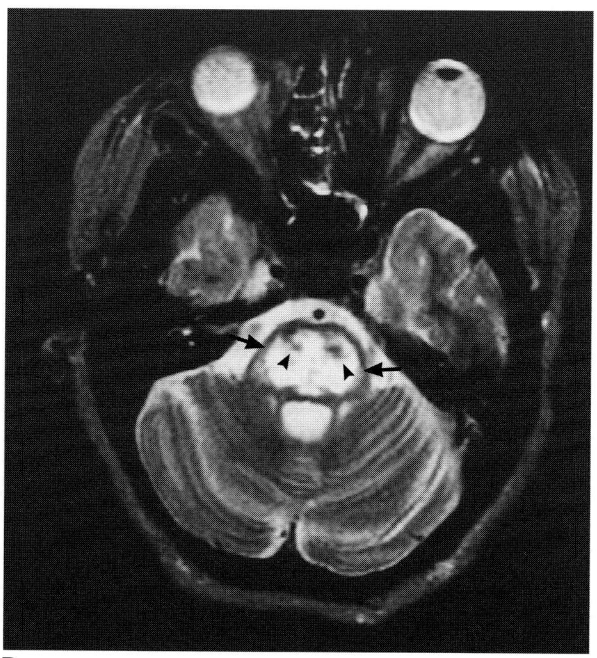

B

A 30-year-old alcoholic woman presented with confusion and disorientation after a grand mal seizure. The patient's serum sodium concentration on admission was 99 mmol per liter. Treatment was initiated with a slow infusion of normal saline, resulting in serum sodium values of 102 mmol per liter 4 hours after admission, 104 mmol per liter at 8 hours, 115 mmol per liter at 12 hours, 118 mmol per liter at 18 hours, and 125 mmol per liter at 24 hours. The patient initially had dysarthria, with slurred speech, and a slow finger-to-nose test on cerebellar examination, although there was no Babinski reflex. During days 2 to 6 with a normal serum sodium concentration, her condition gradually improved, although she interacted slowly with staff members and family, and had difficulty following commands. On the seventh day she became unresponsive to commands and painful stimuli and had a Babinski reflex. Magnetic resonance imaging demonstrated central pontine myelinolysis as a region of prominent low signal intensity on a sagittal T_1-weighted image (Panel A, arrowheads) and high signal intensity on an axial T_2-weighted image (Panel B, arrows). The signal intensity on the periphery of the pons is normal on both images, and there is relative preservation of the corticospinal tracts (Panel B, arrowheads). The patient remained in an unresponsive state for seven weeks, but her sensorium gradually improved until she was fully responsive, alert, and oriented.

Blaine L. Hart, M.D.
R. Philip Eaton, M.D.

University of New Mexico
School of Medicine
Albuquerque, NM 87131

November 9, 1995

Periodic Lateralized Epileptiform Discharges

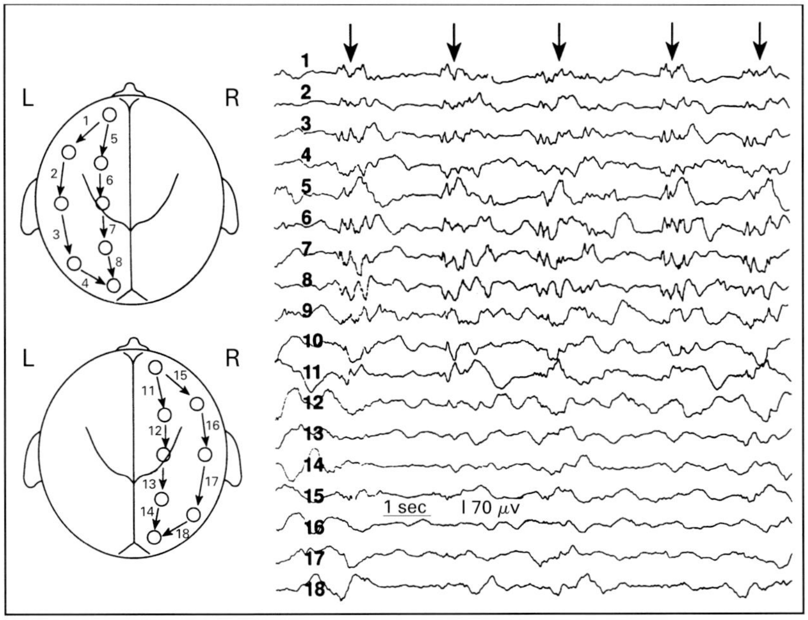

A

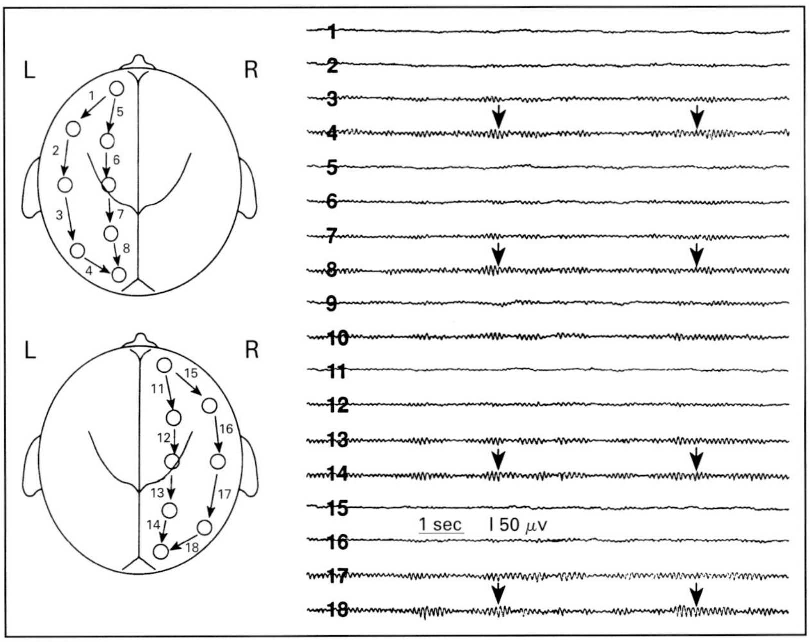

B

Electroencephalography in a 13-year-old boy with fever, altered sensorium, and sudden onset of seizures reveals complex repetitive discharges composed of spiky elements mixed with slower waveforms (Panel A). They are seen diffusely in the left (L) hemisphere (leads 1 to 8), occurring at intervals of approximately 2.5 seconds (arrows). The right (R) hemisphere (leads 11 to 18) shows abnormally slow background activity of 2 Hz per second (delta rhythm) compatible with the presence of acute encephalopathy. For comparison, an electroencephalogram obtained in a normal, awake subject is shown in Panel B. There is normal background activity of 11 to 12 Hz per second (alpha rhythm). This rhythm is predominantly posterior and is evident in leads 4, 8, 14, and 18 (arrows). Note the symmetry in activity between left and right cerebral hemispheres.

The patient was found to have herpes simplex encephalitis, was treated with acyclovir (15 mg per kilogram of body weight per day for 14 days), and made a full neurologic recovery within 6 weeks.

Nathan Watemberg, M.D.
Lawrence D. Morton, M.D.

Medical College of Virginia
Richmond, VA 23298-0211

March 7, 1996

Correspondence

Herpes Simplex Encephalitis

July 18, 1996

To the Editor: Drs. Watemberg and Morton (March 7 issue) describe a case of herpes simplex encephalitis in a 13-year-old boy and present the classic electroencephalographic finding of periodic lateralized epileptiform discharges.[1] Whereas it is gratifying to learn that the boy recovered fully after treatment with 15 mg of acyclovir per kilogram of body weight per day for 14 days, the only studies that have prospectively evaluated intravenous acyclovir for the treatment of herpes simplex encephalitis have used a dosage of 30 mg per kilogram per day (10 mg per kilogram every 8 hours) for 10 days.[2,3] This standard dose of acyclovir should be used for the treatment of herpes simplex encephalitis unless there is evidence from clinical trials that demonstrates the superiority of another dosing regimen.

Stephen D. Shafran, M.D.
University of Alberta
Edmonton, AB T6G 2B7, Canada

1. Watemberg N, Morton LD. Periodic lateralized epileptiform discharges. N Engl J Med 1996;334:634.
2. Sköldenberg B, Forsgren M, Alestig K, et al. Acyclovir versus vidarabine in herpes simplex encephalitis: randomised multicentre study in consecutive Swedish patients. Lancet 1984;2:707-11.
3. Whitley RJ, Alford CA, Hirsch MS, et al. Vidarabine versus acyclovir therapy in herpes simplex encephalitis. N Engl J Med 1986;314:144-9.

To the Editor: The legend to the Image in Clinical Medicine on periodic lateralized epileptiform discharges refers several times to the wave forms shown in the image as having an activity of a certain number of "Hz per second." In the physical sciences, the unit of frequency is the hertz, abbreviated Hz. In primitive units, 1 Hz is equivalent to one cycle per second. The authors were pointing out the dominant frequencies of the wave forms, and the correct usage should have been either "Hz" or "cycles per second" but not "Hz per second."

Nelson Thompson, B.S.
Department of Veterans Affairs
Houston, TX 77030

Dermatology

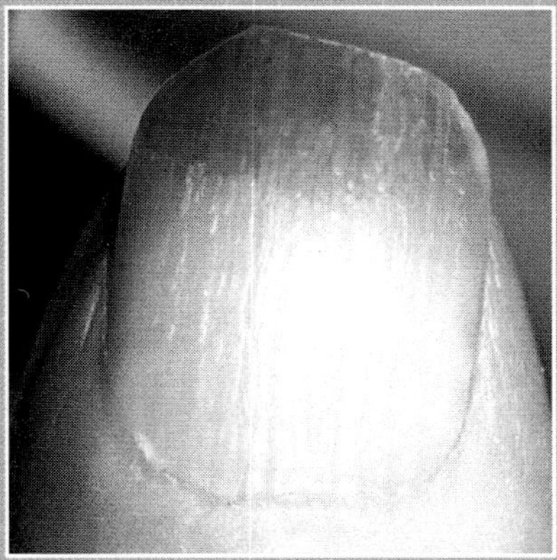

Peutz–Jeghers Syndrome

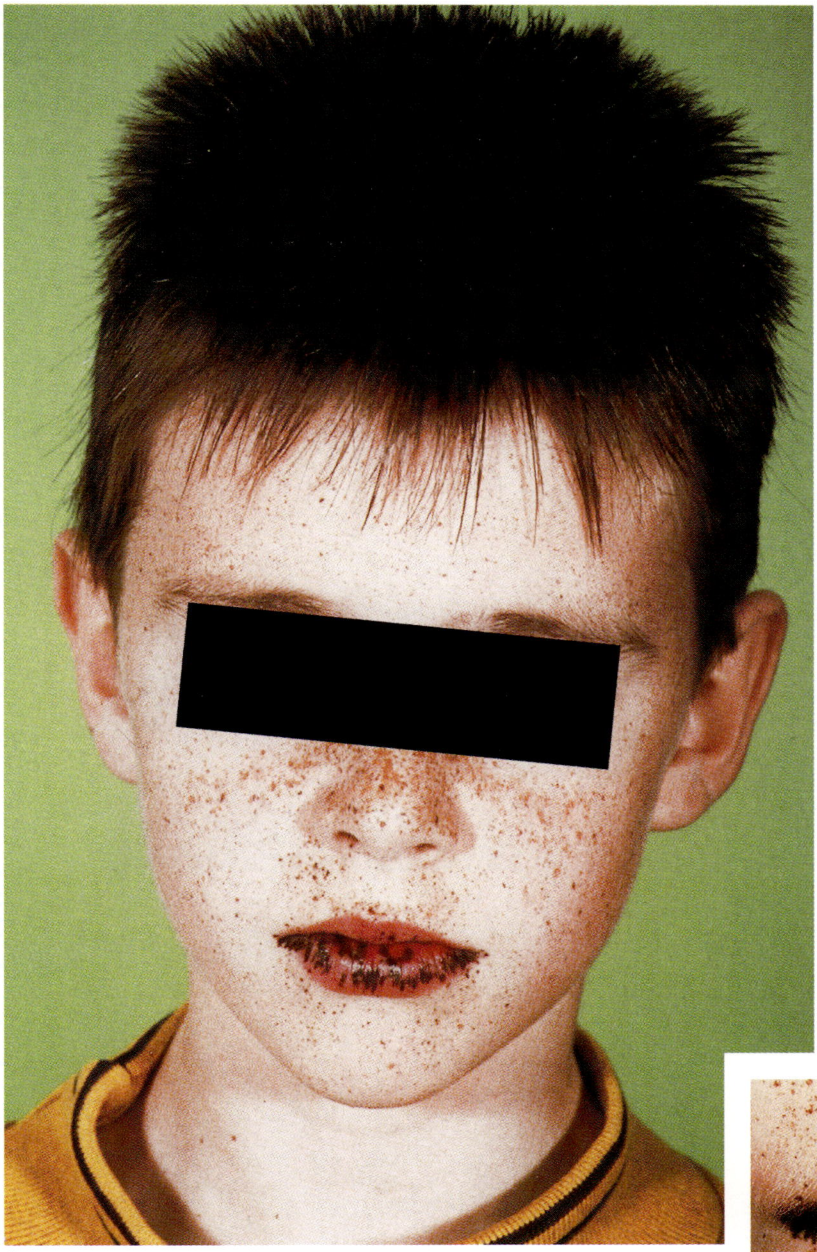

A

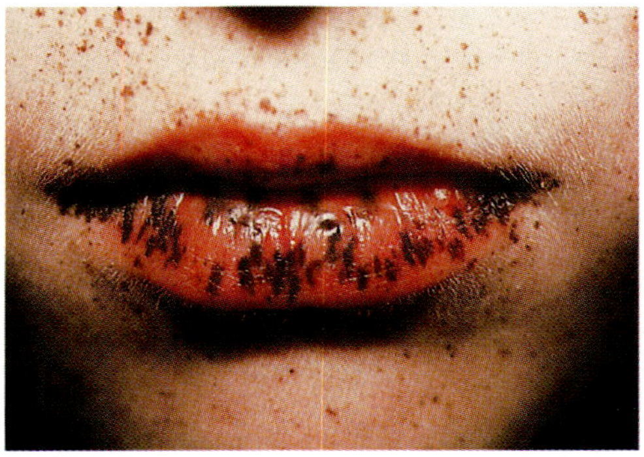

B

Striking examples of facial (Panel A) and lip (Panel B) pigmentation are shown in an eight-year-old boy with Peutz–Jeghers syndrome, an inherited disorder characterized by mucocutaneous pigmentation, gastrointestinal polyposis, and occasionally carcinoma of the colon or duodenum. The patient also had smudgy pigmentation of the fingertips and pigmentation of the mucous membranes of the mouth, but no other manifestations.

Patrick J. Morrison, M.D.
Norman C. Nevin, M.D.

Belfast City Hospital
Belfast BT9 7AB,
Northern Ireland, United Kingdom

September 9, 1993

Meningococcal Purpura

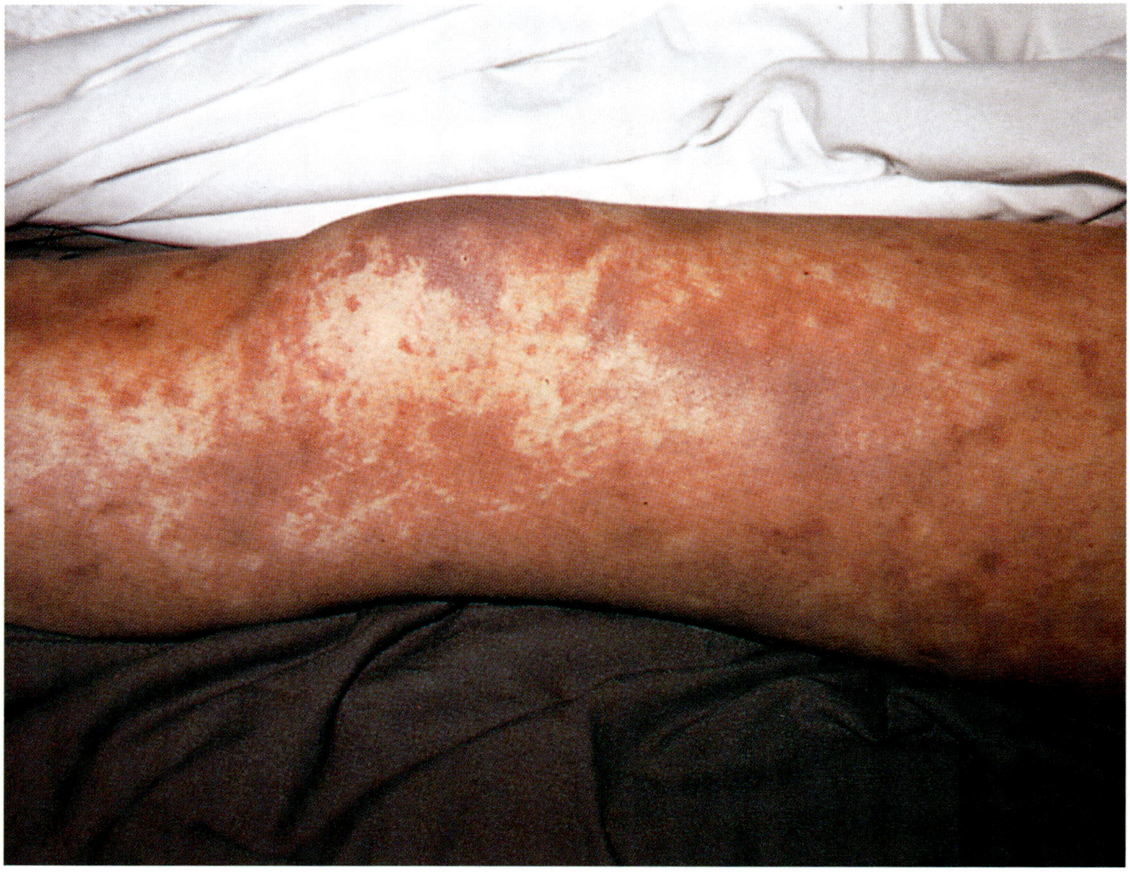

Massive intracutaneous hemorrhages are apparent in a patient with meningococcemia. The bleeding is related in part to thrombocytopenia, which is often part of the syndrome of disseminated intravascular coagulation, and in part to vascular damage caused by the meningococci, which can often be found invading the blood vessels. The lesions shown here are sometimes referred to as "purpura fulminans" and are associated with a high mortality rate.

Michael Barza, M.D.

Tufts University School of Medicine
Boston, MA 02111

January 7, 1993

HIV-Related Herpes Simplex Virus Infection

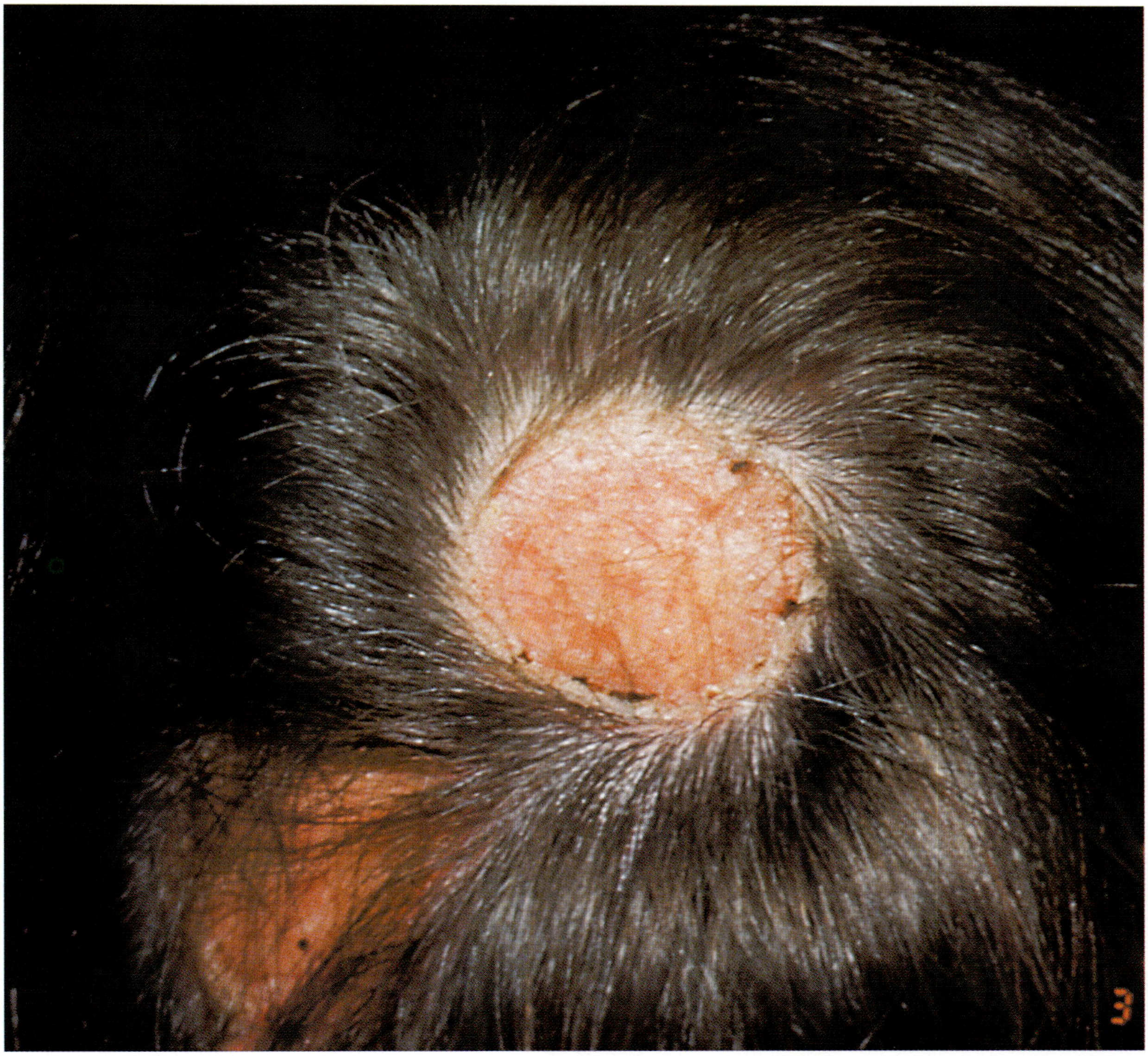

The two ulcerations visible on the scalp of a 41-year-old man with human immunodeficiency virus (HIV) infection had become progressively larger over a two-month period. Herpes simplex virus was cultured from a biopsy specimen, and multinucleated giant cells were seen on histopathological analysis. The lesions resolved after treatment with acyclovir.

Andrew Samel, M.D.
Howard Heller, M.D.

Massachusetts General Hospital
Boston, MA 02114

September 10, 1992

Herpes Zoster

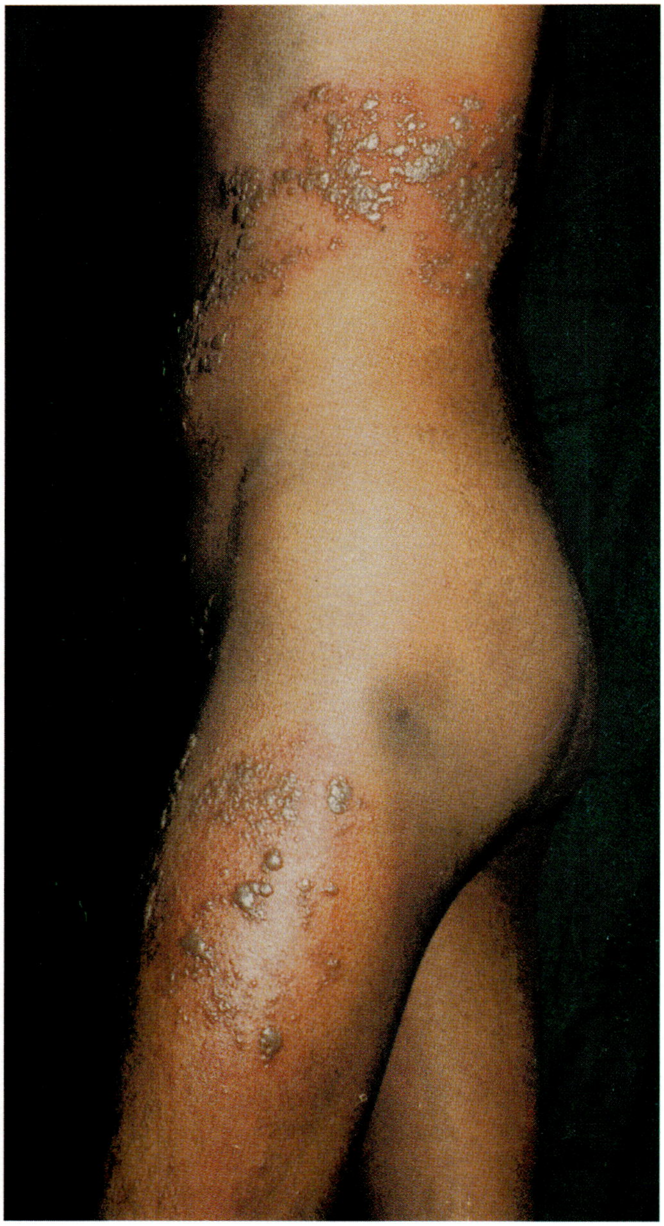

Confluent vesicular lesions of herpes zoster in consecutive dermatomes are visible in two distinct locations in a 20-year-old man with miliary tuberculosis. The patient was being treated with four antitubercular drugs; he also received prednisolone (1 mg per kilogram of body weight per day) because meningeal involvement was suspected. The lesions, accompanied by severe pain, appeared 4 weeks after therapy was begun and healed within 10 days after prednisolone was discontinued. Except for the prednisolone, the patient had no known cause of immunosuppression. He was seronegative for the human immunodeficiency virus. The miliary tuberculosis was cured by drug treatment.

A.G. Kulkarni, M.D.
N.S. Brid, M.D.

Krishna Hospital and Medical Research Centre
Karad, Maharashtra, India 415110

June 22, 1995

Cutaneous Lesions of Disseminated Candidiasis

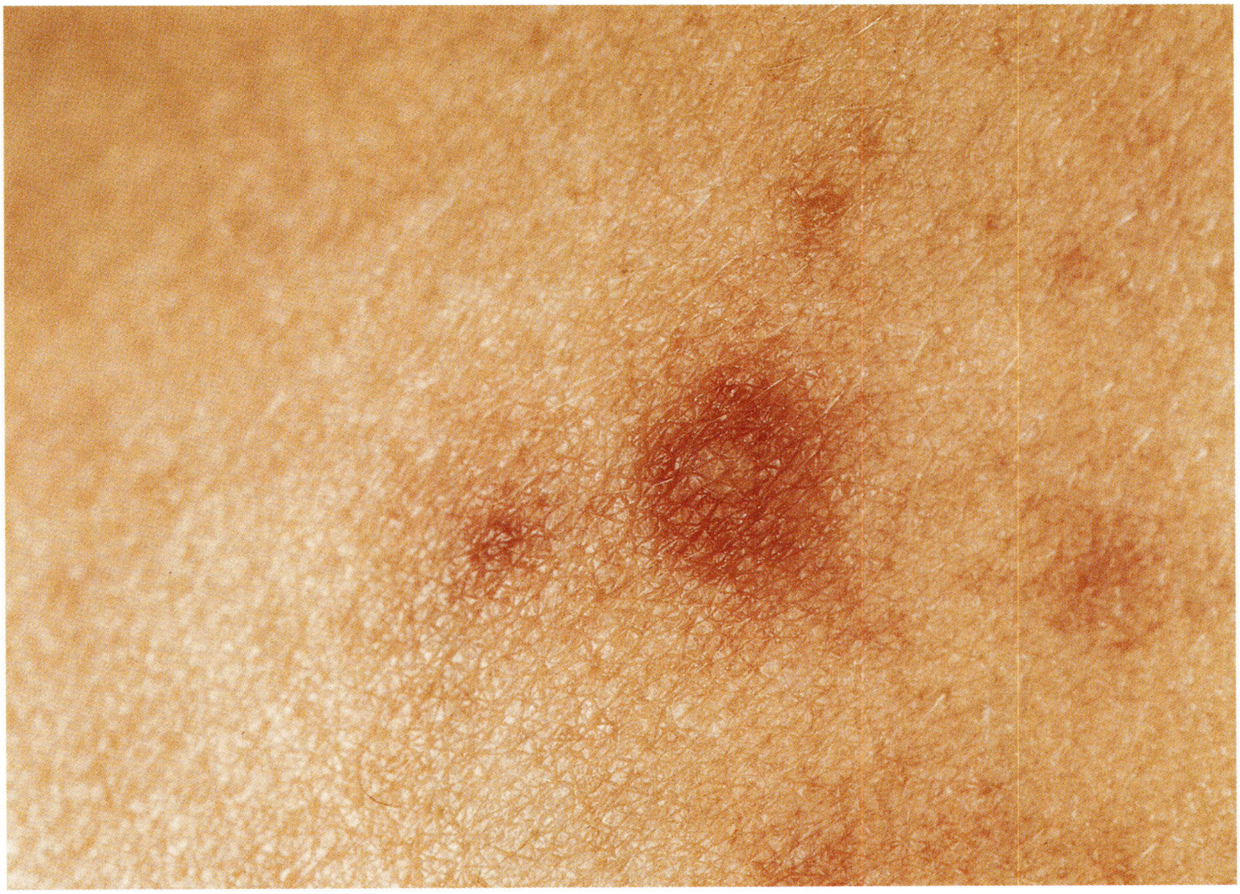

Erythematous papules with pale centers are present on the arm of a 13-year-old boy with neutropenia and Ewing's sarcoma. Blood cultures grew *Candida parapsilosis* and *C. lusitania*. The lesions were widespread and numbered in the hundreds. The patient presented with the skin lesions; myalgias and eye pain followed.

The pustule is the cutaneous sign of disseminated candidiasis in a host capable of leukocytosis. In the absence of circulating neutrophils, pustules do not appear on the skin; as the white-cell count recovers, the lesions may become pustular even as the infection is being treated.

Jeffrey S. Roth, M.D., Ph.D.

580 Park Ave.
New York, NY 10021

Marc E. Grossman, M.D.

Columbia–Presbyterian Medical Center
New York, NY 10032

June 9, 1994

Tinea Capitis

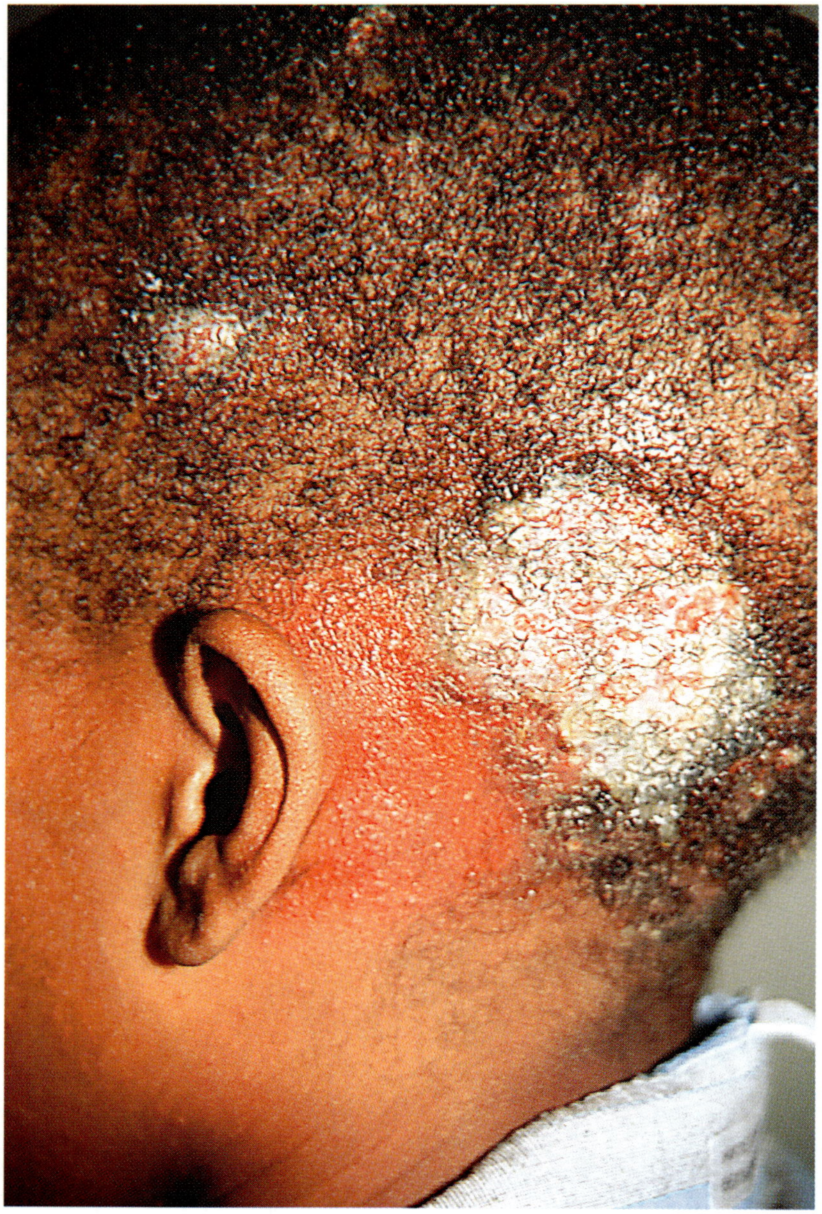

Tinea capitis with kerion formation and cervical adenopathy is shown in an 11-year-old boy who had had the infection for three years. The child had a partial response to a one-month course of griseofulvin and one month of ketoconazole therapy. There was complete resolution after two months of oral griseofulvin and two weeks of tapering corticosteroid therapy.

Del J. DeHart, M.D.

Saginaw Cooperative Hospitals
Saginaw, MI 48602

September 16, 1993

Toxic Epidermal Necrolysis

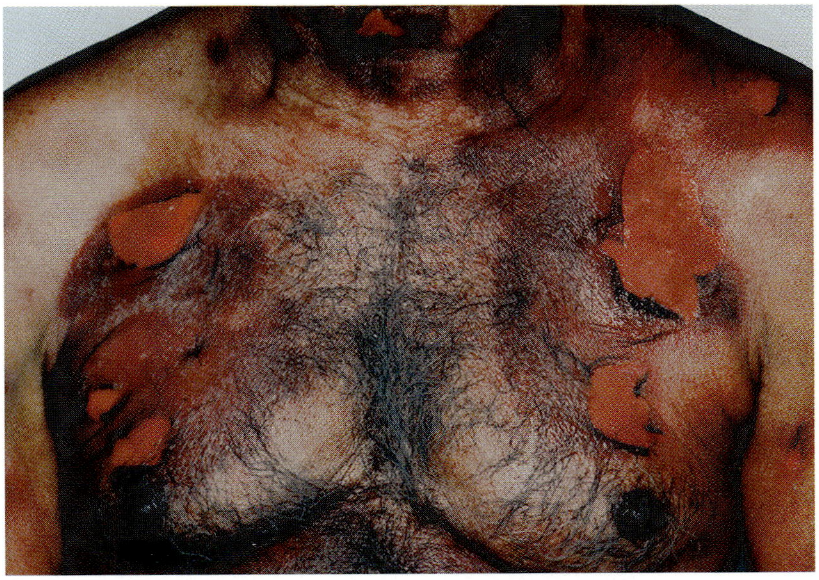

A

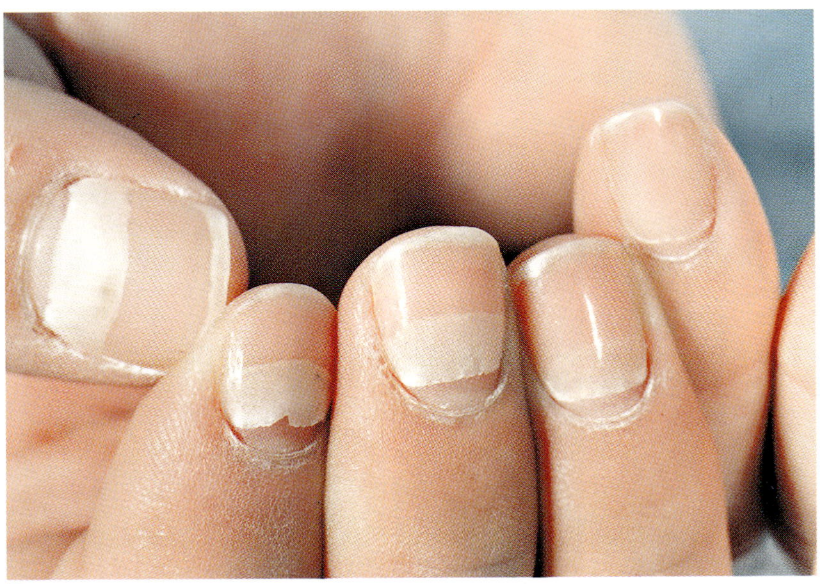

B

A 40-year-old man was hospitalized after the development of toxic epidermal necrolysis on his chest (Panel A). The condition developed three weeks after the initiation of treatment with phenytoin and progressed caudally during a period of three days, involving 50 percent of the skin surfaces, as well as his fingernails (Panel B). The eruption stopped progressing within 48 hours after the phenytoin had been withdrawn. The erythema gradually abated, the erosions healed, and the patient was discharged two weeks later.

Ira A. Pion, M.D.
William Slue

New York University Medical Center
New York, NY 10016

December 14, 1995

Heparin-Induced Skin Necrosis

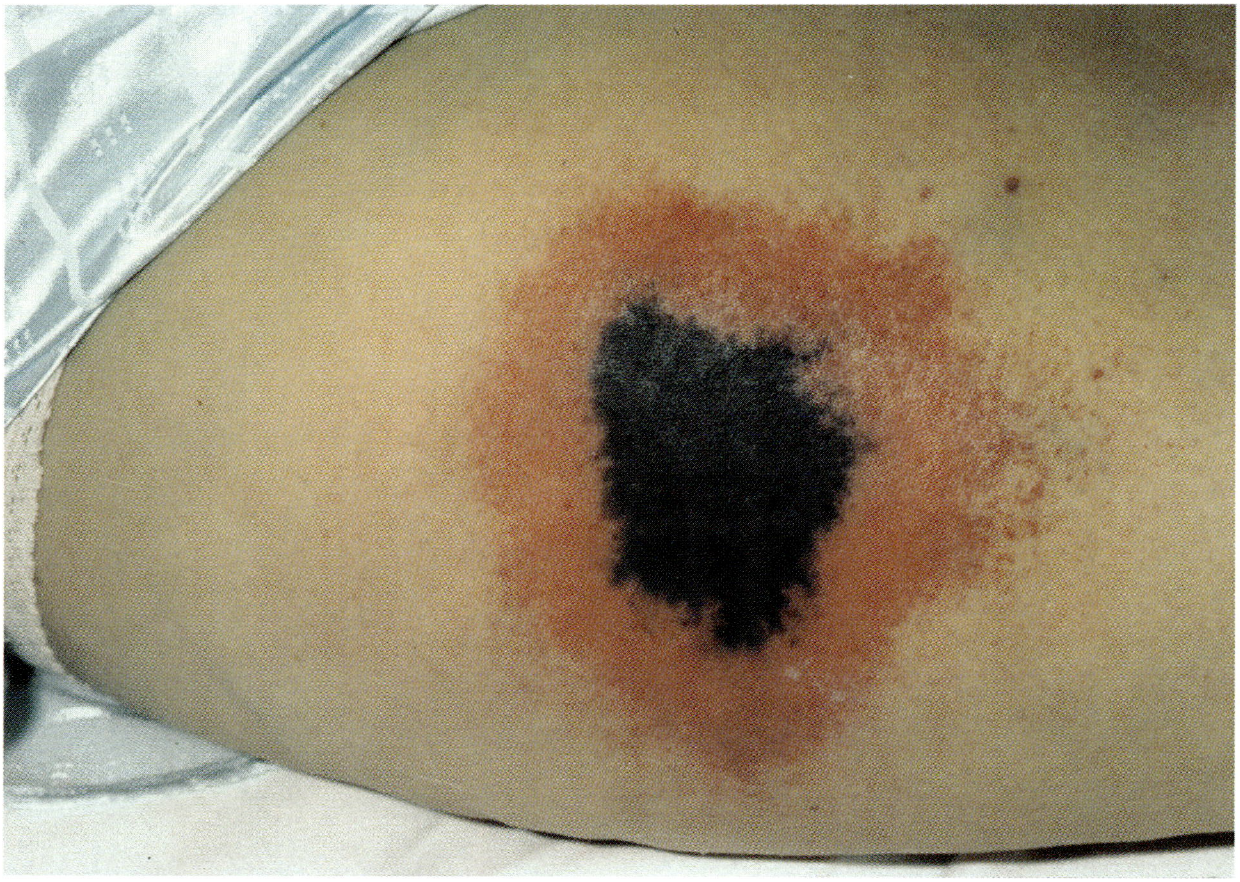

A 36-year-old woman received prophylactic subcutaneous heparin injections after an elective cesarean section. On the fifth postoperative day, subcutaneous edema, redness, and pain developed at the injection site, and heparin was discontinued. The next day, central necrosis of the lesion developed, with a clear line of demarcation between the affected area and surrounding tissue (the diameter of the lesion was 20 cm). The patient did not have thrombocytopenia or thrombotic complications. She also had normal plasma concentrations of protein C and protein S. The lesion later became bullous, with subsequent necrosis of the entire lesion, and skin grafting was required.

G.C.M. Lieve Christiaens, M.D., Ph.D.
H. Karel Nieuwenhuis, M.D., Ph.D.

University Hospital Utrecht
Utrecht, the Netherlands

September 5, 1996

Correspondence

Heparin-Induced Skin Necrosis

February 20, 1997

To the Editor: In the September 5 Image in Clinical Medicine[1] the appearance of the skin lesion described as heparin-induced skin necrosis is also compatible with a diagnosis of ecthyma gangrenosum. The authors do not state whether the heparin injected was sterile or whether cultures of aspirates from the skin lesion grew gram-negative organisms. This information would be useful for the differential diagnosis.

Richard V. McCloskey, M.D.
Centocor
Malvern, PA 19355-1307

1. Christiaens GCML, Nieuwenhuis HK. Heparin-induced skin necrosis. N Engl J Med 1996; 335:715.

To the Editor: With respect to the image of heparin-induced skin necrosis, the authors should have considered other causes, since the initial injections of heparin apparently did not result in similar lesions. The morphology and clinical course of a cutaneous lesion resulting in ulceration requiring skin grafting resemble those of ecthyma gangrenosum observed in cases of *Pseudomonas aeruginosa* septicemia. Was the patient immunosuppressed? Did she have any associated systemic symptoms or neutropenia? Did she receive any antibiotic therapy before or after the appearance of the skin lesion?

Similar lesions are also possible in primary cutaneous infections with *P. aeruginosa* (primary *P. aeruginosa* pyoderma), other gram-negative rods such as *Escherichia coli,* klebsiella, or even fungi. Did the authors perform Gram's staining and culture of the aspirate from the lesion? Secondary infection from a contaminated needle or some other source is always a possibility in hospitals. Biopsy of the lesion might have documented large numbers of bacteria invading the blood vessels, with few inflammatory cells in the case of ecthyma gangrenosum.[1]

Furthermore, the estimations of protein C and protein S mentioned in the report seem irrelevant, since deficiencies of these proteins predispose patients to skin necrosis after warfarin therapy and not heparin. Warfarin given alone in those situations causes a further decrease in protein C or protein S concentrations (since they are dependent on vitamin K), leading to thrombosis of veins and capillaries supplying blood to the skin and resulting in extensive necrosis.

P. Dileep Kumar, M.D.
Sur Central Hospital
Sur, PB 259 Code 411, Oman

1. Pollack M. Pseudomonas infections. In: Isselbacher KJ, Martin JB, Braunwald E, Fauci AS, Wilson JD, Kasper DL, eds. Harrison's principles of internal medicine. 13th ed. Vol. 1. New York: McGraw-Hill, 1994:665-71.

Correspondence Continued

To the Editor: Do the authors know for a fact that heparin was given? Could the patient have received a subcutaneous injection of a vasoactive, vasoconstrictive agent, such as epinephrine?

Frederick G. Schechter, M.D.
University of California, Irvine
Irvine, CA 92717

To the Editor: The image of heparin-induced skin necrosis is a striking and instructive example of this clinical problem. However, the report would have been made more complete by the inclusion of skin-biopsy findings on this bullous lesion for both routine hematoxylin-and-eosin staining and immunofluorescence microscopy to establish the diagnosis.

Despite the clear-cut history of recent heparin injections at the lesion site, the lesion might have had other causes — bullous erythema multiforme, pemphigus vulgaris, and bullous impetigo to name just a few. Since a skin graft was necessary to repair the lesion, a definitive diagnosis is imperative. Histologic findings in heparin-induced necrosis include extensive thrombosis of the dermal and subcutaneous vessels, with hemorrhage and focal epidermal necrosis but no evidence of vasculitis or an inflammatory infiltrate.[1]

Robert Lee Carter, M.D.
1515 Chain Bridge Rd.
McLean, VA 22101

1. Gold JA, Watters AK, O'Brien E. Coumadin versus heparin necrosis. J Am Acad Dermatol 1987;16:148-50.

The authors reply:

To the Editor: We agree with Drs. McCloskey and Kumar that infectious causes should be considered in the differential diagnosis of erythematous, necrotic skin lesions after an injection. In this case there were no indications of an infection, the patient was otherwise healthy and was not immunocompromised, and cultures were negative for pathogens.

With respect to the comment of Dr. Schechter, we believe it is very unlikely that the patient was given an injection of epinephrine instead of heparin. A skin biopsy may be helpful if one is doubtful about the diagnosis of a heparin-induced skin lesion, but it is usually not necessary. Heparin-induced skin lesions at injection sites typically begin five or more days after the initiation of treatment. The lesions may appear as painful erythematous plaques or skin necrosis. Heparin-dependent platelet-activating antibodies may be present. This adverse effect is not uncommon; Warkentin[1] observed it in six patients over a 30-month period.

H. Karel Nieuwenhuis, M.D., Ph.D.
G.C.M. Lieve Christiaens, M.D., Ph.D.
University Hospital Utrecht
3508 GA Utrecht, the Netherlands

1. Warkentin TE. Heparin-induced skin lesions. Br J Haematol 1996;92:494-7.

Quitter's Nail

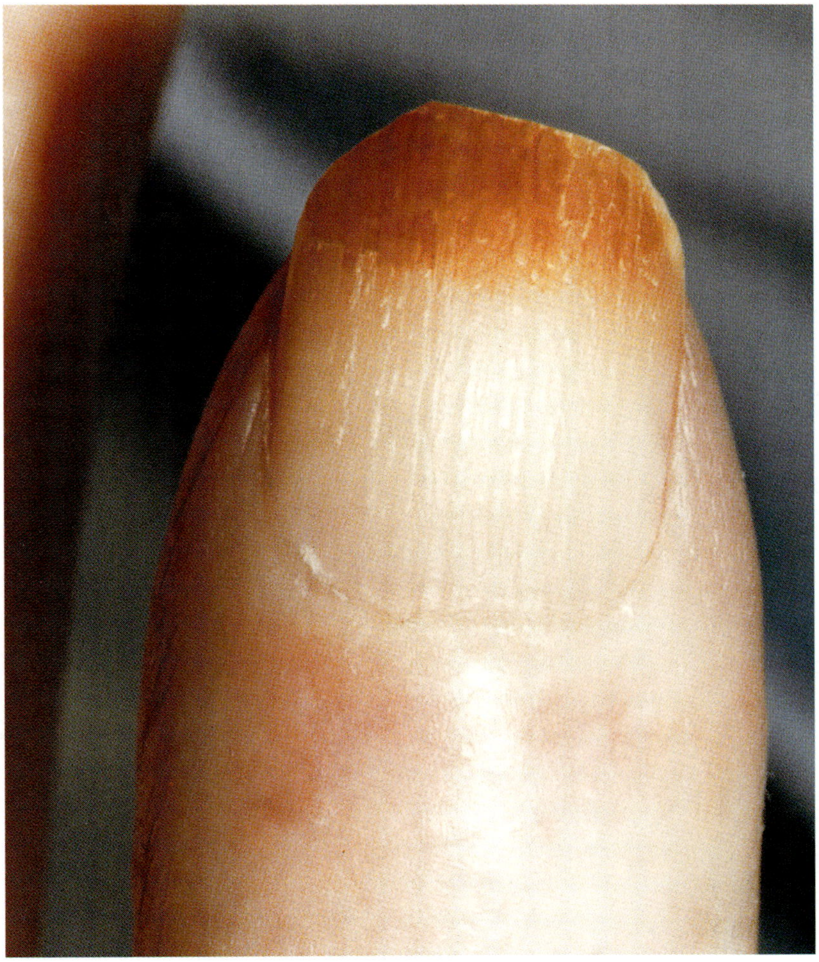

The tip of the fingernail is discolored in a 68-year-old former cigarette smoker who was unable to smoke after sustaining a head injury. Given the rate of nail growth (0.5 to 1.2 mm per week), the tar-stained portion took approximately 9 to 21 weeks to reach its current position.

Abraham Verghese, M.D.

Texas Tech University
El Paso, TX 79905

April 7, 1994

Correspondence

False Positive Quitter's Nail

September 1, 1994

To the Editor: Quitter's nail (April 7 issue)[1] can be a false positive sign of smoking cessation. The same week you illustrated this physical sign, I was pleased to observe it in a patient with asthma who smoked heavily. My joy turned to sorrow, however, when she reported having switched to a "low tar" filter cigarette at the indicated time and was smoking more than ever to sustain her nicotine level!

J.A. Frederick, M.D.
12 Chase Pk.
Logansport, IN 46947

1. Verghese A. Quitter's nail. N Engl J Med 1994;330:974.

Transverse Leukonychia

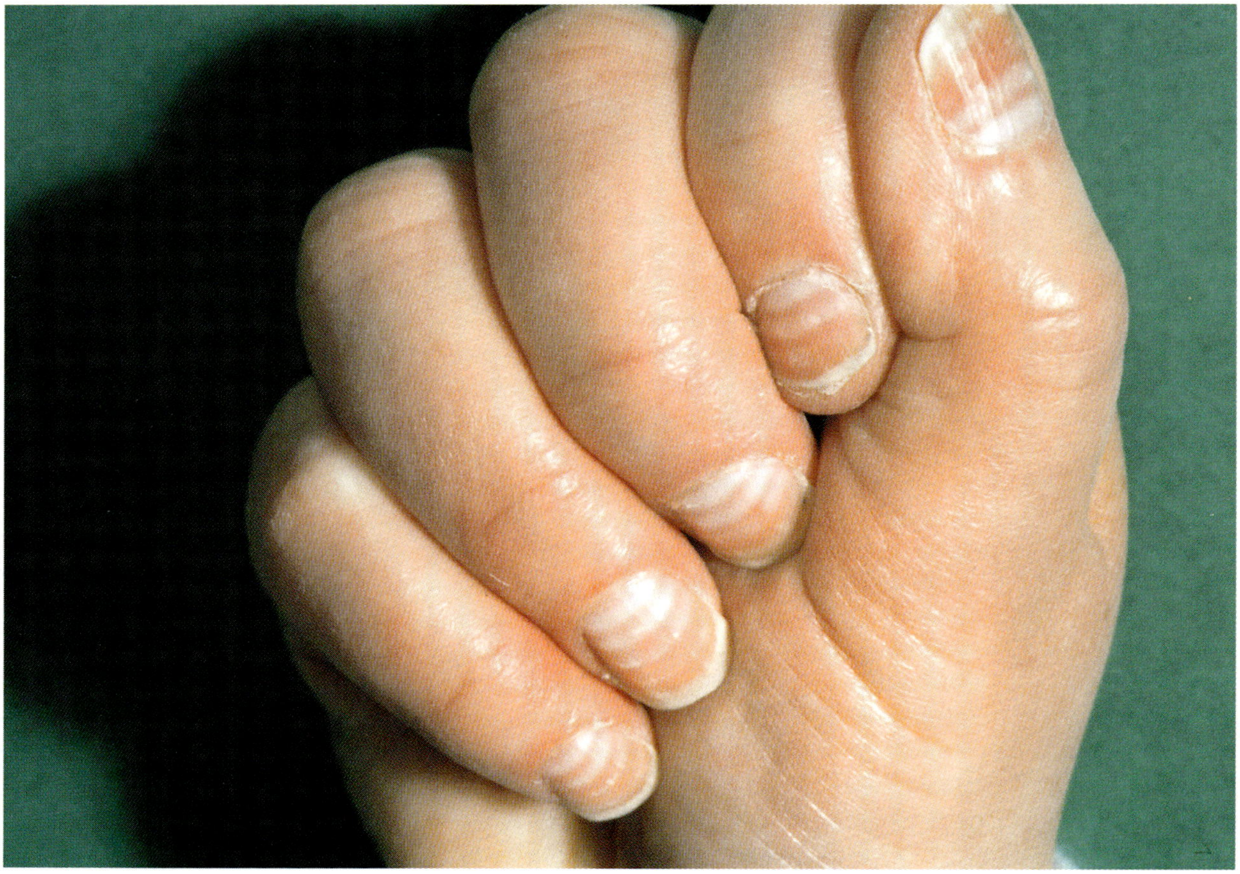

Multiple white lines are present in the fingernails of a patient undergoing anthracycline chemotherapy for metastatic carcinoma of the breast. The spacing of the lines coincides with the three-week intervals between cycles of chemotherapy. The cause of the lines is unclear, but they may be a consequence of abnormal keratinocyte maturation.

David W. Miles, M.R.C.P.
Robert D. Rubens, M.D.

Guy's Hospital
London SE1 9RT, United Kingdom

July 13, 1995

Basal-Cell Carcinoma

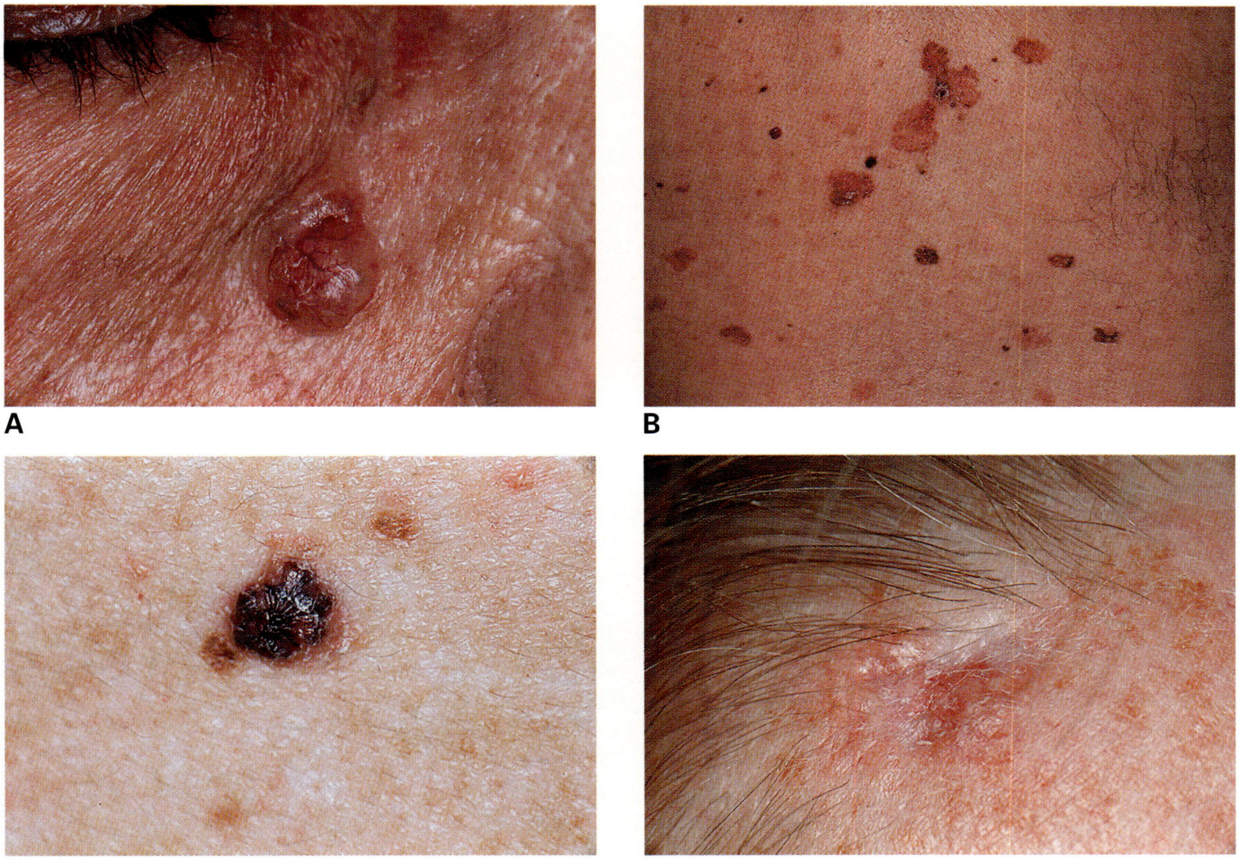

A B C D

Basal-cell carcinoma appears most frequently as a classic pearly papule (Panel A). It can also take other forms. Panel B shows multiple superficial multicentric lesions on a patient's back that may be associated with the ingestion of inorganic arsenic, Panel C shows a single pigmented lesion that can be mistaken for a melanoma, and Panel D shows a cicatricial lesion, present for five years on the forehead of a 29-year-old woman.

Jeffrey S. Dover, M.D.
Richard A. Johnson, M.D.

New England Deaconess Hospital
Boston, MA 02215

August 19, 1993

Malignant Melanoma

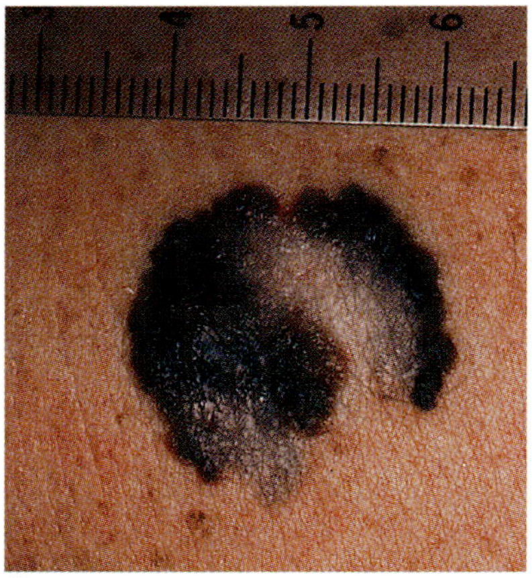

A

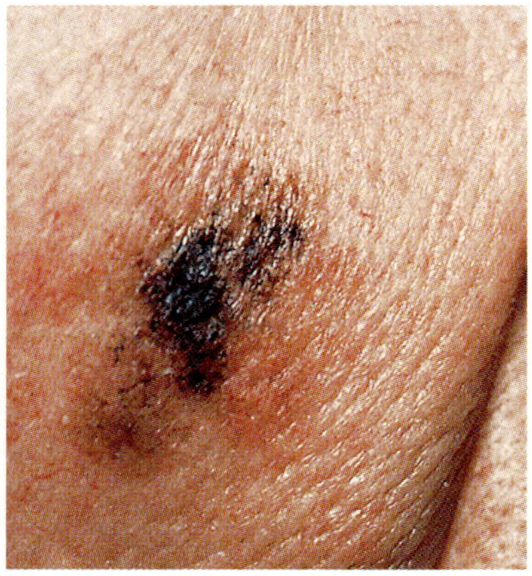

B

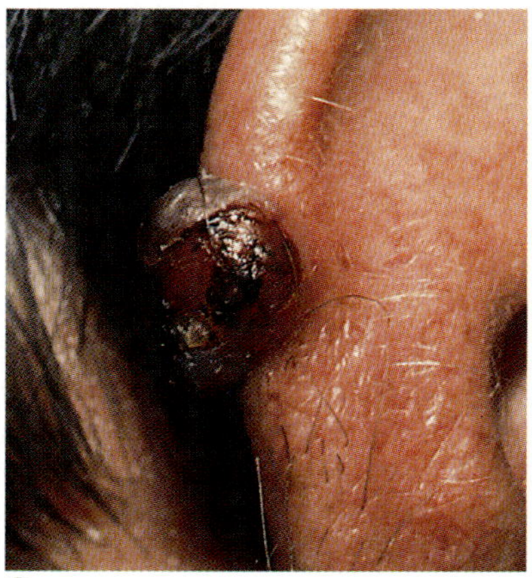

C

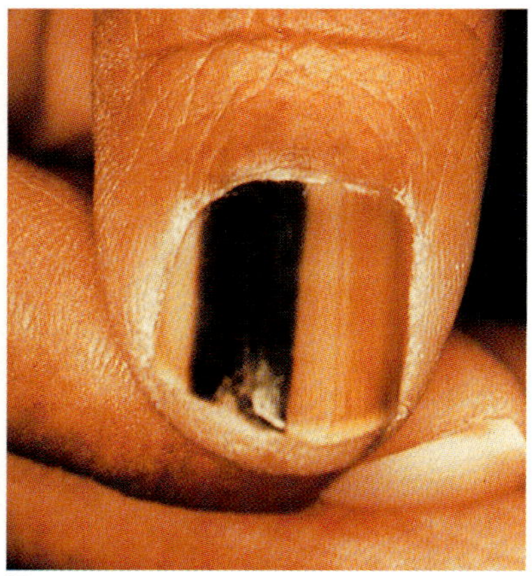

D

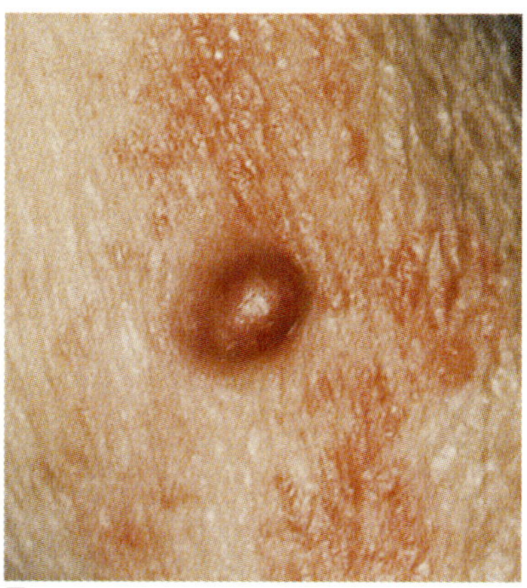

E

There are several recognized variants of malignant melanoma. Panel A depicts a superficial spreading melanoma of the trunk, the type most commonly seen in fair-skinned patients. Panel B shows a lentigo maligna melanoma of the cheek, a type seen most frequently on sun-exposed areas in elderly patients. Panel C shows a nodular melanoma of the helix. The black streak in Panel D is a subungual melanoma of the thumb, a subtype of acral–lentiginous melanoma seen most frequently in Asians and blacks. Panel E shows an amelanotic melanoma on the arm.

Greta C. Zimmerman, D.O.
William J. Grabski, M.D.

Brooke Army Medical Center
Fort Sam Houston, TX 78234

July 21, 1994

Parasites and Insects

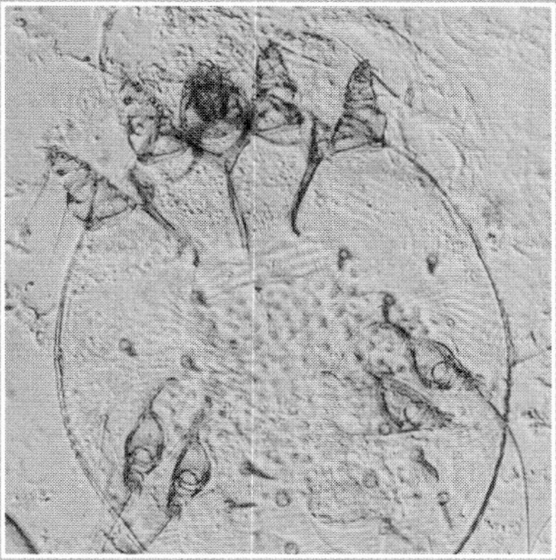

Coiled Larva of Trichinella spiralis

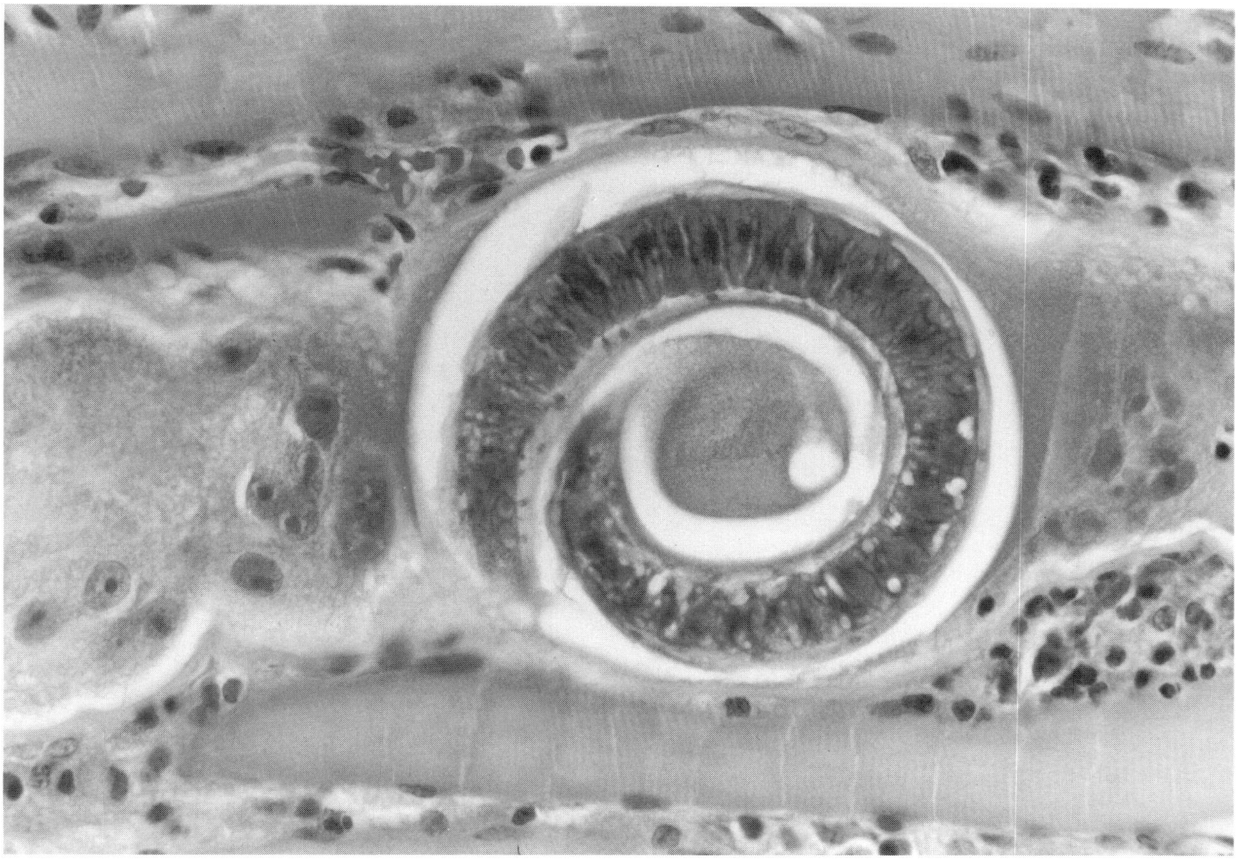

A larva of *Trichinella spiralis* is coiled in a still-living skeletal-muscle cell. The patient contracted trichinosis by eating raw pork in which similar viable larvae were undoubtedly encysted (×828).

David Lacomis, M.D.

University of Massachusetts
Medical Center
Worcester, MA 01655

October 15, 1992

Visceral Leishmaniasis

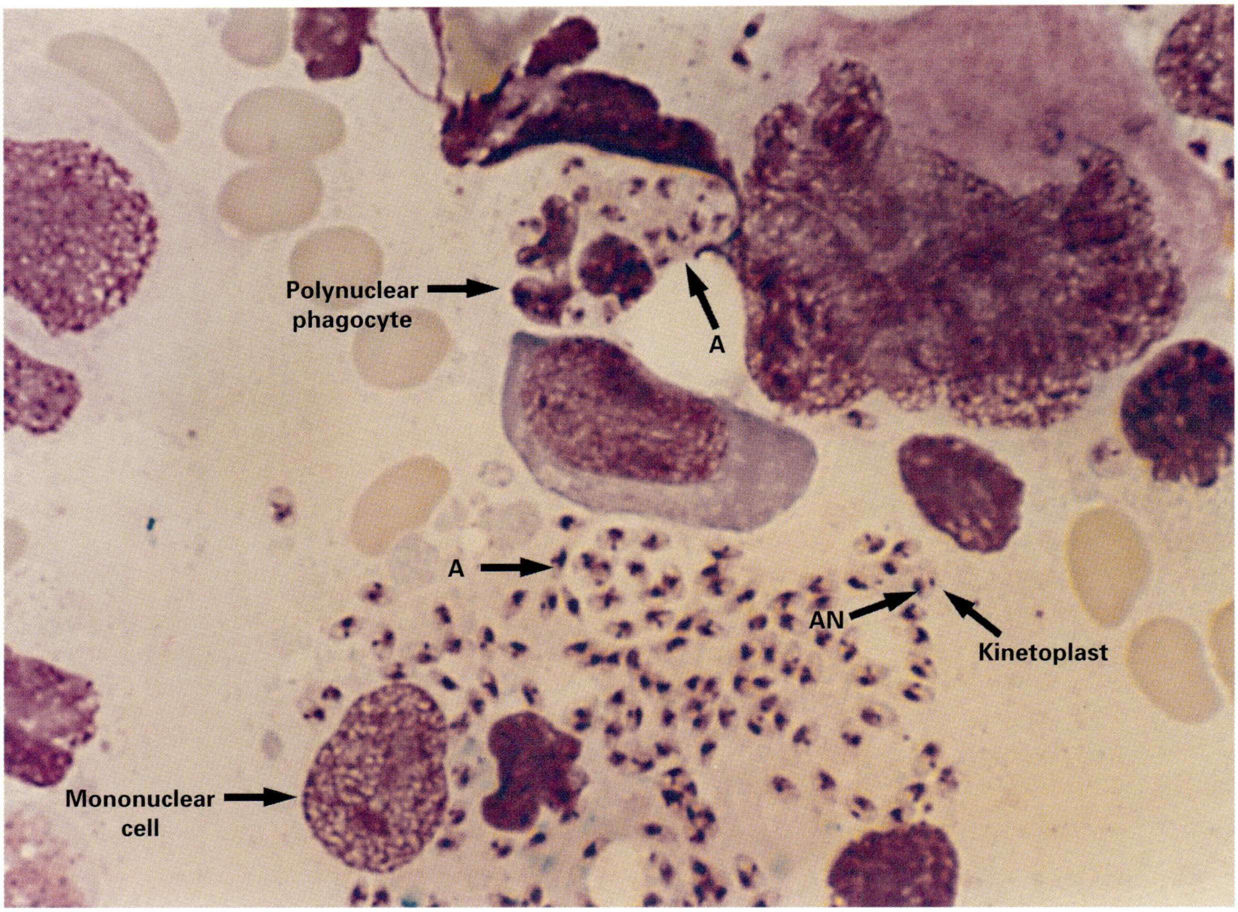

A 72-year-old Spanish woman admitted to the hospital for high fever and leukopenia had neither hepatomegaly nor splenomegaly, as assessed by physical examination and abdominal ultrasonography. A bone marrow aspirate shows intracellular and extracellular amastigotes (A), the form of the leishmania organism that lacks an exteriorized flagellum. The kinetoplast is an independently replicating organelle in the mitochondrion of the organism. The findings in the bone marrow were surprising because of the lack of organomegaly. The patient was treated with pentavalent antimonial compounds for 20 days. At follow-up 10 days later, the leukopenia and fever had resolved. AN denotes amastigote nucleus.

M.J. García Bueno, M.D.
J. Herráez, M.D.

Hospital Campo Arañuelo
10300 Navalmoral, Spain

October 3, 1996

Correspondence

Visceral Leishmaniasis

March 27, 1997

To the Editor: The Image in Clinical Medicine of leishmanial amastigotes (Oct. 3 issue)[1] was striking, and the clinical history was unusual, but I was left with several questions: What was the leishmanial species? Was this woman an immigrant from an area with a different level of endemicity? Was the patient tested for antibodies to the human immunodeficiency virus?

Thomas A. Moore, M.D.
National Institute of Allergy and Infectious Diseases
Bethesda, MD 20892-0425

1. García Bueno MJ, Herráez J. Visceral leishmaniasis. N Engl J Med 1996;335:1034.

The authors reply:

To the Editor: The leishmania shown was not cultured, but the patient's indirect immunofluorescence test was reactive. The test was performed by the National Center of Microbiology, Virology, and Immunology of Majadahonda, which uses promastigotes of *Leishmania infantum,* the only leishmanial species found in Spain.[1] The patient was not from an area with a different level of endemicity. Her test for antibodies to the human immunodeficiency virus was negative.

M.J. García Bueno, M.D.
J. Herraez García, M.D.
Hospital Campo Arañuelo
10300 Navalmoral, Spain

1. Alvar Ezquerra J. Leishmaniasis. In: Farreras, Rozman, eds. Medicina interna. Barcelona, Spain: Mosby-Doyma, 1996:2444-7.

Echinococcal Cyst of the Pericardium

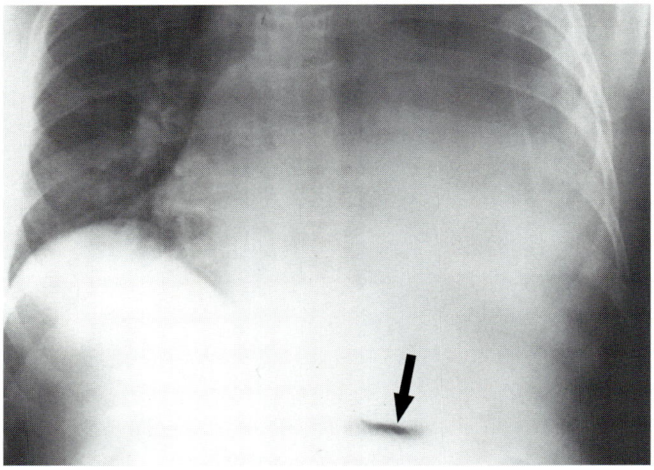

A

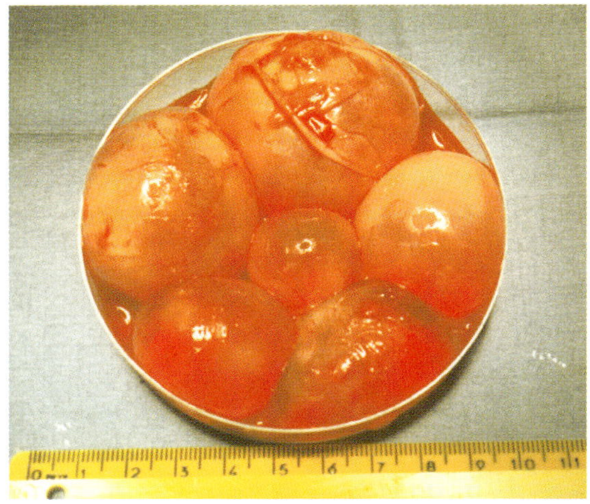

D

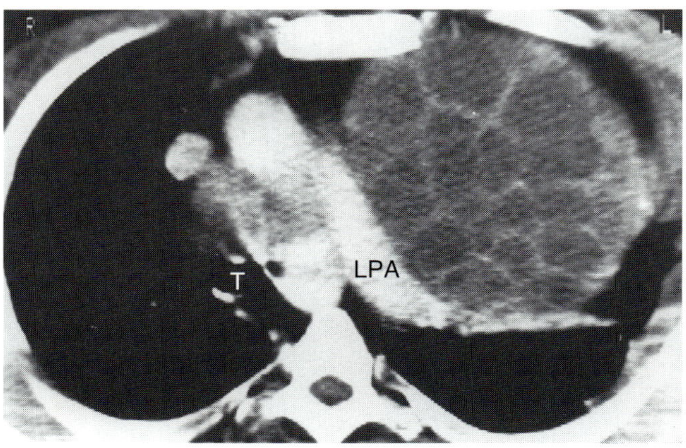

B

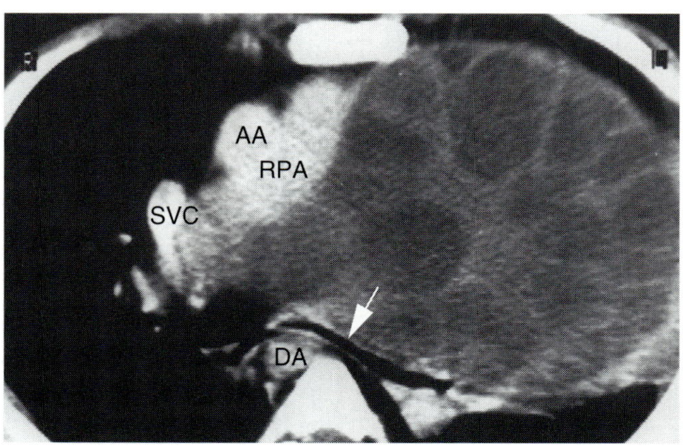

C

A 56-year-old man from Saudi Arabia presented with dyspnea. A chest film (Panel A) revealed a large mass in the left hemithorax, with contralateral mediastinal shift and depression of the gas-filled stomach (arrow). Computed tomography after the injection of intravenous contrast medium (Panels B and C) showed a large multilocular cyst in the left hemithorax with contralateral displacement of mediastinal structures, including the trachea (T), the ascending aorta (AA) and the descending aorta (DA), the superior vena cava (SVC), and the right pulmonary artery (RPA). The left main bronchus (arrow) and left pulmonary artery (LPA) were compressed. Thoracotomy, performed in an attempt to remove the lesion, resulted in decompression and rupture of both the cyst and the left pulmonary artery, and the patient became exsanguinated. The unruptured daughter cysts, some of which are shown in Panel D, contained echinococcus granulosus scolices.

Ferris M. Hall, M.D.

Beth Israel Hospital
Boston, MA 02215

July 20, 1995

Correspondence

Echinococcal Cyst of the Pericardium

December 7, 1995

To the Editor: The patient with a huge hydatid cyst of the pericardium (July 20 issue)[1] died, I suspect, because of the attempted removal of the lesion.

It is always tempting to remove such lesions in toto, in an attempt to avert rupture with local spillage and an inevitable local recurrence. The pathology of the disease, however, argues against an excision strategy. Hydatid cysts of the species *Echinococcus granulosus,* as clearly shown in this instance in the two computed tomographic scans and the photograph of the specimens, create a fibrovascular layer around themselves. This is nothing more than compressed host tissue with no surgical plane between it and the host organ. This layer provides physical support and allows the transfer of nutrients to the spherical cysts of the parasite within the pericystic cavity. Accordingly, hydatid cysts in soft-tissue organs cannot be enucleated, nor can the pericystic layer be removed by excision from within the host organ, without uncontrollable hemorrhage. A more practical surgical approach would be simply to "evacuate" the contents of the pericystic cavity and excise only redundant portions of the pericystic layer. Local recurrence occurs in about 11 percent of cases[2] and can be guarded against by the proper walling off of the surgical field and the judicious use of scolicidal agents, such as 0.5 percent silver nitrate solution.[3]

Farrokh Saidi, M.D.
Modarress Hospital
Tehran, Iran 198446

1. Hall FM. Echinococcal cyst of the pericardium. N Engl J Med 1995;333:165.
2. Mottaghian H, Saidi F. Postoperative recurrence of hydatid disease. Br J Surg 1978;65:237-42.
3. Saidi F, Nazarian I. Surgical treatment of hydatid cysts by freezing of cyst wall and instillation of 0.5 percent silver nitrate solution. N Engl J Med 1971;284:1346-50.

The author replies:

To the Editor: The surgery that was contemplated in this patient was, I believe, simply to evacuate the contents of the pericystic cavity, as suggested by Dr. Saidi. The rupture of the cyst was unintended but probably not unexpected, because thoracotomy collapsed the contiguous lung. This rupture would not normally have been life-threatening. However, the decompression of the cyst resulted in the sudden reexpansion of the compressed left pulmonary artery. This vessel ruptured immediately after the rupture of the cyst. Unfortunately, the patient bled to death on the operating table.

Ferris M. Hall, M.D.
Beth Israel Hospital
Boston, MA 02215-5491

Hydatid Disease of the Liver

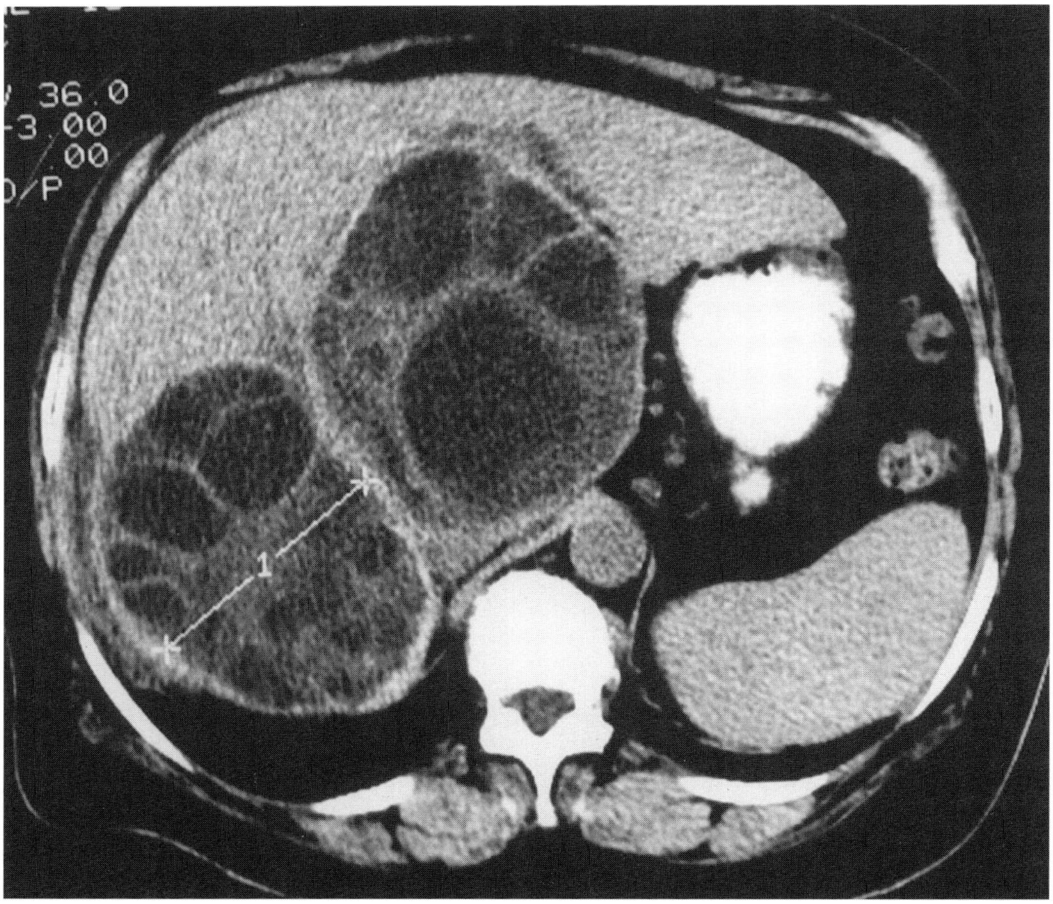

A computed tomographic scan of the liver of a 57-year-old woman reveals large cystic, lobulated structures with daughter cysts, consistent with hydatid disease. The patient had severe abdominal pain and a markedly enlarged, firm, and nodular liver. Her white-cell count was 12,000 per cubic millimeter, with 45 percent eosinophils. A serologic test for echinococcal disease was positive.

Sanjiv Chopra, M.D.

Beth Israel Hospital
Boston, MA 02215

May 20, 1993

Giardia lamblia

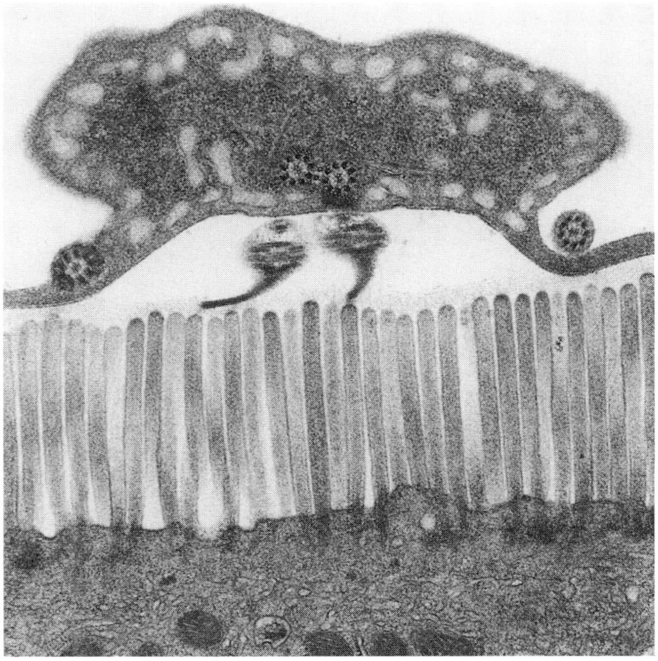

A

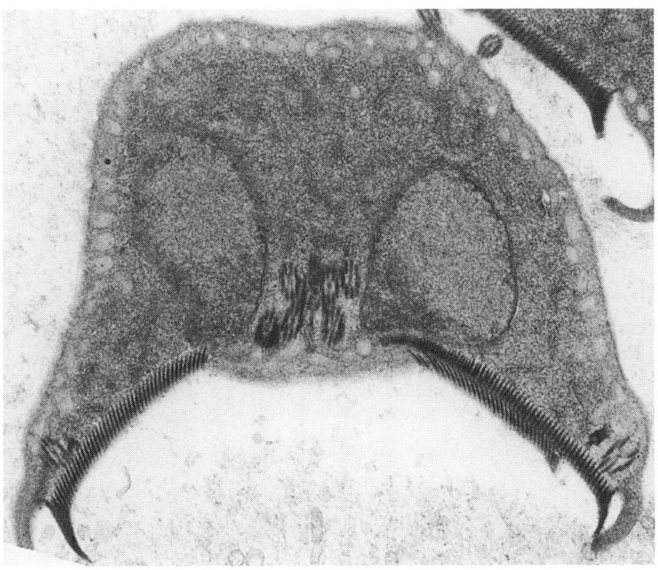

B

Electron micrographs show a duodenal-biopsy specimen from a 29-year-old student of veterinary medicine with a history of fatigue, abdominal pain, and chronic diarrhea that prompted tests for Whipple's disease and Crohn's disease. The appearance of the parasite is typical of *Giardia lamblia*.

Panel A shows a cross-sectional view of the trophozoite form of *G. lamblia* posterior to the ventral suction disk (×19,000). The trophozoite rests outside the glycocalyx of the microvillous border of a duodenal epithelial cell. Its paired central flagella are in contact with the underlying epithelial cells (the continuity of the flagella is not evident in this view), and there are two dorsal flagella resting above the two lateral cytoplasmic flanges. A row of peripheral absorptive vesicles and tubules is present in the cytoplasm. Cross sections of two microtubular axonemes, with the constant microtubular arrangement of nine plus two characteristic of flagella (and cilia), are centered in the ventral cytoplasm above the extracellular portions of the paired central flagella.

Panel B shows a cross-sectional view at the level of two large nuclei in the cytoplasm and the ventral, striated, adhesive suction disk by which the organism attaches to epithelial cells (×10,200). Eight microtubular axonemes (oblique sections of microtubule-containing intracellular portions of flagella) are located in the cytoplasm (six between the nuclei and two adjacent to the lateral cytoplasmic flanges). Note the row of cytoplasmic vesicles under the dorsal absorptive surface.

Ann M. Dvorak, M.D.

Beth Israel Hospital
Boston, MA 02215

April 8, 1993

Norwegian Scabies in a Patient with AIDS

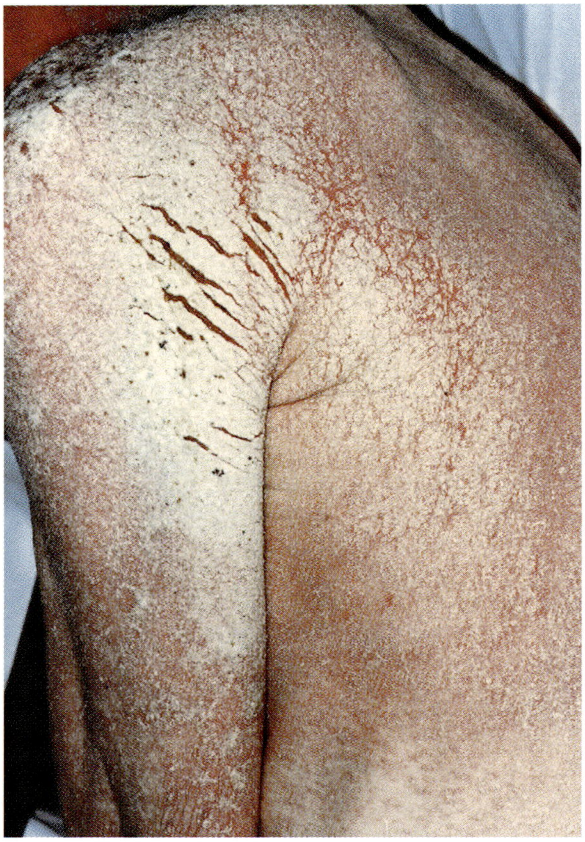

A

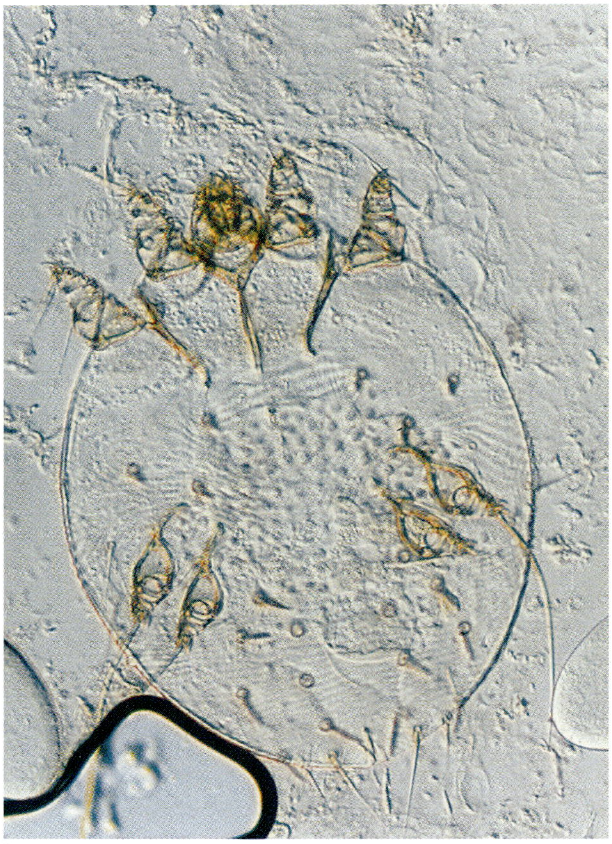

B

A diffuse, nonpruritic, erythematous, macular rash developed in a 43-year-old man with the acquired immunodeficiency syndrome (AIDS) and a CD4+ cell count of 22 per cubic millimeter. Initially, the rash was attributed to a drug eruption (due to either phenobarbital or ciprofloxacin). Approximately one week after the patient discontinued these medications, however, the rash progressed to form hyperkeratotic plaques on the chest, back, shoulders, elbows, and thighs. Panel A shows these hyperkeratotic plaque-like lesions in the shoulder region, where marked fissuring developed. Skin scrapings from multiple body sites revealed abundant scabies mites. Panel B shows a single scabies mite, *Sarcoptes scabiei* (×1100). The patient was treated with five applications of 5 percent permethrin cream over a two-week period, and the skin lesions resolved completely.

David H. Spach, M.D.
Thomas R. Fritsche, M.D., Ph.D.

University of Washington
Seattle, WA 98122

September 22, 1994

Correspondence

Scabies

March 2, 1995

To the Editor: The Images in Clinical Medicine entitled "Norwegian Scabies in a Patient with AIDS" (Sept. 22 issue)[1] are superb, but I take issue with the use of the term "Norwegian" scabies. "Crusted" scabies is appropriate,[2] whereas "Norwegian" is truly derogatory and should be discarded, just as "mongolism" has been replaced by "Down's syndrome."

Lawrence Charles Parish, M.D.
1819 J.F. Kennedy Blvd.
Philadelphia, PA 19103

1. Spach DH, Fritsche TR. Norwegian scabies in a patient with AIDS. N Engl J Med 1994; 331:777.
2. Parish LC, Lomholt G. Crusted scabies: alias Norwegian scabies. Int J Dermatol 1976; 15:747-8.

To the Editor: The hyperkeratotic plaque-like lesions of Norwegian scabies shown in a patient with AIDS[1] are very representative. Since 1983, we have diagnosed Norwegian scabies in 6 of 1100 patients with AIDS. We reported an outbreak of common scabies that originated in 2 patients with AIDS who had Norwegian scabies, affecting a total of 35 people.[2]

In our experience, the treatment of such severe scabies needs to be more intensive and prolonged than is suggested by Spach and Fritsche. To soften the hyperkeratotic lesions and allow the entry of lindane or permethrin, we suggest a whole-body application of either, although we prefer lindane and have not observed any toxic effects with its use. The lotion is administered twice a day as a bath, followed by salicylic acid and petroleum-jelly ointment, further applications of lindane, and petroleum jelly when severe scaling develops. The lindane lotion may need to be applied twice a day for three days each week over a three-week period.

Once Norwegian scabies is cured, no prophylaxis is necessary, although if a complete resolution is not achieved, a nosocomial outbreak may occur such as the one we described a few years ago.[2]

Bonaventura Clotet, M.D.
Guillem Sirera, M.D.
Carles Ferrandiz, M.D.
Hospital Universitari "Germans Trias i Pujol"
08916 Badalona, Spain

1. Spach DH, Fritsche TR. Norwegian scabies in a patient with AIDS. N Engl J Med 1994; 331:777.
2. Sirera G, Rius F, Romeu J, et al. Hospital outbreak of scabies stemming from two AIDS patients with Norwegian scabies. Lancet 1990;335:1227.

Correspondence Continued

The authors reply:

To the Editor: We thank Dr. Parish for his comments about the term "Norwegian scabies" and agree that "crusted scabies" is more appropriate. Although this change in terminology was proposed in 1976,[1] most articles since then have continued to refer to Norwegian scabies. Our use of the term was in no way intended to be derogatory. Instead, we chose the term because it is still used predominantly in the medical literature and thus was more likely to be recognized by the diverse readers of the *Journal.*

The experience of Dr. Clotet and colleagues points up an extremely important aspect of this disorder. At least six additional outbreaks have been described,[2,3] and no clearly optimal treatment regimen has been established.[2] Although our patient had complete resolution of his scabies (with no recurrence) after five total-body treatments of permethrin, we agree that in some instances more aggressive therapy may be required. Our patient also received keratolytic agents before the permethrin treatment; these agents are generally recommended in patients with hyperkeratotic lesions, to improve the penetration of the scabicide. Experience has shown that patients with substantial skin damage may have more systemic absorption of lindane and that lindane-associated neurotoxic effects may develop as a result. Because one would expect increased systemic absorption of lindane through the deep cutaneous fissures that often occur in patients with this type of scabies, we would caution against using lindane in patients with such fissures. Moreover, in one outbreak of common scabies that originated in a patient with Norwegian (crusted) scabies, resistance to lindane was documented in seven patients.[3] To the best of our knowledge, no resistance has been associated with permethrin treatment thus far.

David H. Spach, M.D.
Thomas R. Fritsche, M.D., Ph.D.
University of Washington
Seattle, WA 98122

1. Parish LC, Lomholt G. Crusted scabies: alias Norwegian scabies. Int J Dermatol 1976; 15:747-8.
2. Lam S, Brennessel D. Norwegian scabies and HIV infection — case report and review of the literature. Infect Dis Clin Pract 1993;3:169-73.
3. Purvis RS, Tyring SK. An outbreak of lindane-resistant scabies treated successfully with permethrin 5% cream. J Am Acad Dermatol 1991;25:1015-6.

Ascaris lumbricoides

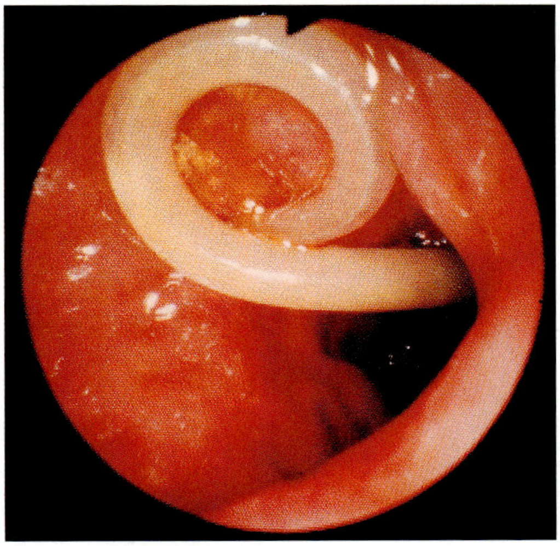

A

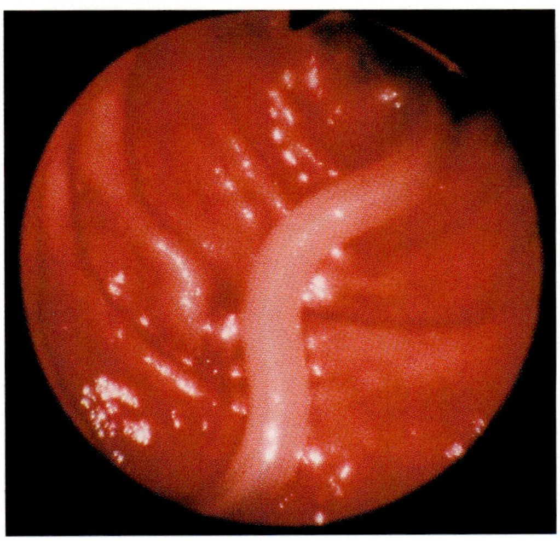

B

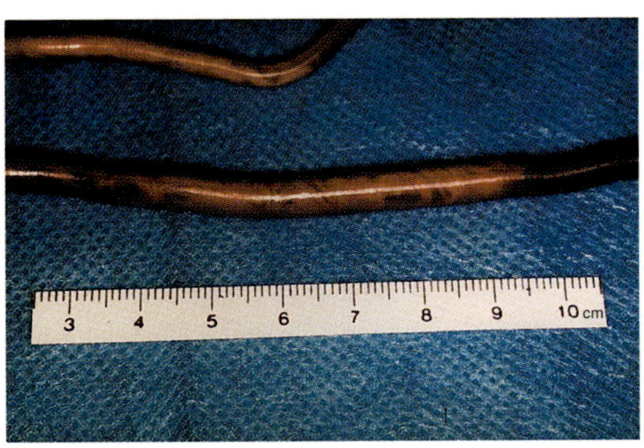

C

Upper endoscopy was performed in a 19-year-old man from Afghanistan because of four days of watery diarrhea and dysphagia without abdominal pain. Stool examination revealed no parasitic ova, and cultures were negative for bacterial pathogens. Endoscopy revealed an erosive inflammation of the terminal esophagus. In the duodenum, two worms (Panels A and B) were removed with biopsy forceps — one a female (length, 28 cm) and the other a male (length, 18 cm) *Ascaris lumbricoides.* Both worms are shown after removal (Panel C). After treatment with mebendazole, the patient passed several worms in the feces. It is unusual to diagnose ascariasis during upper endoscopy, because the worms live in lower parts of the small intestine, but they may migrate and can enter the common bile duct and cause obstruction.

Hermann Fuessl, M.D.

Munich University
80336 Munich, Germany

August 4, 1994

Pinworms

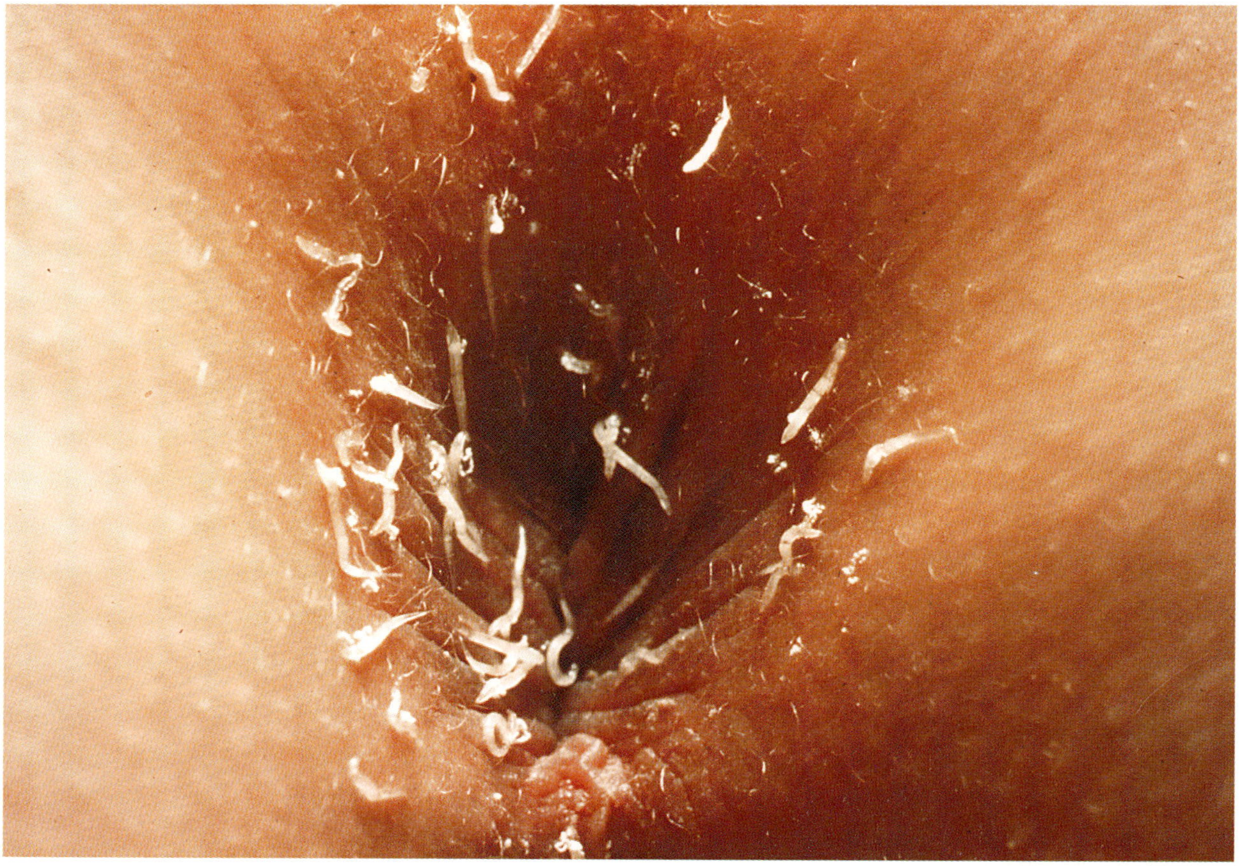

Female pinworms (*Enterobius vermicularis*) are shown leaving the anus of a five-year-old child who presented with crying, restlessness, and abdominal pain at 11 p.m. Female worms leave the rectum during the night and deposit eggs on the perianal skin, producing pruritus.

Martin Weber, M.D.

Children's Hospital
Hannover Medical School
3000 Hannover 61, Germany

April 1, 1993

Strongyloides stercoralis *Infestation*

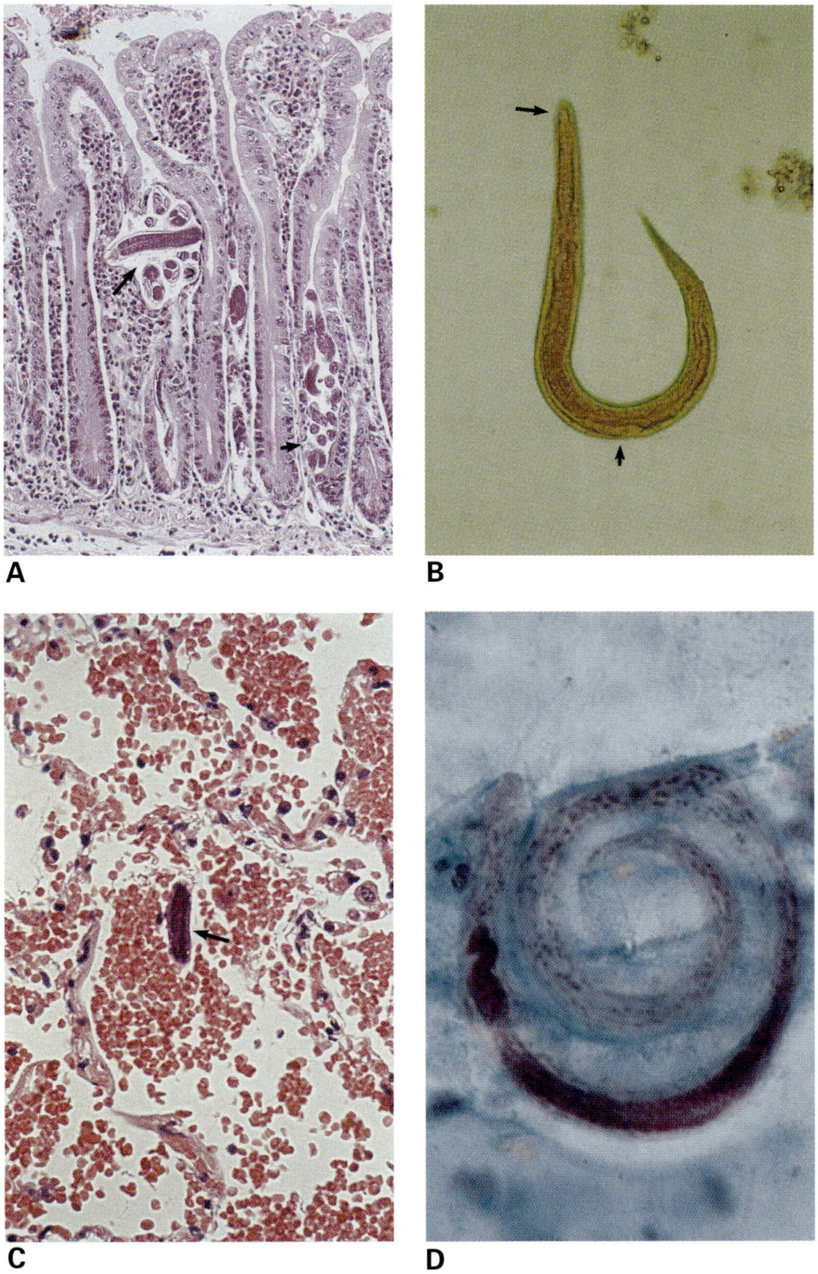

Strongyloides stercoralis infection occurs when filariform larvae from the soil penetrate the skin, pass through the circulation to the lungs, enter the airways, and are then swallowed. In the small-intestinal mucosa, the larvae mature into adults (Panel A, long arrow) and deposit eggs that release first-stage rhabdoid larvae (Panel A, short arrow; hematoxylin and eosin, ×105). These larvae are the usual diagnostic feature in the stool specimen (Panel B; iodine stain, ×505) and are identified by their short buccal cavity (long arrow) and prominent genital primordium (short arrow).

Immunosuppression, particularly that associated with excess levels of corticosteroids, can lead to a marked acceleration of autoinfection and dissemination and result in the hyperinfection syndrome, which is often manifested as hemorrhagic bronchopneumonia, hemorrhagic enteritis, gram-negative sepsis, or meningitis. During hyperinfection, migrating larvae (Panel C, arrow; hematoxylin and eosin, ×380) cause intraalveolar hemorrhage, and larvae may be seen on cytologic examination of respiratory secretions (Panel D; Papanicolaou's stain, ×615).

Jeoffry Brennick, M.D.
Anthony Mattia, M.D.

Massachusetts General Hospital
Boston, MA 02114

May 2, 1996

Sting of the Fire Ant (Solenopsis)

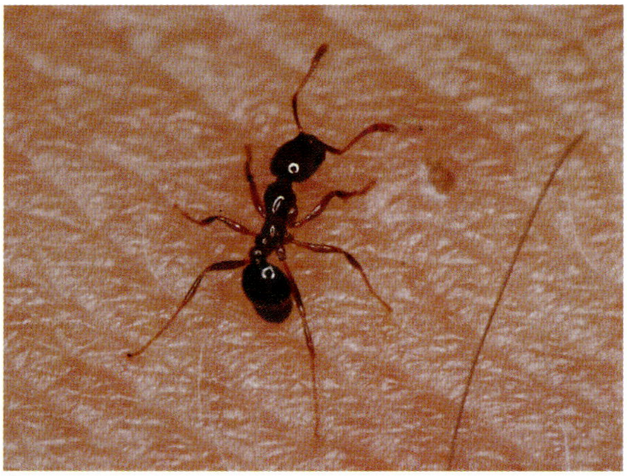

A

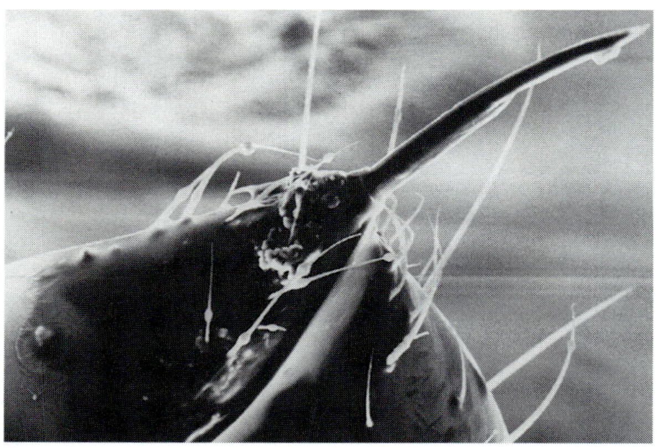

B

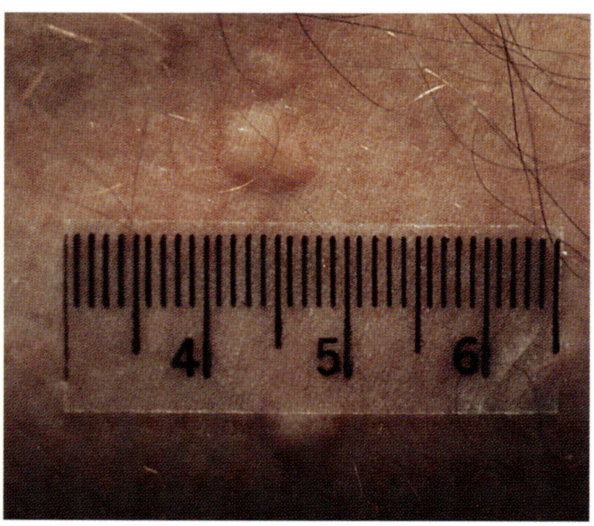

C

Panel A shows the fire ant with body arched, stinging and injecting venom through the stinger (a modified ovipositor) in its distal abdomen (×30). Panel B is a scanning electron micrograph of the stinger (×90). Panel C shows the wheal-and-flare response that occurred 10 minutes after envenomation (×30); it is often accompanied by a severe burning sensation. The scale is in millimeters.

Leon Kundrotas, M.D.

Wilford Hall U.S. Air Force Base Medical Center
Lackland AFB, TX 78236

October 28, 1993

Miscellaneous

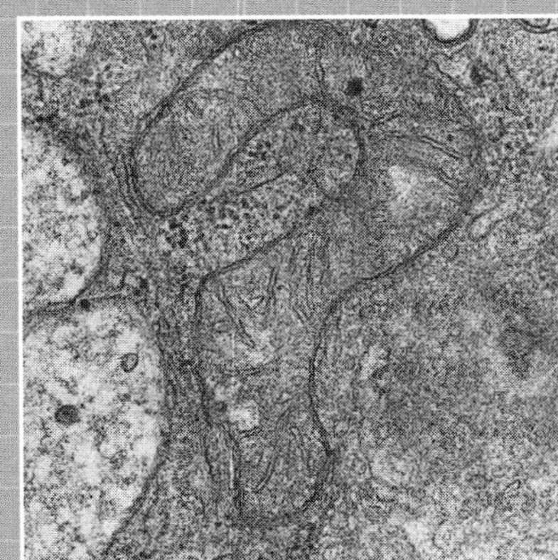

A Morphologic Question

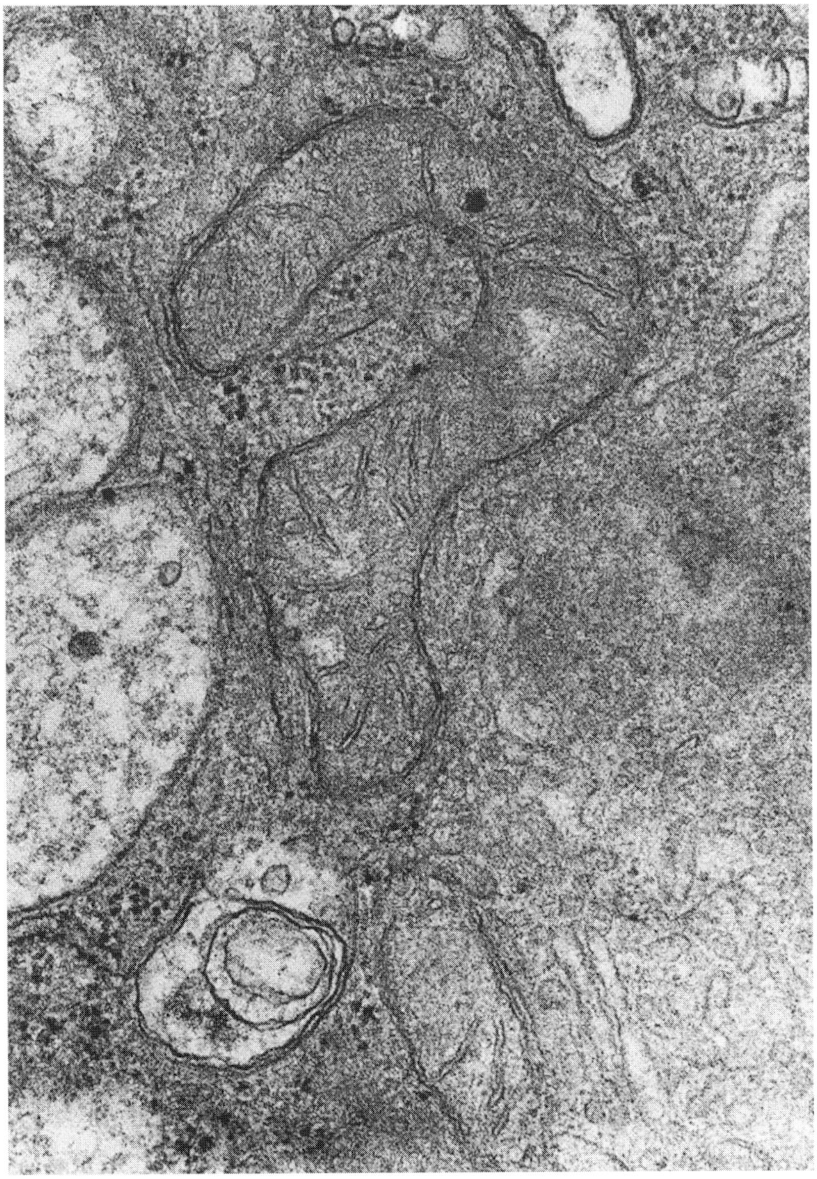

A mitochondrion of a murine peritoneal macrophage is shown after exposure to peptidoglycan (×20,000).

Marc R. Barnard, M.S.
Alan D. Michelson, M.D.

University of Massachusetts
Medical Center
Worcester, MA 01655

October 19, 1995

California Bigfoot

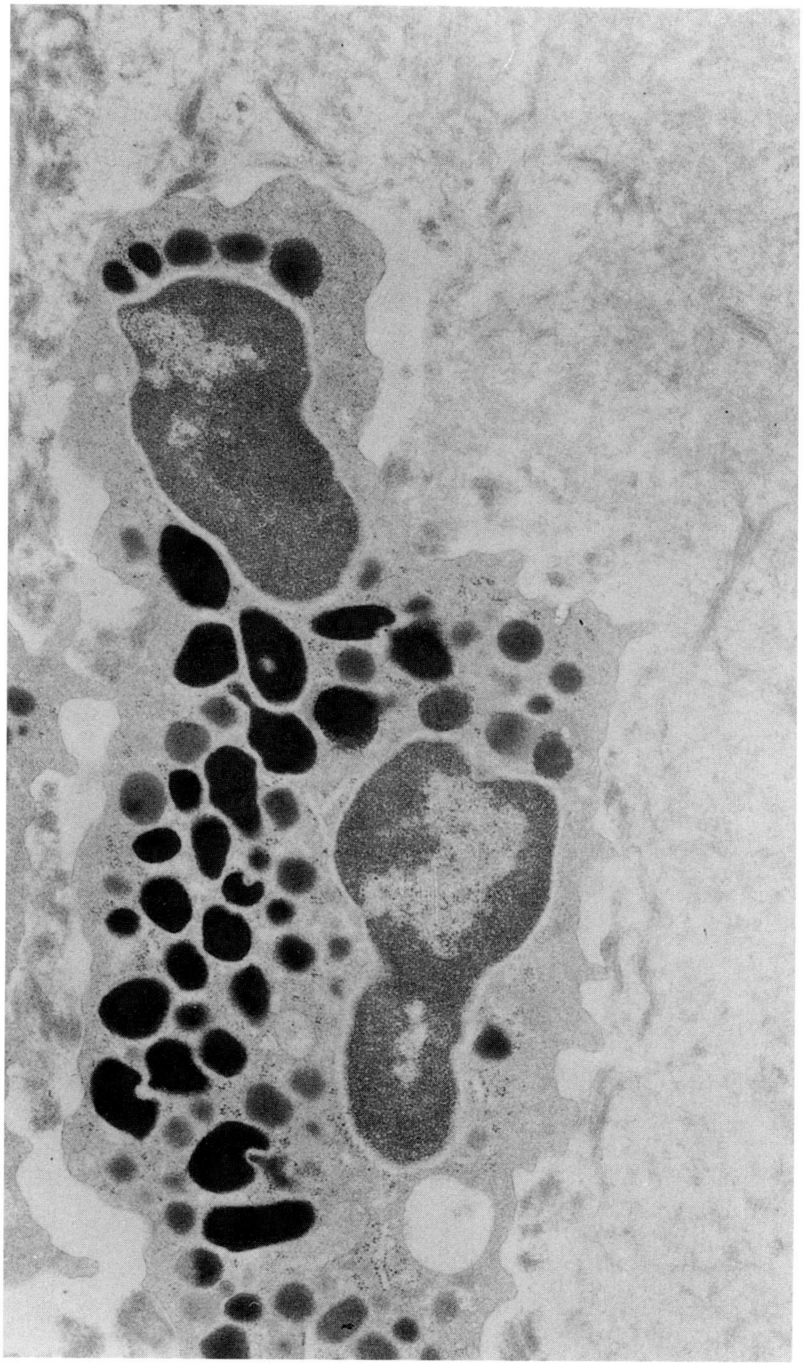

An electron micrograph shows a neutrophilic leukocyte from an acute bacterial inflammatory reaction in the peritoneal cavity of a rabbit. Two segments of the nucleus can be seen, as well as a cytoplasm full of granules that contain antibacterial and lysosomal enzymes (×12,000).

Dorothy F. Bainton, M.D.

University of California,
San Francisco
San Francisco, CA 94143

December 22, 1994

A Fetal Yawn

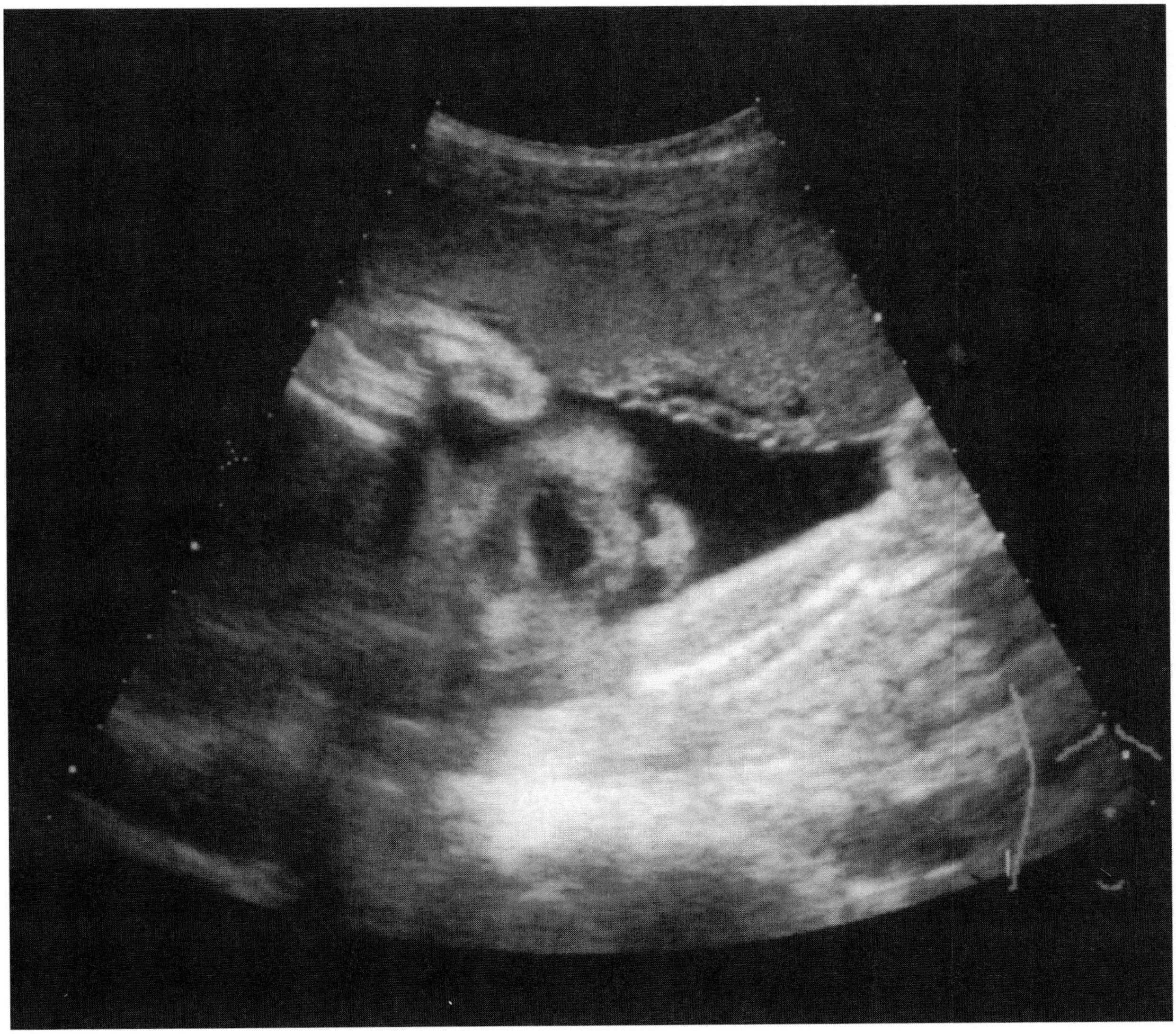

Fetal facial expressions are sometimes seen during ultrasonography. This yawning fetus, studied at 34 weeks' gestation, was born vigorous and healthy at term.

Robert S. Egerman, M.D.
Donald S. Emerson, M.D.

University of Tennessee, Memphis
Memphis, TN 38103

November 14, 1996

Massive Obesity Simulating Lymphedema

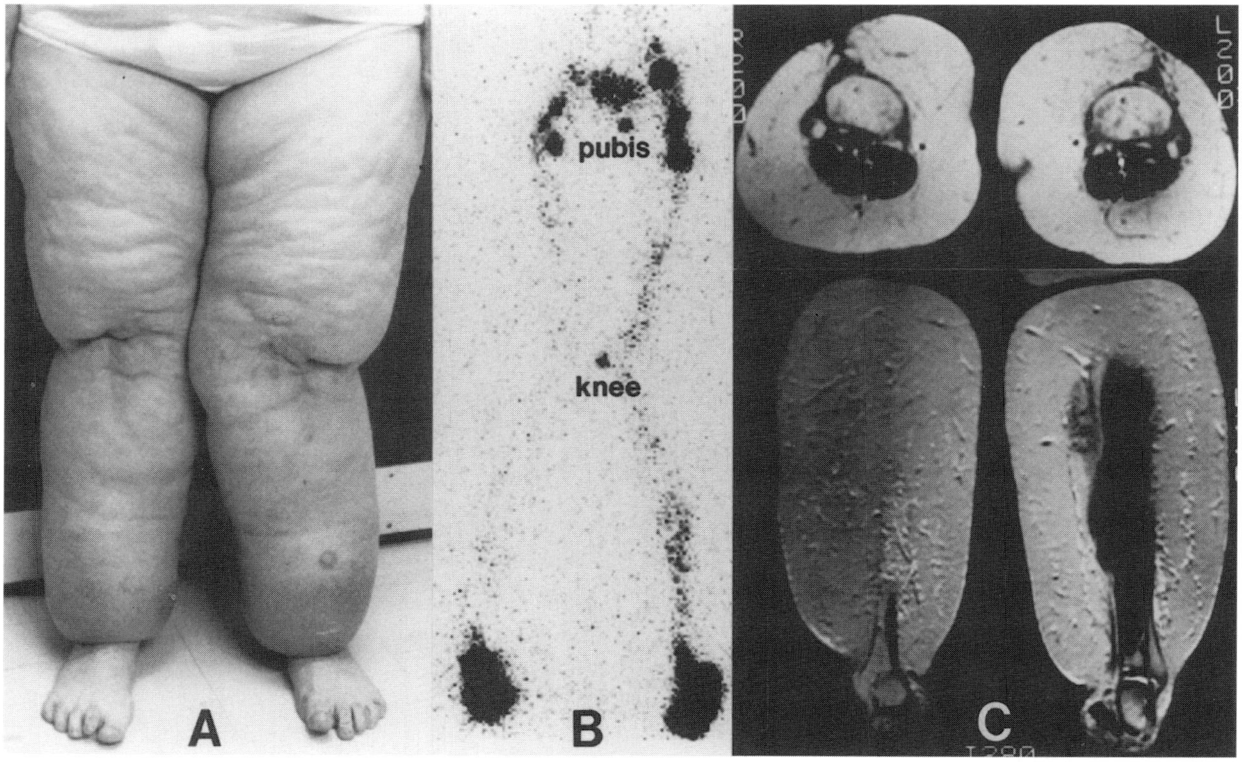

Panel A shows massive obesity of the lower legs of a 64-year-old woman. Note the bilateral symmetric, non-pitting swelling of the legs with sparing of the feet, which can be mistaken for lymphedema. In Panel B, a radionuclide lymphangiogram taken 30 minutes after the injection of ^{99m}Tc-labeled human albumin demonstrates normal lymphatic vessels and regional lymph nodes with prompt cephalad migration of the radionuclide. In Panel C, transaxial (above) and coronal (below) magnetic resonance images confirm the presence of diffuse subcutaneous fat deposits without the accumulation of free fluid. The irregular high-intensity subcutaneous signals on the coronal images represent venous varicosities.

Marlys H. Witte, M.D.
Charles L. Witte, M.D.

University of Arizona
Health Sciences Center
College of Medicine
Tucson, AZ 85724

December 31, 1992

Correspondence

Massive Obesity Simulating Lymphedema

May 20, 1993

To the Editor: The images of massive obesity simulating lymphedema (Dec. 31 issue)[1] are quite impressive. The photograph clearly shows the condition of lipomatosis of the legs, also known as lipedema. When confined to the thighs, the condition is known as "riding-breeches thighs." When involving the whole leg, it is known as either "billiard-table legs" or "stovepipe legs." If lymphedema were the cause of this degree of leg swelling, there would also be pitting or spreading edema on the dorsum of either foot in response to pressure, with the chronic skin changes of hyperkeratosis and increased skin markings. None of these signs are evident in the photograph. What were the indications for lymphangiography and magnetic resonance imaging when the correct diagnosis could be made by physical examination?

Victor Loughlin, B.Sc., F.R.C.S.
Lagan Valley Hospital
Lisburn BT28 1JP, Northern Ireland

1. Witte MH, Witte CL. Massive obesity simulating lymphedema. N Engl J Med 1992; 327:1927.

The authors reply:

To the Editor: Dr. Loughlin is correct that the term "lipedema" is often applied to the peculiar condition this patient had. The magnetic resonance images show that the term is a misnomer, because edema is not present. The patient was given the diagnosis of lymphedema several years before we first saw her. She was being vigorously treated with external pneumatic compression at another hospital to no avail. She was scheduled to undergo a debulking operation for intractable lymphedema. Lipedema bears a superficial resemblance to lymphedema, which also occasionally spares the dorsum of the foot. Little is known about the underlying pathophysiology of lipedema with regard to peripheral lymphatic function, the composition of soft tissues, and the presence or absence of true edema.[1] Because of the ease, accuracy, and safety of intradermal isotope lymphography (also called lymphangioscintigraphy) in demonstrating lymph dynamics[2] and the unique capability of magnetic resonance imaging to delineate soft-tissue composition, including fluid entrapment,[3] we deemed it appropriate to perform these imaging studies.

We sought to diagnose definitively what we suspected clinically and to direct the approach to the patient's long-term treatment. The images establish that in lipedema the peripheral lymphatic system is normal, soft tissue swelling consists solely of fat, and subcutaneous edema is notably absent.

Marlys H. Witte, M.D.
Charles L. Witte, M.D.
University of Arizona Health Sciences Center
Tucson, AZ 85724

1. Lofferer O, Mostbeck A. Lipoedema. In: Földi M, Casley-Smith JR, eds. Lymphangiology. Stuttgart, Germany: Schattauer, 1983:736.
2. McNeill GC, Witte MH, Witte CL, et al. Whole-body lymphangioscintigraphy: preferred method for initial assessment of the peripheral lymphatic system. Radiology 1989;172: 495-502.
3. Case TC, Witte CL, Witte MH, Unger EC, Williams WH. Magnetic resonance imaging in human lymphedema: comparison with lymphangioscintigraphy. Magn Reson Imaging 1992;10:549-58.

Index